SHASHANK R. PINNAPIREDDY, Ph.D
Dept. of Pharmaceutics & Biopharmaceutics,
University of Marburg.
Robert-Koch-Str. 4, Marburg-35037, Germany
Tel: 049/6421-2825883
email:shashank.pinnapireddy@yahoo.com

D1617653

BRITISH
MEDICAL BULLETIN

VOLUME FORTY-FIVE
1989

CHURCHILL LIVINGSTONE
EDINBURGH, LONDON, MELBOURNE AND NEW YORK

CHURCHILL LIVINGSTONE
Medical Division of Longman Group UK Limited

Distributed in the United States of America by Churchill Livingstone Inc., 1560 Broadway, New York, NY 10036, and by associated companies, branches and representatives throughout the world.

© The British Council 1989

All rights reserved. No part of this publication may be reproduced, stored in a retrieval system, or transmitted in any form or by any means, electronic, mechanical, photocopying, recording or otherwise, without the prior written permission of the copyright owner, or a licence permitting restricted copying in the United Kingdom issued by the Copyright Licensing Agency Ltd, 33–34 Alfred Place, London WC1E 7DP.

ISSN 0007-1420
ISBN 0 443 04198 9

Growth Factors

Scientific Editor: *M D Waterfield*

Introduction *M D Waterfield*	317
Growth factors in embryogenesis *J K Heath and A G Smith*	319
Haemopoietic growth factors *T M Dexter*	337
Regulatory factors in lymphoid development *J J T Owen and E J Jenkinson*	350
T cells and lymphokines *M Feldmann, M Londei and C Haworth*	361
Cytokine regulation of B-cell growth and differentiation *R E Callard*	371
Tumour necrosis factor *F R Balkwill*	389
Epidermal growth factor and transforming growth factor α *A W Burgess*	401
Transforming growth factors β *J J Hsuan*	425
Fibroblast growth factors *A Baird and P A Walicke*	438
Platelet-derived growth factors: A family of isoforms that bind to two distinct receptors *C-H Heldin and B Westermark*	453
Structural and functional analysis of insulin-like growth factors *D R Clemmons*	465
Scatter factor and other regulators of cell mobility *M Stoker and E Gherardi*	481
Neuropeptides as growth regulators *P J Woll and E Rozengurt*	492
Erythropoietin *G R Johnson*	506
Signal transduction pathways in mitogenesis *E Rozengurt*	515
Early gene induction by growth factors *J R Woodgett*	529
Growth factor receptors *M D Waterfield*	541
Structure-function relationships of growth factors and their receptors *N McDonald, J Murray-Rust and T Blundell*	554
Altered growth regulation in cancer *M D Waterfield*	570
Haemopoietic growth factors: their role in acute myeloblastic leukaemia *N G Testa and T M Dexter*	582
Clinical use of growth factors *M H Bronchud and T M Dexter*	590
Index	600

1989 Vol. 45 No. 2

Professor Waterfield chaired the committee which included Dr E Rozengurt, Professor T M Dexter and Professor M Feldmann that planned this number of the *British Medical Bulletin*. We are grateful to them for their help, and particularly to Professor Waterfield who acted as Scientific Editor for the number.

British Medical Bulletin is published by Churchill Livingstone for The British Council, 10 Spring Gardens, London SW1A 2BN

Introduction

M D Waterfield
Ludwig Institute for Cancer Research, Middlesex Hospital/University College Branch, London, UK

One of the most exciting achievements of the medical research community has been the characterization of a diverse family of signal molecules, the growth factors, which are involved in the control of cell growth and differentiation and may play a crucial role in cancer and other diseases. The origins of this research lies in the studies of S. Cohen, R. Levi-Montalchini, D. Metcalf and others who first used complex biological assays to characterize epidermal and nerve growth factors and the colony stimulating factors respectively, and then stimulated many groups to establish methods for elucidation of both their biological role and mechanism of molecular action through specific receptors. Particularly important to the development of the field has been the ability to work with characterized single peptide species which has in many cases only been possible since the advent of molecular biology. Thus in the last five years it has been possible to isolate and produce for the research community many factors which might never have been available in large amounts if cDNA cloning techniques and expression methods had not been developed. The availability of pure factors and of modern molecular and cellular techniques have firmly established the central role of these signal molecules in all aspects of biology. The realization that the factors trigger, through specific receptors, the generation of second messengers and hence intracellular enzyme cascades and that these can be subverted by oncogenes or tumour promoters at particular sensitive points, has unified diverse fields of cancer research and generated new insight into the mechanisms which may be operating in the disease. In addition these studies have stimulated the introduction of novel methods for manipulating growth factor induced signal cascades which could be important in many diseases.

It seems clear that a large number of growth factors remain to be characterized and it is to be expected that the understanding of their receptor signal transduction mechanisms will allow the design of specific antagonists. It remains to be seen whether the selectivity of these antagonists will be useful for therapeutic manipulation because many distinct differentiated cell types may respond to the same factor with fundamentally different consequences. This crosstalk probably reflects the modulation of a cell's response, in developmental time and location, by a panel of synergistically acting factors. The unravelling of these complex responses is an enormously challenging task.

The whole growth factor field is at a very exciting stage because we will see in the next few years answers to questions of basic research which have therapeutic implications. This volume describes current knowledge of the structure and function of the major growth factors and provides both an overview and also exquisite detail of the role of these factors in biology and medicine. This should make it possible for the general reader and the specialist to derive from this text a current assessment of the knowledge available both for specific factors and also of their role in development, in cancer and in other diseases.

Growth factors in embryogenesis

John K Heath
Austin G Smith
Cancer Research Campaign Group, Department of Biochemistry, University of Oxford, Oxford, UK

> The growing appreciation that embryonic material is a rich source of growth factors underlies increasing interest in the role of growth factors in early development. These developments have arisen from a desire to understand fundamental embryological processes; the control of differentiation and the generation of form. One expectation of this research is the discovery of new forms of regulatory agent with novel biological and therapeutic potential. Furthermore, there is a direct relationship between growth and differentiation processes in early development and pathological processes in the adult; for example, the behaviour of tumour cells has historically been compared to that of embryonic cells and regenerative processes in the adult such as angiogenesis, wound healing and fracture repair may be considered to recapitulate events that occur in the normal course of embryogenesis. An understanding of the mechanisms that underlie these fundamental processes in normal development may therefore lead to a concomitant understanding of related pathological events in the adult.

Direct identification and analysis of growth factors in mammalian embryonic material has been a difficult task due to the inaccessibility and small size of the developing embryo. However, progress in recent years has been aided by three important technical developments: the increasingly detailed structural and biological characterization of growth factors isolated from adult sources; the availability of cell lines derived directly from mammalian embryos (particularly pluripotent embryonic stem cells) as a resource for experimental analysis; and finally, the appreciation that growth factors and their cellular response systems are not confined to mammals but are present and active in a diversity of species, including those whose embryonic stages are genetically and experimentally more accessible than mammals. It is beginning to emerge from the combination of these approaches that growth factors (and related molecules) are agents that not only control cell proliferation but also regulate developmental decisions. This adds to the growing awareness that many growth factors are multifunctional regulatory molecules exerting diverse biological effects dependent upon the identity of the target cell with which they interact (see Ref. 1 for review).

In this article we focus on four sets of growth factors—the insulin-like growth factors, differentiation inhibitory activity/leukaemia inhibitory factor, the fibroblast growth factors and the transforming growth factor beta family. This focus reflects the fact that more is known about the action of these agents in developing systems than other factors. Nevertheless, our understanding of this field is far from complete. It will be clear to the reader that whilst something is known of the embryonic expression and biological action of these factors in some systems, a full appreciation of the action of these agents awaits the experimental manipulation of their expression and action in vivo.

INSULIN-LIKE GROWTH FACTORS (IGFs)

The IGFs (also known as somatomedins) were amongst the first growth factors both to be biochemically characterized[2-4] and to be implicated in embryonic development.[5] IGF-I and IGF-II are small polypeptides of 67 amino acids ($M_r = 7500$). They share 62% sequence identity and are structurally homologous to proinsulin. IGFs are mitogenic for a variety of mesoderm-derived cells in vitro (reviewed in Ref. 6). They are (unusually for growth factors) present in significant quantities in plasma due to their secretion by the liver, but are also produced locally in many tissues. The IGFs thus appear to function both in the classical endocrine manner and locally within tissues in the paracrine/autocrine mode associated with other growth factors. Aspects of IGFs are covered in detail in the chapter by Clemmons, this Issue.

The major role of IGF-I appears to be in the growth of young mammals. IGF-I production is regulated primarily by pituitary growth hormone whose growth-promoting activity on skeletal tissues it, in turn, mediates.[7,8] Growth hormone, like other classical endocrine hormones, is not required for prenatal growth and development, however, since normal human neonates are observed which have a congenital absence of the pituitary, and rat fetuses can develop normally following hypophysectomy in utero (reviewed in Ref. 9).

In fact, IGF-I is present only at very low levels in the rat fetus (though expression is higher in the human; see below). By contrast, IGF-II is relatively abundant in fetal and neonatal rat serum and levels decline post-natally when IGF-I production increases.[5] Moreover, whereas adult fibroblasts secret IGF-I, fetal fibroblasts release IGF-II.[8] This developmentally regulated reciprocal pattern of expression gave rise to the hypothesis that IGF-II is the fetal counterpart of IGF-I and functions as a specific embryonic/fetal growth factor.[5] While such a rigid distinction between the IGFs can no longer be sustained, a wide body of evidence has accumulated indicating that IGF-II is indeed likely to play an important role in embryogenesis.

The presence of IGF-II mRNA has been demonstrated in a variety of embryonic and fetal tissues by Northern analysis and in situ hybridization. Beck et al.[10] have investigated the distribution of IGF-II transcripts in rat embryos from early somite stages to full term. High level continuous expression detected in the yolk sac and liver is presumably the source of circulating immunoreactive IGF-II protein.[5] Transcripts also persist throughout development in myoblasts, myotubes and skeletal muscle. IGF-II message is observed transiently in many mesodermally-derived tissues as they undergo differentiation and in the endoderm-derived gut and broncheal epithelia at specific stages in development. In such tissues expression is greatly reduced in mature differentiated cells. In the mid-gestation human fetus, IGF-II mRNA is found more widely in tissues and organs of both mesodermal and endodermal origin, where it appears to be localized exclusively to connective tissue and mesenchyme.[11] In contrast to the rat, low levels of IGF-I message are also present in the human fetus, with a similar tissue distribution to IGF-II transcripts.[11,12] This difference may reflect developmental distinctions between rodents and humans, or arise from an evolutionary divergence of IGF function between the species.

The mapping of gene transcripts provides an essential framework for formulation of hypotheses on the functions of growth factors in embryogenesis. However, critical evaluation of the possible roles of IGFs in development requires, in addition to identification of potential sites of synthesis, information on the distribution of IGF polypeptides and their cognate binding proteins and cellular receptors. Unfortunately, whilst secretion of IGF has been detected by explants of both rodent[12,13] and human[14] embryonic tissues, a detailed immunohistochemical localization of IGF-I and -II during embryogenesis has not yet been published. Secreted IGFs are found in association with specific binding proteins.[15,16] The latter may modulate biological activity both by prolonging the half-life of free IGF, and by directly inhibiting or promoting interaction with particular target cells (reviewed in Ref. 17). Cell surface IGF receptors are of two structurally distinct types,[18] both of which bind IGF-I and -II but may mediate different biological responses.[19] IGF binding proteins and receptors have been demonstrated in extra-embryonic and embryonic tissue[12,13] but their precise cellular distribution has not been determined. Functional IGF receptors are expressed by embryonal carcinoma (EC) cells,[20] which share many properties in common with early embryo cells,[21] and IGF binding proteins have been detected in mouse blastocysts.[13] These observations suggest that pluripotential embryo cells may be responsive to IGF-II very early in development.

In conclusion, circulating IGF-II secreted by the yolk sac and fetal liver may serve a generalized growth-promoting function throughout embryogenesis. However, the temporal and tissue-specific patterns of expression of the IGF-II message by cells anatomically integrated into developing tissues and organs are consistent with an additional role in autocrine and/or paracrine regulatory processes associated with morphogenesis. This may entail interaction with other growth factors, notably TGF-β (see below), with which IGFs can synergise in vitro.[22] At present the embryological data is essentially descriptive and therefore circumstantial. As with other growth factors, direct demonstration of embryonic function will require generation of specific perturbations of the expression of IGFs and their receptors in transgenic animals.

POLYPEPTIDE FACTORS CONTROLLING EMBRYONIC STEM CELL DIFFERENTIATION

Embryonic stem (ES) cells are cell lines established directly from implantation stage mouse embryos.[23,24] They retain the unique ability, even after prolonged periods in culture, to contribute functional differentiated progency to all tissues, including the germ line, following reincorporation into a host blastocyst.[25] Consequently ES cells may be employed as cellular vectors for generating transgenic animals (reviewed in Ref. 26). They also provide a population of normal, pluripotential, early embryo cells in an experimentally accessible form and can be exploited to identify and characterize novel factors involved in the regulation of embryonic growth and differentiation.[27]

ES cells undergo rapid 'spontaneous' differentiation when cultured in isolation. Such differentiation is traditionally prevented by maintaining the stem cells on feeder layers of mitotically inactivated embryonic fibroblasts.[28] Differentiation can also be inhibited, however, by culture in medium conditioned by preincubation with buffalo rat liver (BRL) cells. The latter secrete a diffusible factor termed Differentiation Inhibitory Activity (DIA) which suppresses differentiation of ES cells.[29] The effect of DIA is fully reversible and without any compromise of developmental capacity: germ-line chimaeras have been obtained from ES cells after extended culture in the absence of feeders and presence of BRL cell-conditioned medium as a source of DIA (Ref. 30, and Smith & Beddington, unpublished).

The action of DIA is attributable to a single polypeptide which has recently been purified.[31] It is a glycoprotein of apparent $M_r = 43\,000$ generated by extensive glycosylation of a core polypeptide of apparent $M_r = 20\,000$. Purified DIA inhibits ES cell differentiation at concentrations as low as 0.2 ng/ml (10pM), confirming that its activity is hormonal in nature rather than mere fulfillment of some nutritional or metabolic requirement. DIA thus constitutes a novel bioregulatory factor which exerts negative control over the differentiation of pluripotent embryo cells.

The effect of DIA does not appear to be mediated via direct intervention in the cell cycle, since ES cells continue to multiply rapidly for some time after withdrawal from DIA and the onset of overt cellular differentiation. Furthermore, DIA is not mitogenic for fibroblasts and is structurally dissimilar to characterized fibroblast mitogens.

The production of DIA by BRL cells derived from adult liver[32] and of related activities by a variety of heterologous cell types[29,33,34] suggests that its actions may not be confined to the peri-implantation embryo, but might also be manifest in other stem cell systems. Evidence that this may indeed be the case, at least for myeloid cells is provided by the finding that DIA can sustain proliferation of a factor-dependent Mo-MuLV-transformed lymphoma cell line Da-1a.[31] This property is shared by a recently characterized lymphokine, known variously as human interleukin for Da cells (HILDA, Ref. 35) owing to its action on Da-1a cells, and leukaemia inhibitory factor (LIF, Ref. 36) because it induces differentiation with concomitant inhibition of proliferation of M1 myeloid leukaemia cells. Full length complementary DNA clones for HILDA/LIF encode a polypeptide of $M_r = 20 000$.[37,38] This is heavily glycosylated to give a mature species of apparent $M_r = 35–55 000$ depending on cellular source. HILDA/LIF is thus similar in structure to DIA. Moreover, recombinant HILDA/LIF reproduces the biological activity of DIA, suppressing differentiation of ES cells in the absence of feeders.[31,39] Inhibition of differentiation is apparent at concentrations of purified HILDA/LIF down to 10pM and ES cells maintained in medium supplemented with HILDA/LIF retain the capacity to contribute normally to chimaeric animals. The action of HILDA/LIF appears to be initiated via binding to specific, high affinity, cell surface receptors expressed by ES cells. DIA can interact with the same receptors.[31] HILDA/LIF is thus closely related, if not identical, to DIA in structure, function, potency and receptor reactivity.

DIA/HILDA/LIF provides a clear example of the differentiation regulatory action of polypeptide factors. Significantly, differentiation can either be induced or inhibited depending upon the target cell. The activity on pluripotential ES cells demonstrates that polypeptide factors may be important regulatory agents at even the earliest stages of development. Finally it should be noted that DIA/HILDA/LIF is active on two, apparently unrelated cellular systems, the embryonic stem cells and cell lineages in haemopoiesis. This conjunction of haemopoietic and embryonic stem cell regulatory activities is an exciting new development. The availability of recombinant factor should greatly facilitate the routine culture and experimental manipulation of ES cells. This is likely to prove particularly valuable in the genetic alteration of ES cells prior to transgenesis, most notably in attempts to introduce predetermined modifications into the germ-line via homologous recombination or 'gene targetting'.[40] Use of DIA/HILDA/LIF may also enable the isolation of ES cells from other species, including agricultural livestock. Primitive ectoderm is the embryonic counterpart of ES cells (reviewed in Ref. 41) and gives rise to all tissues of the fetus in addition to most of the extra-embrionic membranes. The primitive ecotoderm proliferates rapidly after implantation, then differentiates at the primitive streak stage. DIA/HILDA/LIF may well regulate the switch between self-renewal and differentiation in vivo as in vitro. The potential functions of DIA/HILDA/LIF in normal haemopoiesis and other developing tissues have yet to be determined, but the molecular probes now available can be used to map embryonic expression and to generate transgenic animals for functional analyses.

THE FIBROBLAST GROWTH FACTOR FAMILY

The prototype members of the fibroblast growth factor family are acidic fibroblast growth factor (aFGF) and basic fibroblast growth factor (bFGF). These factors were first identified in nervous tissue and their biological activity defined by their ability to support the proliferation of fibroblasts and vascular endothelial cells in vitro.[42] These properties have been used to support the suggestion that a major function of aFGF and bFGF is regulation of angiogenesis in vivo.[43] A review of the FGFs is presented in the Chapter by Baird & Walicke, this Issue.

A characteristic biochemical feature of acidic and basic FGF is a strong affinity for heparin; indeed, heparin affinity chromatography has become a standard procedure in their purification. Both aFGF bFGF are between 15 000–17 000 Kd in molecular mass; the variation in forms found in various tissues seems to depend on proteolytic processing at the N-terminus. The gene structures of aFGF and bFGF are known[44,45] and this information has revealed the surprising feature that neither gene has a functional secretory signal sequence, suggesting that either these factors do not normally escape from the cell or some unusual secretory mechanism is employed.

More recently, several additional genes encoding molecules with significant sequence homology to the fibroblast growth factor prototype genes have been identified. These have all been discovered by virtue of their association with naturally-occurring or experimentally-induced tumours. Two groups independently identified a transforming oncogene by transfection of tumour cell (Kaposi's sarcoma or stomach tumour) DNA into NIH/3T3 cells. This gene (ks[46] or hst[47] encodes a $M_r = 24\,000$ protein (hereafter called K-FGF) with significant amino acid sequence homology to the aFGF and bFGF prototypes with the important addition of a functional secretory signal sequence. Experimental expression of *K-FGF* in heretologous systems reveals that it is made as a glycosylated prohormone, secreted, and proteolytically cleaved to form the mature secreted protein.[48] Similar fibroblast transfection techniques have also led to the isolation, from bladder tumour DNA, of FGF-5[49] another FGF-like gene with a functional secreted signal sequence. The final member of the 'FGF family' of growth factors whose structure is known is *int-2*,[50] which was identified as a gene whose expression was activated in a significant proportion of mammary tumours of mice infected with the mouse mammary tumour virus MMTV. The MMTV provirus in these tumours was found to have integrated at sites flanking the *int-2* gene, thereby activating its expression in the tumour.[51] The association between *int-2* and *K-FGF* extends beyond sequence homology since the two genes are located very close to each other on chromosome 11 and are co-amplified in certain stomach and vulval carcinoma cells lines.[52]

There is a clear association between the activity of members of the FGF gene family and tumourgenesis in the adult. But what is their biological function in the normal organism? Several lines of evidence point to an important function of the FGF-gene family in regulating cell behaviour and differentiation during normal development in vivo.

The first piece of evidence comes from studies of the pattern of expression of these genes in the course of normal embryogenesis. In particular, *K-FGF* and *int-2* expression seems to be specifically activated in early mammalian embryonic development. Wilkinson et al.[53] showed by in situ hybridization techniques that the *int-2* gene exhibits a remarkable tissue-specific pattern of expression during early development. It is first expressed transiently in cells undergoing gastrulation in the primitive streak of the early post-implantation embryo and subquently expression becomes localized in the developing hindbrain and pharyngeal pouches. There is accordingly a correlation between *int-2* expression and certain sites of cellular differentiation and specification in the embryo. *K-FGF* expression has also been found in cells derived from the early mammalian embryo; *K-FGF* transcripts and functional *K-FGF* protein are expressed by pluripotential ES and EC cells. In this system *K-FGF* expression ceases as the cells differentiate away from the stem cell state (Heath et al., in preparation). This suggests that *K-FGF* may be expressed by pluripotent stem cells in the early post-implantation embryo. Although these findings suggest a link between the expression of specific members of the FGF-family of growth factors and embryonic regulatory processes, evidence for their physiological function in early mammalian development is lacking.

Direct evidence for the importance of FGF-like factors in controlling embryonic differentiation comes, however, from an unexpected source; the early amphibian embryo. One of the key differentiation events in early amphibian development is the differentiation of mesodermal cell types (principally muscle, notochord and blood cells) in the animal pole cells of the embryo as a result of signals emanating from cells in the vegetal pole of the embryo. The existence of vegetal hemisphere-derived mesoderm-inducing signals can be shown by cutting the embryo into animal and vegetal halves; in the absence of vegetal pole cells the animal halves form epidermal structures. When recombined with vegetal pole cells extensive mesodermal differentiation in the animal hemisphere occurs (Fig. 1). This inductive signalling effect of vegetal pole cells can be reproduced by exposing the isolated animal pole to bovine bFGF.[54] A growth factor can therefore mimic the effect of the inductive signal that occurs in normal

Mesoderm Induction in Amphibians

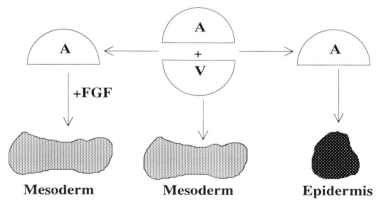

Fig. 1 Mesoderm induction in *Xenopus*. The embryo is dissected into animal (**A**) and vegetal (**V**) pieces. Culture of animal poles in the absence of vegetal tissue results in differentiation into epidermis (right hand side). Recombination of animal and vegetal halves produces structures with extensive mesodermal differentiation (centre). Exposure of animal poles to fibroblast growth factors (FGF) produces a similar mesodermal pattern to that found in the presence of vegetal tissue (left hand side).

development. Significantly, FGF-like factors have no discernible effect on cell multiplication in the early stages of amphibian development. The mesoderm-inducing effect of basic FGF has led to an investigation of the action of other members of the FGF-family in this system. Human *K-FGF* and mouse *int-2* synthesized in vitro also induce mesodermal differentiation in animal pole explants (Paterno, Gillespie, Slack & Heath, submitted), although with marked differences in potency. In particular, *int-2* has been found to be a relatively weak mesoderm induction agent compared to bFGF, aFGF or *K-FGF*. Thus, although mesoderm induction can be considered a characteristic feature of the FGF family of growth factors, the indications are that important differences in potency and activity between members of the family exist.

This phenomenon of mesoderm induction has several general consequences. Firstly it shows that molecules identified as mitogens may act to regulate differentiation in early development; these agents may be key intercellular signalling molecules in the complex web of inductive interactions between cells required to form the body of the developing embryo. Secondly, it demonstrates a remarkable conservation of signalling mechanisms across species. The *Xenopus* homologue of the bFGF gene is, in fact, very similar to its mammalian counterpart.[55,56] This type of evolutionary conservation and action across taxonomic boundaries may indicate that growth factor-like agents may have an ancient and fundamental role in controlling differentiation processes in the development of many species.

THE TRANSFORMING GROWTH FACTOR BETA FAMILY

The multiple biological activities of the transforming growth factor beta (TGF-β) family emphasizes the multi-functional role of polypeptide regulatory factors in development which is reviewed in the chapter by Hsuan, this Issue. The prototype factor in this family, TGF-β1, was first identified by virtue of its ability, when acting in concert with other growth factors such as transforming growth factor alpha, to induce the anchorage independent growth of mouse cell lines,[57] thereby mimicking the behaviour of transformed or tumourogenic cells. TGF-β1 is a homodimeric molecule composed of two disulphide-linked $M_r = 12\,500$ chains[58] which is secreted in an inactive latent form as a complex with other proteins.[59] Latent TGF-β1 may be biologically activated experimentally by exposure to acid conditions but the exact mechanisms of activation in vivo are unclear. This requirement of TGF-β1 for activation post-secretion may be an important feature of its action since, in principle, it provides a mechanism for modulating or targeting the biological action of TGF-β1 in vivo.

TGF-β1 was first identified in media conditioned by various virally transformed cell lines, but it has subsequently become clear that TGF-β1 can be isolated from a range of normal tissues, especially those rich in extracellular matrix such as the kidney, placenta or bone. TGF-β1 is, however, also expressed in the developing embryo. Heine et al.[60] in an immunolocalization study showed that TGF-β1 deposition in the embryo was widespread, but especially marked in tissues undergoing morphogenesis or modelling such as the salivary gland, palate, face and teeth. Sandberg et al.[61] and Lehnert & Ackhurst[62] have also localized TGF-β1 transcripts by *in situ* hybridization techniques to the growth plates of cartilage and the epithelia overlying mesenchyme in developing organs such as thymus, thyroid and tooth. It must be emphasized, however, that these current studies fail to distinguish between active and latent forms of TGF-β1 and a more exact definition of the sites of TGF-β1 activity in embryogenesis awaits the development of methods which discriminate between these forms. Nevertheless the general picture that emerges from these localization studies is a close association of TGF-β1 expression in the embryo with sites of morphogenesis and tissue modelling.

The biological functions of TGF-β1 are complex. Although first identified as an agent which co-operated with mitogens to induce anchorage independent growth in vitro it is clear that the biological actions of TGF-β1 encompass mitogenicity, inhibition of cell growth[63], induction of differentiation and inhibition of differentiation (reviewed in Ref. 1) depending upon the identity of the target cell type. However despite the apparently bewildering variety of biological effects observed, a major theme in the action of TGF-β1 is beginning to emerge—It exerts a pronounced effect on the deposition of extracellular matrix components. This was first indicated by the experiments of Roberts et al.[64] who showed that injection of TGF-β1 into mice caused local fibrosis at the site of injection. These observations have been subsequently extended to reveal that TGF-β1 has a pronounced effect on the expression extracellular matrix components such as collagen Type I,[65] the integrins which bind extracellular matrix components to the cell surface[66] and the enzymes which degrade extracellular matrix components and their inhibitors.[57] The general trend of these effects is to induce, or stabilize the deposition of extracellular matrix components. This remarkable effect of TGF-β1 on extracellular matrix deposition may well account for the localization in sites of tissue modelling in embryos and strongly indicates an important role for TGF-β1 in morphogenetic processes.

TGF-β1 is the prototype member of what is emerging as a large multigene family exhibiting strong associations with embryonic development. These new members of the family have been identified from diverse species and sources and fall into two basic categories: (a) genes with strong overall relatedness to TGF-β1; and (b) genes with regions of TGF-β1 homology embedded within apparently unrelated amino acid sequences. Two examples of category (a) TGF-βs have been recently described; TGF-β2[68] and TGF-β3.[69] These genes were isolated on the basis of their overall similarity to TGF-β1. TGF-β2 is, in fact, identical to epithelial cell growth inhibiting factor originally described by Holley.[70,71] Little information exists, at the present time, on the embryonic expression of TGF-β2 and 3 and it will be interesting to see the extent of co-expression of these related genes in vivo. In neither case has it been established if these new TGF-β-like agents exist in latent forms like TGF-β1.

The biological actions of these new members of the TGF-β family seem qualitatively similar to TGF-β1 but, as in the case of the FGFs, intriguing quantitative differences emerge when the action of these factors is examined in more detail. TGF-β2 is for example significantly more potent than TGF-β1 in inhibiting the multiplication of haemopoetic stem cells.[72] Furthermore, TGF-β2 is biologically active in the *Xenopus* mesoderm induction system described above,[73] albeit at relatively high concentrations, whereas TGF-β1 is almost inactive in the same assay. Again we see that related members of a regulatory factor family exhibit subtle differences in potency in different assay systems. A final, provisional, member of the TGF-β-like peptides is the *Xenopus* mesoderm-inducing factor isolated from the medium of the *Xenopus* cell line XTC by Smith.[74] This factor is a potent mesoderm-inducing agent in its own right and seems considerably more active than TGF-β1 or TGF-β2. Nevertheless, this factor is not only unrelated to the potent FGF-like mesoderm inducing agents but has a heterodimeric structure of two chains approximately $M_r = 12\,500$,[75] a feature shared with the TGF-β-like agents described above. The exact relationship of this factor to the known TGF-βs, and its action in mammalian systems will be of interest.

The category (b) members of the TGF-β family represent a class of genes encoding regulatory factors, isolated by independent means which contain stretches of sequence relatedness to TGF-β1. These genes include the reproductive hormones the activins and inhibins[76] as well as two gene products with significant functions in embryonic development. Mullerian Inhibitory Substance (MIS) is a $M_r = 74$–$70\,000$ factor secreted by the undifferentiated gonads during mammalian embryogenesis which inhibits the female pathway of secondary sexual differentiation at a critical stage of embryonic development. Its action is at least partly responsible for the development of male secondary sexual characteristics and it is therefore a key differentiation regulatory factor in embryonic sexual development. Molecular cloning and sequence analysis of the MIS gene[77] reveals a distinct C-terminal domain with significant homology to TGF-β1. An interesting issue that arises is that whilst MIS is isolated as a monomeric protein, all the other TGF-β-like proteins are biologically active as homo- or heterodimers. It is unclear whether MIS requires dimerisation for full biological activity, or exists in a latent complex.

The second example of a TGF-β related gene with significant action in development was found by classical developmental genetic analysis of insects. *Decapentaplegic* (DPP-C) is a gene complex in *Drosophila* required for establishment of dorsal-ventral pattern and morphogenesis of the imaginal disks. A cDNA encoding an open reading frame from this complex encodes a potential protein of $M_r = 66\,000$, whose carboxyterminal region contains a domain with significant sequence relatedness to TGF-β1[78] Although little is known about the protein product of this gene, the region of TGF-β homology is flanked by dibasic amino acid residues, suggesting that a protein approximately the same size as TGF-β1 could be formed from the precursor by proteolytic processing. Furthermore, the positioning of cysteine residues in the predicted DPP-C protein is well preserved compared to the TGF-β prototype, suggesting the possibility that the protein may form a dimer. The unexpected existence of genes with homologies to TGF-β in distant phyla indicates that the TGF-β family of agents is ancient in evolution and the discovery of more members of this group must be anticipated.

CONCLUSIONS

This review of growth factor action in development, although highlighting the fragmentary nature of knowledge in this field has revealed some important common themes. Firstly it is clear that polypeptide regulatory factors function in development to control developmental specification, differentiation and morphogenesis as well as simply coordinating the growth of the embryo. Secondly these agents seem to fall into related families of factors with similar overall structure. Where information is available it seems that individual members are highly conserved between species yet multiple genes exist with overlapping functions within a species. This implies that each member of the gene family has distinct, but related, biological functions. This is beginning to be confirmed in the case of the FGF and TGF-β families. Thirdly, we have discussed several cases where growth factors exhibit precise tissue specific expression in early development, but this is not confined to a single cell lineage or anatomical site. This suggests that the same signals are 're-used' several times in development. Finally, it is clear that the same agent may elicit very different biological responses in different cell types. This argues that the response to growth factor signals in development is itself developmentally regulated.

ACKNOWLEDGEMENTS

We are grateful to Peter Rathjen & Dylan Edwards for their comments on this paper. The authors research is supported by the Cancer Research Campaign.

REFERENCES

1 Sporn M, Roberts A. Peptide growth factors are multifunctional. Nature 1988; 332: 217–218
2 Rinderknecht E, Humbel R. The amino acid sequence of human insulin-like growth factor-I and its structural homology with insulin. J Biol Chem 1978; 253: 2769–2773
3 Rinderknecht E, Humbel R. Primary structure of human insulin-like growth factor-II. FEBS Letts 1978; 89: 283–286
4 Marquardt H, Todaro GJ, Henderson LE, Oroszlan S. Purification and primary structure of a polypeptide with multiplication stimulating activity from rat liver cell cultures. J Biol Chem 1981; 256: 6859–6865
5 Moses AC, Nissley SP, Short PA et al. Increased levels of multiplication stimulating activity, an insulin-like growth factor, in foetal rat serum. Proc Natl Acad Sci USA 1980; 77: 3649–3653
6 Froesch ER, Schmid C, Schwander J, Zapf J. Actions of insulin-like growth factors. Ann Rev Physiol 1985; 47: 443–467

7 Schoenle E, Zapf J, Humbel RE, Froesch ER. Insulin-like growth factor I stimulates growth in hypophysectomized rats. Nature 1982; 296: 252–253
8 Adams SO, Nissley SP, Handwerger S, Rechler MM. Developmental patterns of insulin-like growth factor-I and -II synthesis and regulation in rat fibroblasts. Nature 1983; 302: 150–153
9 Underwood LE, D'Ercole AJ. Insulin and somatomedins/insulin-like growth factors in fetal and neonatal development. Clin Endocrinol Metab 1984; 13: 69–89
10 Beck F, Samani NJ, Penschow JD, Thorley B, Tregear JW, Coghlan JP. Histochemical localization of IGF-I and -II mRNA in the developing rat embryo. Development 1987; 101: 175–184
11 Han VKM, D'Ercole AJ, Lund PK. Cellular localization of somatomedin (insulin-like growth factor) messenger RNA in the human fetus. Science 1987; 236: 193–197
12 Heath JK, Shi W-K. Developmentally regulated expression of insulin-like growth factors by differentiated murine teratocarcinomas and extraembryonic mesoderm. J Embryol Exp Morphol 1986; 95: 193–212
13 Smith EP, Sadler TW, D'Ercole AJ. Somatomedins/insulin-like growth factors, their receptors and binding proteins are present during mouse embryogenesis. Development 1987; 101: 73–82
14 D'Ercole AJ, Hill DJ, Stain AJ, Underwood LE. Tissue and plasma sometamedin-C/insulin-like growth factor I concentrations in the human fetus during the first half of gestation. Pediatr Res 1986; 20: 253–255
15 Zapf J, Schoenle E, Jagars G, Sand I, Grunwald J, Froesch ER. Inhibition of the action of non-suppressible insulin-like activity on isolated rat fat cells by binding to its carrier protein. J Clin Invest 1979; 63: 1077–1084
16 Knauer DJ, Smith GL. Inhibition of biological activity of multiplication-stimulating activity by binding to its carrier protein. Proc Natl Acad Sci USA 1980; 77: 7252–7256
17 Baxter RC, Martin JL. Binding proteins for the insulin-like growth factors: structure, regulation and function. Prog Growth Factor Res 1989: In press
18 Massague J, Czech MP. The subunit structure of two distinct receptors for insulin-like growth factors I and II and their relationship to the insulin receptor. J Biol Chem 1982; 257: 5038–5045
19 Mottola C, Czech MP. The type II insulin-like growth factor receptor does not mediate increased DNA synthesis in H-35 hepatoma cells. J Biol Chem 1984; 259: 12705–12713
20 Heath JK. Regulation of murine embryonal carcinoma cell proliferation and differentiation. Cancer Surveys 1983; 2: 141–164
21 Evans MJ, Lovell-Badge RH, Stern PL, Stinnakre M-G. In: Le Douarin N, ed., Cell Lineage, Stem Cells and Determination Paris: INSERM, 1979: pp. 115–129
22 Massague J, Kelly B, Mottola C. Stimulation by insulin-like growth factors is required for cellular transformation by type β transforming growth factor. J Biol Chem 1985; 260: 4551–4554
23 Evans MJ, Kaufman MH. Establishment in culture of pluripotential cells from mouse embryos. Nature 1981; 292: 154–156
24 Martin GR. Isolation of a pluripotent cell line from early mouse embryos cultured in medium conditioned by teratocarcinoma stem cells. Proc Natl Acad Sci USA 1981; 78: 7634–7636
25 Bradley A, Evans M., Kaufman MH, Robertson E. Formation of germ-line chimaeras from embryo-derived teratocarcinoma cells lines. Nature 1984; 309: 255–256
26 Robertson EJ. Pluripotential stem cells as a route into the mouse germ line. Trends Genet 1986; 2: 9–13

27 Heath JK, Smith AG, Wills AJ, Edwards DR. In: De Laat S, Mummery C, Bluemink J, eds. Cell to Cell Signalling in Mammalian Development. Berlin: Springer-Verlag, 1989: In Press
28 Martin GR, Evans MJ. In: Sherman MI, Solter D, eds. Teratomas and Differentiation Town: Publisher 1975: pp. 169–187
29 Smith AG, Hooper ML. Buffalo rat liver cells produce a diffusible activity which inhibits the differentiation of murine embryonal carcinoma and embryonic stem cells. Dev Biol 1987; 121: 1–9
30 Hooper ML, Hardy K, Handyside A, Hunter S, Monk M. HPRT-deficient (Lesch-Nyhan) mouse embryos derived from germline colonization by cultured cells. Nature 1987; 326: 292–294
31 Smith AG, Heath JK, Donaldson DD, Wong GG, Moreau J, Stahl M, Rogers D. Inhibition of pluripotential embryonic stem cell differentiation by purified polypeptides. Nature 1989; 326: 197–200
32 Coon H. Clonal culture of differentiated rat liver cells. J Cell Biol 1968; 39: 29
33 Smith TA, Hooper ML. Medium conditioned by feeder cells inhibits the differentiation of embryonal carcinoma cells. Exp Cell Res 1983; 145: 458–462
34 Koopman P, Cotton RGH. A factor produced by feeder cells which inhibits embryonal carcinoma cell differentiation. Exp Cell Res 1984; 154: 233–242
35 Moreau J-F, Bonneville M, Godard A, Gascan H, Gruart V, Moore MA, Soulillou JP. Characterization of a factor produced by human T cell clones exhibiting eosinophil-activating and burst-promoting activities. J Immunol 1987; 138: 3844–3849
36 Hilton DJ, Nicola N, Gough NM, Metcalf D. Resolution and purification of three distinct factors produced by Krebs ascites cells which have differentiation-inducing activity on murine myeloid leukemic cell lines. J Biol Chem 1988; 263: 9238–9243
37 Moreau J-F, Donaldson D, Bennett F, Witek-Giannotti J, Wong GG, Clark SC. Leukaemia inhibitory factor is identical to the myeloid growth factor human interleukin for DA cells. Nature 1988: 326: 201–204
38 Molecular cloning and expression of cDNA encoding a murine myeloid leukaemia inhibitory factor (LIF). EMBO J 1988; 6: 3995–4002
39 Williams RL, Hilton DJ, Pease S, et al. Myeloid leukaemia inhibitory factor (LIF) maintains the developmental potential of embryonic stem cells. Nature 1988: 326: 194–197
40 Thomas K, Capecchi M. Site-directed mutagenesis by gene targeting in mouse embryo-derived stem cells. Cell 1987; 51: 503–512
41 Evans MJ, Kaufman MH. Pluripotential cells grown directly from normal mouse embryos. Cancer Surveys 1983; 2: 185–206
42 Vlodavsky I, Johnson L, Greenburg G, Gospodarwicz D. Vascular endothelial cells maintained in the absence of fibroblast growth factor undergo structural and functional changes that are incompatible with their in vivo differentiated properties. J Cell Biol 1979; 83: 468–486
43 Folkman J, Klagsbrun M. Angiogenic factors. Science 1987; 235: 442–447
44 Abraham J, Mergia A, Whang J et al. Nucleotide sequence of a bovine clone encoding the angiogenic protein, basic fibroblast growth factor. Science 1986; 233: 545–548
45 Jaye M, Howk R, Burgess W et al. Human endothelial cell growth factor: Cloning, nucleotide sequence and chromosome location. Science 1986; 233: 541–545
46 Delli Bovi P, Curatola A, Kern F, Greco A, Ittman M, Basilico C. An oncogene isolated by transfection of Kaposis's sarcoma DNA encodes a growth factor that is a member of the FGF family. Cell 1987; 50: 729–737
47 Taira M, Yoshida T, Miyagawa K, Sakamoto H, Terada M, Sigmura T. cDNA sequence of human transforming gene hst and identification of the coding

sequence required for transforming activity. Proc Natl Acad Sci USA 1987; 84: 2980–2984
48 Delli-Bovi P, Curatola A-M, Newmark K, et al. Processing, secretion and biological properties of a novel growth factor of the fibroblast growth factor family with oncogenic potential. Mol Cell Biol 1988; 8: 2933–2941
49 Zhan X, Bates B, Hu X, Goldfarb M. The human FGF-5 oncogene encodes a novel protein related to fibroblast growth factors. Mol Cell Biol 1988; 8: 3487–3495
50 Dickson C, Peters G. Potential oncogene produce related to growth factors. Nature 1987; 326: 833
51 Dickson C, Smith R, Brookes S, Peters G. Tumourgenesis by mouse mammary tumour virus: proviral activation of a cellular gene in the common integration site int-2. Cell 1984; 37: 529–536
52 Yoshida M, Wada M, Satoh H, et al. Human HST1 gene maps to chromosome band 11q13 and coamplifies with the Int-2 gene in human cancer. Proc Natl Acad Sci USA 1988; 85: 4861–4864
53 Wilkinson D, Peters G, Dickson C, MacMahon A. Expression of the FGF-related proto-oncogene int-2 during gastrulation and neurulation in the mouse. EMBO J 1988; 7: 691–695
54 Slack J, Darlington B, Heath J, Godsave S. Mesoderm induction in early xenopus embryos by heparin-binding growth factors. Nature 1987; 326: 197–200
55 Kimmelman D, Kirschner M. Synergistic induction of mesoderm by FGF and TGF-β and the identification of an mRNA coding for FGF and the early xenopus embryo. Cell 1987; 51: 869–877
56 Kimelman D, Abraham J, Haaparanta T, Palisi T, Kirshner M. The presence of fibroblast growth factor in the frog egg: Its role as a natural mesoderm inducer. Science 1988; 242: 1053–1056
57 Anzano M, Roberts A, Smith J, Sporn M, DeLarco J. Sarcoma growth factor from conditioned medium of virally transformed cells is composed of both type α and type beta transforming growth factors. Proc Natl Acad Sci USA 1983; 80: 6264–6269
58 Derynck R, Jarrett R, Chen E, et al. Human transforming growth factor beta complementary DNA sequence and expression in normal and transformed cells. Nature 1985; 316: 701–705
59 Lawrence D, Pircher R, Jullien P. Conversion of a high molecular weight latent TGF-β from chicken embryo fibroblasts into a low molecular weight active TGF-beta under acidic conditions. Biochem Biophys Res Commun 1984; 133: 1026–1034
60 Heine U, Munoz E, Flanders K, et al. The role of TGF-β in the development of mouse embryo. J Cell Biol 1987; 105: 2861–2876
61 Sandberg M, Vurio T, Hirovan H, Alitalo K, Vurio E. Enhanced expression of TGF-β and fos mRNAs in the growth plates of human long bones. Development 1988; 102: 461–123
62 Lehnert S, Ackhurst R. Embryonic pattern of TGF beta type-1 RNA suggests both paracrine and autocrine mechanisms of action. Development 1988; 104: 263–273
63 Roberts A, Anzano M, Wakefield L, Roche N, Stern D, Sporn M. Type beta transforming growth factor: a bifunctional regulator of cell growth. Proc Natl Acad Sci USA 1985; 83: 119–123
64 Roberts A, Sporn M, Assoian R, et al. Transforming growth factor β: rapid induction of fibrosis and angiogenesis in vivo and stimulation of collagen formation in vivo. Proc Natl Acad Sci USA 1986; 83: 4167–4171
65 Penttinen R, Kobiyashi S, Bornstein P. Transforming growth factor β increases mRNA for matrix proteins both in the presence and the absence of changes in mRNA stability. Proc Natl Acad Sci USA 1988; 85: 1105–1108

66 Ignotz R, Massague J. Cell adhesion protein receptors as targets for TGF-β action. Cell 1987; 51: 189–193
67 Edwards D, Murpohy G, Reynolds J, Docherty A, Angel P, Heath J. TGF-β modulates the expression of collagenase and TIMP. EMBO J 1987; 6: 1899–1902
68 deMartin R, Haendler B, Hofer-Warbinek R, Gaugitsch H, Wrann M, Schlusener H, Seifert J, Bodmer S, Fontana A, Hofer E. Complementary DNA from human gliobastoma derived T cell supressor factor: a novel member of the transforming growth factor beta gene family. EMBO J 1987; 6: 3673–3672
69 ten Dijke P, Hansen P, Iwata K, Pieler C, Foulkes G. Identification of another member of the transforming growth factor beta gene family. Proc Natl Acad Sci USA 1988; 85: 4715–4719
70 Holley R, Bohlen P, Fava R, Baldwin J, Kleeman G, Armour R. Purification of kidney epithelial cell growth inhibitor. Proc Natl Acad Sci USA 1980; 77: 5989–5992
71 Tucker R, Shipley G, Moses H. Growth Inhibitor from BSC-1 cells closely related to platelet type β transforming growth factor. Science 1984; 226: 705–707
72 Ohta M, Greenberger J, Ankelsaria P, Bassols A, Massague J. Two forms of transforming growth factor beta distinguished by multipotential haemopetic cells. Nature 1987; 329: 539–541
73 Rosa F, Roberts A, Danielpour D, Dart L, Sporn M, Dawid I. Mesoderm induction in amphibians: the role of TGF-β2-like factors. Science 1988; 239: 783–785
74 Smith JC. A mesoderm inducing factor is produced by a Xenopus cell line. Development 1987; 99: 3–14
75 Smith JC, Yaqoob M, Symes K. Purification, partial characterisation and biological effects of the XTC mesoderm-inducing factor. Development 1988; 103: 591–600
76 Mason A, Hayflick J, Ling N, Esch F, Ueno N, Ying S, Guillemin R, Niall H, Seeburg P. Complementary DNA sequences of ovarian follicular fluid inhibin show precursor structure and homology with transforming growth factor beta. Nature 1985; 318: 659–663
77 Cate R, Mattalanio R, Hession C, et al. Isolation of the bovine and human genes for Mullerian inhibiting substance and expression of the human gene in animal cells. Cell 1986; 45: 685–698
78 Padgett R, Johnston D, Gelbart M. A transcript from a drosophila pattern gene homologous to the transforming growth factor beta family. Nature 1987; 325: 81–84

Haemopoietic growth factors

T M Dexter
Paterson Institute for Cancer Research, Christie Hospital and Holt Radium Institute, Manchester, UK

> The growth and development of mature blood cells in vitro is supported by a series of glycoproteins with a range of biological activities. Many of these growth factors have been molecularly cloned, purified to homogeneity, and their biological effects determined on various target cells. Some of these growth factors promote the proliferation and differentiation of multipotent stem cells; others are more restricted in their action and, when used alone, can support only the development of lineage-restricted progenitor cells. When used in combinations however, the spectrum of target cells supported by these growth factors can be considerably enlarged. Furthermore, other molecules (which are not themselves growth promoters for multipotent stem cells) can synergise with these growth factors and permit primitive cells to undergo proliferation and development. These findings are likely to have major therapeutic implications.

THE HAEMOPOIETIC SYSTEM

All mature blood cells are derived from stem cells which arise during embryonic development. These stem cells, which in the adult are located in the bone marrow, are able to proliferate and either produce more stem cells (a process called self-renewal) or give rise to more differentiated cells (a process known as commitment).[1,2] Such committed progenitor cells can then undergo further proliferation and development to produce the mature blood cells (Fig. 1).

The developmental potential of stem cells has been investigated using unique radiation-induced chromosome marker analysis and

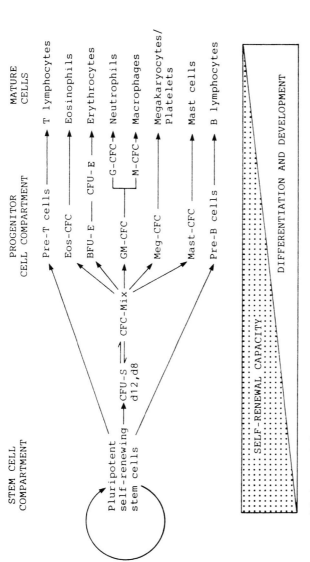

Fig. 1 The structure of the haemopoietic system

CFU-S, cells able to form colonies in the spleens of potentially lethally irradiated mice. Those cells producing colonies 12 days post transplantation are more primitive than the cells forming colonies 8 days post injection; CFC-Mix, multipotent cells with an ability to produce colonies in vitro containing cells of various myeloid lineages; GM-CFC, bipotent cells able to produce both macrophages and neutrophils. These give rise to neutrophil restricted (G-CFC) and macrophage restricted (M-CFC) progenitor cells; BFU-E, primitive erythroid progenitor cells which undergo proliferation and development in vitro to produce cells (CFU-E) which can respond to erythropoietin. Subsequent proliferation and development of the CFU-E result in the production of mature erythrocytes; Eos-CFC, progenitor cells which give rise to colonies in vitro containing mature eosinophils; Meg-CFC, diploid progenitor cells which proliferate and develop into polyploid megakaryocytes in vitro; Mast-CFC, progenitor cells developing in vitro into mast cells. The production and development of all these cells takes place in the bone marrow. Pre-T cells migrate to the thymus, where they proliferate and develop into mature immune-reactive T-lymphocytes. Pre B cells' develop in the bone marrow.

more recently by exploiting the ability of retroviruses to insert randomly into the genome.[3-5] Both these techniques of clonal analysis have clearly demonstrated that some stem cells are pluripotent with respect to their ability to give rise to *all* the various cell components of the lymphoid and myeloid lineages. However, these studies have also shown that the 'stem cell' compartment is heterogenous and should be considered as a developmental continuum. For example, cells have been detected which show varying degrees of lineage-restriction (being able to produce only myeloid or only lymphoid cells) and self-renewal ability. Because of this, it has been difficult to accurately quantify the numbers and concentration of pluripotent stem cells in the bone marrow. A rough estimate, however, can be gained from the finding that transplantation of 30 000 mouse bone marrow cells into a potentially lethally irradiated recipient will fully reconstitute the haemopoietic system and allow the animal to live a normal lifespan. Clearly, 30 000 cells contain at least one (and probably more) 'reconstitution units' equivalent to stem cells.[6]

A second, more readily quantified, assay for 'stem cells' is the spleen colony forming assay; which measures the ability of primitive cells (CFU-S) to lodge in the spleen.[7] Subsequent clonal proliferation and developmental of these cells results in the formation of spleen nodules (colonies), some of which contain only cells of one cell lineage while others contain cells of several cell lineages, including cells with the ability to give rise to lymphoid as well as myeloid cells. Evidence indicates, therefore, that at least some of the CFU-S overlap with the pluripotent stem cells while others are more developmentally restricted (so called committed multipotent, bipotent or unipotent cells).[8]

Lineage-restricted haemopoietic progenitor cells can also be detected using in vitro assay systems.[2] Some cells, for example, can undergo clonal proliferation and development in soft-gel culture systems to produce colonies containing all the different mature myeloid cells (erythrocytes, neutrophils, macrophages, eosinophils, mast cells and megakaryocytes). These progenitor cells are known as CFC-Mix. Heterogeneity is also found within the CFC-Mix population, in that the colonies produced may be lacking in one or more of the cell types classified above. It has not been determined, however, if this represents an *intrinsic* fixed heterogeneity of the CFC-Mix population or is a reflection of the assay systems used and arises as a consequence of stochastic processes acting upon a homogenous cell population. Both mechanisms are probably operating since, as stressed above, the haemopoietic system is best viewed as a continuum of cells in various stages of differentiation, lineage-commitment and development. This is emphasized by the finding that other progenitor cells can be assayed in vitro by their ability to produce: large (BFU-E) or small (CFU-E) clones of mature erythroid cells; megakaryocytes (Meg-CFC); eosinophils (Eos-CFC); or neutrophils and macrophages (GM-CFC). The GM-CFC (a biopotent cell) further gives rise to macrophage-restricted and neutrophil-restricted progenitor cells.

The end result of this process is that the appropriate numbers of mature cell types are produced to meet the animals needs at any one time. Because the majority of the mature cells have only a short-life span (for example, neutrophils persist for only a few hours), mature cells must be continually generated. Clearly, the haemopoietic system is organised to ensure that this regenerative capacity persists throughout life and that sufficient flexibility exists to maintain normal steady state blood cell production while still allowing extra production of one or more types of cells required in situations of stress (such as bleeding, hypoxia or severe infections).

ROLE OF GROWTH FACTORS IN HAEMOPOIESIS

Relatively little is known of the mechanisms underlying differentiation and self-renewal of stem cells. Evidence suggests, however, that 'decisions' are made on a stochastic basis with a probability which reflects the nature and metabolic state of the cell (the presence of specific cell surface receptors, cell cycle status and so on) and environmental influences. These external influences are many and diverse, encompassing interaction of developing haemopoietic cells with extracellular matrix molecules, with a variety of stromal cells and with growth factors.[9]

Haemopoietic growth factors comprise a family of glycosylated polypeptides, many of which have been defined by their ability to support the growth and development of colonies of haemopoietic cells of various lineages in vitro, usually using soft-gel culture systems. For this reason, they have been termed 'colony stimulating factors' (CSF's).[10] Some of the haemopoietic growth factors, however, were initially defined in other assay systems, and are referred to as 'interleukins'.[11] Historically, those growth factors were ill defined factors present in media conditioned by the growth of certain cells.[12] In the past few years, however, most of these activities have been purified to homogeneity, molecularly cloned and the gene products expressed in suitable prokaryotic vector systems.[13] The availability of large amounts of purified recombinant material has facilitated in vivo testing in pre-clinical and clinical situations as described elsewhere in this Issue (*see* Bronchud & Dexter, this Issue) and has allowed structure/function studies to be carried out and the various target cells determined in vitro. Furthermore, recent advances in cell sorting techniques have provided highly enriched populations of multipotential stem cells and lineage-restricted progenitor cells.[14,15] Since these sorted cell populations are essentially free of accessory cells, it is now possible to examine the direct effects of growth factors on defined target cells. In this way, both direct stimulatory activities and synergistic activities have been found (Fig. 2).

INTERLEUKIN-3

Interleukin-3,[16] also commonly referred to as Multi-CSF, is a multilineage stimulating factor which supports the growth of myeloid and mast cell lines and the in vitro survival, growth and differentiation of multipotent stem cells (CFU-S and CFC-Mix) as well as committed progenitor cells (GM-CFC, BFU-E, Meg-CFC and Eos-CFC). It will also support the growth of some pre-B cell lines. Both the murine and the human IL-3 genes have been molecularly cloned and although the stimulatory activities are species restricted, there is 29% homology at the amino acid level. In both species, IL-3 is produced by activated T-cells and murine IL-3 is also produced from a myelomonocytic leukaemia cell line, WEH1-3B (which is apparently auto-stimulated by the growth factor). Indeed, the suspicion that IL-3 (and also M-CSF and GM-CSF) may not only be important in the control of normal haemopoietic cells but also significant in haemopoietic disorders and leukaemias, is indicated by several findings (*see* Testa & Dexter, this Issue).

GRANULOCYTE/MACROPHAGE COLONY STIMULATING FACTOR (GM-CSF)

Initially it was thought that the action of GM-CSF was restricted to the GM-CFC and Eos-CFC. Recent work using recombinant material, however, has shown that at higher concentrations, GM-CSF can also recruit proliferation in a proportion of the CFC-Mix, BFU-E and Meg-CFC. In other words, it has a biological activity

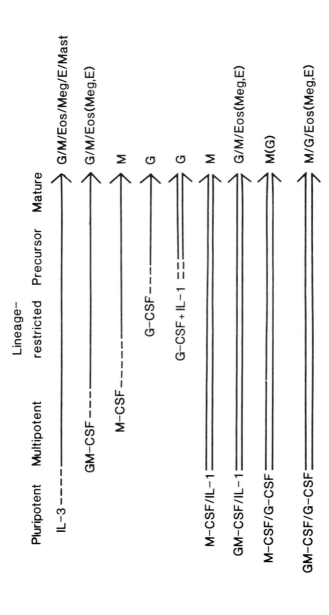

Fig. 2 The target cells of growth factors
Growth Factors: IL-3, Interleukin-3; IL-1, Interleukin-1; GM-CSF, ganulocyte/macrophage colony stimulating factor; G-CSF, granulocyte colony stimulating factor; M-CSF, macrophage colony stimulating factor. Mature cells produced: G, neutrophils; M, macrophages; Eos, eosinophils; Meg, megakaryocytes; E, erythroid.

showing extensive (but not complete) overlap with IL-3.[13] Both the human and the murine genes have been molecularly cloned[17] and although the products show about 50% homology at the amino acid level, their activities are species restricted. Unlike IL-3, GM-CSF can be produced from a wide range of normal cell types including activated T cells, endothelial cells and connective tissue cells and is constitutively produced by a variety of malignant cells.

GRANULOCYTE COLONY STIMULATING FACTOR (G-CSF)

Initial reports described human G-CSF as a pluripoietin,[18] stimulating the growth and development of multipotent cells as well as lineage-restricted granulocyte/macrophage and erythroid progenitor cells. These early studies were performed with unfractionated marrow cells, however, and subsequent work demonstrated that if T-cells and macrophages were first removed from the marrow, G-CSF stimulated the growth and development of only neutrophil progenitor cells. In other words, G-CSF acts directly on the G-CFC but indirectly can recruit more primitive cells presumably by acting in concert with factors released from T cells and/or macrophages.[19] These 'synergistic' interactions will be described more fully later.

The human and murine gene products show 70–80% homology at the amino acid level and unlike the situation with IL-3 and GM-CSF there appears to be no species restriction in biological activity: human G-CSF is an effective stimulus for murine precurser cells.

MACROPHAGE COLONY STIMULATING FACTOR (M-CSF)

As the name suggests, this growth factor has a stimulatory effect on progenitor and precurser cells of the macrophage lineage.[10,20] Since previous work showed little or no additive effect upon colony development in vitro when a combined stimulus of GM-CSF and M-CSF were used, it was thought that the target cells (the GM-CFC) were essentially the same. Recent data, however, indicate that although there is some overlap in the responding cell population, this is by no means extensive.[21] Several experimental protocols have been described where additive effects upon colony development are seen when these two growth factors are combined. It seems likely, then, that M-CSF preferentially recruits a sub-population of progenitor cells which are restricted to macrophage development. Apart from acting on progenitor cells, however, M-CSF can also promote proliferation in morphologically mature macrophages.

The human and mouse gene products show extensive homology at the amino acid level and (as with G-CSF) the human product is active upon murine cells.[22,10] Unlike IL-3, GM-CSF and G-CSF (which are single polypeptide chains), M-CSF consists of a dimer of two identical polypeptide subunits, each with a molecular weight of 14 500. Although all four growth factors are glycosylated in their native form, the sugar groups do not appear to be essential for activity since active material is produced by material synthesized by cells in the presence of tunicamycin, or following treatment of growth factors with various glycosidases. Furthermore, recombinant (non-glycosylated) IL-3, GM-CSF and G-CSF produced in bacteria appears to be as active (in vivo as well as in vitro) as native glycosylated material. In the case of M-CSF, biological activity is only seen with the dimeric form: treatment with mercaptoethanol abolishes activity.

STRUCTURAL/EVOLUTIONARY RELATIONSHIPS

IL-3, GM-CSF, G-CSF and M-CSF are present as single copy genes. In view of their overlapping biological activities it might be anticipated that they are part of a gene family—evolving from a common primordial gene. This does not appear to be the case however, since they share no significant homology and the molecules differ markedly in their predicted secondary structure. Of potential interest, however, is that there does appear to be some degree of conservation in the first few amino acids at the N-terminus (for IL-3, GM-CSF and IL-1) on the putative signal peptide. Perhaps this is a common structural feature for factors active on haemopoietic cells.[23]

It is also significant that three of these genes (IL-3, GM-CSF and M-CSF) are clustered on the distal portion of the long arm of chromosome 5 in humans (a region which also includes the putative receptors for M-CSF, the c-*Fms* proto-oncogene) (*see* Ref. 24). Chromosome deletions or translocation at this site are commonly associated with myeloid leukaemias and myelodysplastic syndromes. Similarly, the gene for G-CSF has been localised on human chromosome 17 adjacent to a site included in translocation associated with acute promyelocytic leukaemia.[25] These associations between chromosome locations, deletions and translocations, with haemopoietic disorders are unlikely to be trivial.

Apart from showing no homology with each other, these myeloid cell growth factors also show no homology with lymphoid-active factors such as IL-2 and IL-1 nor with growth factors active on epithelial cells and mesenchyme such as EGF and PDGF.

It appears, then, that IL-3, GM-CSF, G-CSF and M-CSF have evolved independently. This is further emphasised when the receptors for these growth factors are considered. Data strongly suggest that there are specific high affinity receptors for the CSF's and that each CSF can bind to only one receptor.[26,27] Furthermore, estimates of receptor numbers on responding target cells have given values of between 100 and 500 for IL-3, GM-CSF and G-CSF and somewhat higher for M-CSF (up to about 15 000 on mature macrophages).[20,28] However only 5 to 10% of these receptors need to bind the growth factors to elicit a substantial proliferative effect. But the presence of such low receptor numbers also raises formidable problems in purifying and chracterising the receptors themselves and it is for this reason that structural information on the receptors (with the exception of c-*Fms*, the M-CSF receptor) is lacking.

SYNERGISTIC ACTIVITIES

The range of target cells stimulated by IL-3, GM-CSF, G-CSF and M-CSF perhaps suggests that myelopoiesis is regulated solely by modulation in the production of these different activities. The situation, however, is clearly much more complex: several molecules have now been described which do not, by themselves, stimulate growth and development of myeloid progenitor cells but can nonetheless show dramatic synergistic effects when combined with the CSF's.

Interleukin-4, for example, is a growth factor for T cells and B cells and can also sustain the in vitro proliferation of some mast cell lines[29-31] and continuously growing factor-dependent haemopoietic progenitor cell lines, acting synergistically with IL-3. In common with the CSF's, IL-4 is also produced from activated murine and human T cells.

Interleukin-5, also known as BCGF-II and eosinophil differentiation factor, stimulates proliferation and immunoglobulin secretion of activated B lymphocytes and induces differentiation of eosinophils.[32] It does not, however, act directly as a growth stimulus on the eosinophil progenitor cells (Eos-CFC).

Interleukin-6, previously described as plasmocytoma growth factor of BSF-2, facilitates the growth of plasmocytoma cells and hybridomas and has recently been shown to possess synergistic activities on primitive multipotent myeloid cells when used in combination with CSF's.

It appears, therefore, that many factors which were initially described for their effects upon various lymphoid cell population can also influence the growth of myeloid cells. In other words, 'lineage-restriction' of growth factors may not be as strict as first imagined. This is emphasised in studies using Interleukin-1 (IL-1).

IL-1 has many and diverse effects upon B and T lymphocytes (see articles by Feldmann et al. and by Callard, this Issue), but many other types of cells, including macrophages, connective tissue cells and endothelial cells, have receptors for and can respond to IL-1. Recently IL-1 has been shown to be identical with a factor termed haemopoietin-1;[33] which was recognised by its ability to facilitate the response of primitive cells to apparently 'lineage-restricted' molecules such as M-CSF.[21] However, the problem with many of these studies is that the cell population used as targets were heterogeneous, and the possibility of indirect effects mediated by activation of accessory cells could not be ruled out. To circumvent this problem, we have recently examined the effects of IL-1 on a highly enriched population of d12 CFU-S, i.e. on self-renewing, multipotent stem cells, which had been effectively depleted of contaminating cells using a fluorescence activated cell sorter (=FACS-BM).[14] The results of these experiments can be summarised as follows: (1) Between 4 and 40% of the FACS-BM cells produce mixed myeloid colonies in vitro in the presence of IL-3, i.e. at least some and perhaps all multipotent cells have receptors for and can respond to IL-3; (2) IL-1 alone is not a growth factor—in its presence the FACS-BM cells die; (3) GM-CSF, when used alone, stimulates about 30% of the number of colonies seen with IL-3—this supports other data indicating that at least some stem cells can respond to GM-CSF; (4) M-CSF, on its own, is a relatively poor stimulus for colony development and the colonies produced may well represent lineage-restricted progenitor cells which have been co-fractionated with CFU-S; (5) G-CSF, used alone, gave only a few colonies; (6) When IL-1 was combined with IL-3, no difference in the number of colonies was seen. When IL-1 was combined with either GM-CSF or M-CSF, however, a marked synergy was found and colony number approached that seen in IL-3. In other words, these growth factor combinations are apparently recruiting more primitive cells than can respond to either of the CSF's alone. The fact that the colony forming cells being stimulated by these factors represent essentially the same cells as respond to IL-3 is strongly indicated by the finding that no additive effects are seen i.e. if IL-1 plus M-CSF are combined with IL-3, colony number does not exceed that found in IL-3 alone. Of some importance, however, is that the *end result* is different. In IL-3, mixed myeloid colonies develop: but in M-CSF plus IL-1, all the colonies contain only macrophages.

These results are of importance for two reasons. First, the data suggest that primitive cells have cell surface receptors for most (if not all) of the growth factors (although, in order to respond, they may need a combination of stimuli). Second, the pattern of development seen suggests that the outcome of a response is determined largely by the factors present in the environment and not by an intrinsic stem cell 'responsive' or 'unresponsive' state. Such 'combination' therapy is already producing useful results in experimental animal systems[34] and the data clearly have wide implications on the conduct of future clinical/preclinical trials.

ACKNOWLEDGEMENTS

The authors work is supported by the Cancer Research Campaign, UK.

REFERENCES

1 Metcalf D, Moore MAS. Haemopoietic Cells. Amsterdam: North Holland, 1971
2 Metcalf D. Haemopoietic Colonies. Berlin: Springer-Verlag, 1977
3 Abramson S, Miller RG, Phillips RA. The identification in the adult bone marrow of pluripotent and restricted stem cells of the myeloid and lymphoid systems. J Exp Med 1979; 145: 1567–1579
4 Lemischka IR, Raulet DH, Mulligan RC. Developmental potential and dynamic behaviour of hematopoietic stem cells. Cell 1986; 45: 917–927
5 Snodgrass R, Keller G. Clonal fluctuations within the haematopoietic system of mice reconstituted with retrovirus infected cells. EMBO J 1987; 6: 3955–3960
6 Dexter TM. Stem cells in normal growth and disease. Br Med J 1987; 295: 1192–1194
7 Till JE, McCulloch EA. A direct measurement of the radiation sensitivity of normal mouse bone marrow cells. Radiat Res 1961; 14: 215–222

8 Dexter TM, Spooncer E, Schofield R, Lord BI, Simmons P. Haemopoietic stem cells and the problem of self-renewal. Blood Cells 1984; 10: 315–339
9 Dexter TM, Spooncer E. Growth and differentiation in the haemopoietic system. Ann Rev Cell Biol 1987; 3: 423–441
10 Metcalf D. The haemopoietic colony stimulating factors. Elsevier, Amsterdam; 1984
11 Ihle JN, Rebar L, Keller J, Lee JC, Hapel AT. Interleukin-3: possible roles in the regulation of lymphocyte differentiation and growth. Immunol Rev 1982; 63: 5–32
12 Dexter TM. The message in the medium. Nature 1984; 309: 746–747
13 Metcalf D. The granulocyte macrophage colony stimulating factors. Science 1985; 229: 16–22
14 Heyworth CM, Ponting ILO, Dexter TM. The response of haemopoietic cells to growth factors: developmental implications of synergistic interactions. J Cell Science 1988 (In Press)
15 Lord BI, Spooncer E. Isolation of haemopoietic spleen colony forming cells. Lymphokine Res 1986; 5: 59–72
16 Moore MAS. Interleukin-3: an overview. In: Schrader JW, ed. Interleukin-3: the panspecific hemopoietin. Lymphokines, Vol.15, New York: Academic Press, 1988: pp.219–280
17 Gough NM, Burgess AW. The genes for granulocyte-macrophage colony stimulating factor and multi-colony stimulating factor (IL-3) In: Guroff G, ed. Oncogenes, genes and growth factors. New York: Wiley, 1987: pp.165–197
18 Welte K, Platzer E, Lu L et al. Purification and biochemical characterisation of human pluripotent hematopoietic colony-stimulating factor. Proc Natl Acad Sci 1985; 82: 1526–1530
19 Souza LM, Boone TC, Gabrilove J et al. Recombinant human granulocyte colony stimulating factor: effects on normal and leukaemic myeloid cells. Science, 1986; 232: 61–65
20 Stanley ER, Guilbert J. Methods for the purification, assay, characterisation and target cell binding of a colony stimulating factor (CSF-1). J Immunol Methods, 1981; 445: 253–289
21 Stanley ER, Bartocci A, Patinkin D, Rosendaal M, Bradley TR. Regulation of very primitive multipotent hemopoietic cells by hemopoietin-1. Cell, 1986; 45: 667–674
22 Wong GG, Temple IA, Leary AL et al. Human CSF-1: molecular cloning and expression of 4-kb cDNA encoding the human urinary protein. Science, 1987; 235: 1504–1508
23 Clark-Lewis I, Schrader JW. Molecular structure and biological activities of P cell stimulating factor (Interleukin-3). In: Lymphokines, Vol. 15, New York: Academic Press, 1988: pp.1–37
24 LeBeau M, Epstein ND, O'Brien SJ et al. The interleukin-3 gene is located on human chromosome 5 and is deleted in myeloid leukemias with a deletion of 5q. Proc Natl Acad Sci 1887; 84: 5913–5917
25 Simmers RN, Webber LM, Shannon MF et al. Localisation of the G-CSF gene on chromosome 17 proximal to the breakpoint in the t(15;17) in acute premyelocytic leukemia. Blood 1987; 70: 330–332
26 Nicola NA, Peterson L. Identification of distinct receptors for two hemopoietic growth factors (granulocyte colony stimulating factor and multipotential colony stimulating factor) by chemical cross-linking. J Biol Chem 1986; 261: 12384–12389
27 Walker F, Nicola NA, Metcalf D, Burgess AW. Hierarchial down-modulation of hemopoietic growth factor receptors. Cell 1985; 43: 269–276
28 Bartelmez SH, Stanley ER. Synergism between hemopoietic growth factors (HGF's) detected by their effects on cells leaving receptors for a lineage specific HGF: assay for hemopoietin-1. J Cell Physiol 1985; 122: 370–378

29 Hamaguchi Y, Kanakura Y, Fujita J et al. Interleukin-4 as an essential factor for in vitro clonal growth of murine connective tissue type mast cells. J Exp Med 1987; 165: 268–283
30 Lee F, Yokota T, Otsuka T et al. Isolation and characterisation of a mouse interleukin cDNA clone that expresses B-cell stimulating factor inactivities and T-cell and mast-cell-stimulating activities. Proc Natl Acad Sci 1986; 83: 2661–2664
31 Noma Y, Sideras P, Naito T et al. Cloning of cDNA encoding the murine lgGl induction factor by a novel strategy using SP6 promoter. Nature 1986; 319: 640–642
32 Sanderson CJ, O'Garra A, Warren DJ, Klaus GBB. Eosinophil differentiation factor also has B-cell growth factor activity: proposed name interleukin-4. Proc Natl Acad Sci 1986; 83: 437–440
33 Mechizuki DY, Eisenman JR, Conlon PJ et al. Interleukin-1 regulates hematopoietic activity, a role previously associated to hemopoietin-1. Proc Natl Acad Sci 1987; 84: 5267–5271
34 Moore MAS, Warren D, Souza L. In vivo and in vitro action of G-CSF and IL-1 in myelosuppressed mice. J Cell Biochem 1988 (In Press)

Regulatory factors in lymphoid development

J J T Owen
E J Jenkinson
Department of Anatomy, Medical School, University of Birmingham, UK

> The process of T lymphocyte maturation within the thymus involves a complex series of differentiation events involving T cell receptor gene rearrangement and expression. A beginning has now been made at defining the growth and differentiation signals required for these events. An additional level of complexity is provided by the selection of the repertoire of T cell specificities so that the pool of peripheral T cells available for interaction with antigens is 'shaped' by the thymus.
>
> The maturation of stem cells to B lymphocytes takes place in association with bone marrow stromal cells. Large numbers of newly-formed B cells can now be generated in vitro on stromal cell layers. Stromal cells capable of supporting B lymphopoiesis have now been cloned and, recently, a growth factor (IL-7) which acts on early B cells has been identified.

The aim of this review is to highlight recent advances in knowledge of the factors which regulate the development of lymphocytes from haemopoietic stem cells. With the realization that this phase of development involves the rearrangement and expression of the genes which code for the antigen recognition receptors, work in this field has grown considerably in recent years and we can provide only a selective view of the literature. Although there are similarities between the development of T and B lymphocytes, they are quite distinct cell types with different functions and so we have treated them separately.

SIGNALS IN T-LYMPHOCYTE ONTOGENY

Introduction

The importance of the thymus in the generation of T lymphocytes has been known for some years and was first demonstrated by the observation that neonatal thymectomy in rodents resulted in severe immune deficiency.[1] More recently, studies on nude mice and rats, which have congenital defects of thymic development resulting in an alymphoid thymus have confirmed the sparse development of T lymphocytes in the absence of a lymphoid thymus.[2] The thymus is a complex organ made up of a framework of epithelial cells (derived from the pharyngeal pouches) which is colonised by stem cells which migrate into the organ at an early stage of development (Fig. 1). These stem cells give rise to the lymphocytes of the thymus and various other elements of the thymic stroma, in particular macrophages and dendritic cells. This phase of stem cell migration is followed by two further major phases (Fig. 2), the first of which involves the proliferation and differentiation of the progeny of the lymphoid stem cells whilst the final phase is concerned with the selection of the antigen receptor repertoire of lymphocytes so that autoreactive T cells are eliminated.

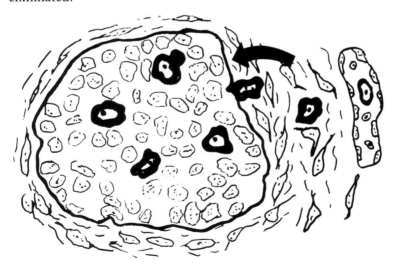

Fig. 1 Stem cells migrate from blood vessels through the mesenchyme which surrounds the thymus and enter the epithelial thymic primordium. Epithelial cells form a major component of the thymus but macrophages and dendritic cells (derived from migrant precursor cells) also contribute to the stroma.

Migration of stem cells to the thymus

The early development of the thymus is characterised by the migration of large blast-like cells from adjacent blood vessels into the thymic stroma after crossing the basement membrane which surrounds the thymic primordium (Fig. 1). These stem cells are known to migrate into the developing thymus in waves suggesting that there is some regulatory control which determines their rate of entry. Indeed, evidence has been produced that the thymic primordium releases chemotactic factors which attract stem cells to it.[3] Perhaps these factors are elaborated and released according to the demand for stem cells and this would explain not only the wave phenomenon but also the continued, albeit low, input of stem cells into the adult thymus. These observations suggest that thymic stem cells are not an autonomous self renewing population.

Thymic stem cells are known to originate from haemopoietic tissues such as fetal liver and bone marrow[4] but their precise identification has proved to be difficult. Various procedures have been used to enrich thymic stem cells, based for example on their

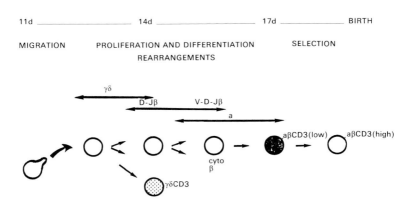

Fig. 2 An outline of the events occurring within the thymus of the mouse embryo (from day 11 of gestation to birth) is shown. γδ and αβ cells are probably separate cell lineages although they may be derived from a common stem cell type. Rearrangements of the T cell receptor genes proceed through the phase of cell proliferation. Expression of various surface antigens e.g. Thy1, CD4, CD8 also occurs at this time. Immediately prior to the appearance of cells with surface αβCD3 receptors, cells can be detected which express cytoplasmic β chains (cytoβ). Newly formed αβCD3$^+$ cells have low levels of receptors, express both CD4 and CD8 antigens and are immunologically immature. A transitional stage is presumed to occur during which some of these cells increase their level of receptor expression and become CD4$^+$ or CD8$^+$ only.

low buoyant density. However, no definitive cell marker has been identified which would allow the purification of thymic stem cells to homogeneity. Recent studies[5] have provided support for the proposal[6] that the stem cells that migrate into the thymus are multipotential with regard to haemopoietic differentiation and their development into T cells is determined by the thymic environment. This is an area where further research is required.

Proliferation and differentiation of stem cells within the thymus

The phase of migration is followed by the proliferation and differentiation of lymphoid cell precursors within the thymic stroma (Fig. 2). This phase is accompanied by the appearance of various glycoproteins on the surface of the developing cells and these molecules can be identified by various monoclonal antibodies. The Thy-I molecule appears early in the ontogeny of lymphocytes within the mouse embryo thymus and continues to be expressed at high levels during the phases of intrathymic lymphopoiesis dropping to lower levels on mature T lymphocytes. The CD5 molecule is also present from an early stage of ontogeny within the mouse thymus and before the appearance of the CD8 and CD4 molecules which are expressed on the majority cellular population of the thymus namely the small cortical thymocytes. In fact, recent evidence indicates that the expression of CD8 slightly proceeds that of CD4[7] so that a population of immediate precursors of so-called 'double positive' cells ($CD4^+$ $CD8^+$) can be detected by expression of CD8 only. The functional significance of CD4 and CD8 expression on 'double positive' thymocytes is unclear but the expression of these molecules on 'single positive' CD4 only and CD8 only mature T cells, which are thought to be derived from the 'double positive' cells, is important in strengthening the interactions between T cell receptors and target antigens.

Another molecule which is expressed quite early in thymic development is CD2 and this is potentially of considerable functional interest because of its known involvement in activation of T cells in the periphery. In addition to CD4 and CD8 expression, small cortical lymphocytes also express the CD1 antigen which can be detected by means of monoclonal antibodies in the human thymus. The functional significance of this expression is as yet unknown.

During these phases of development it is known that the important process of rearrangement of the T cell receptor genes is initiated. Two types of T cell receptor have been identified. One is made up of γ and δ chains, the other of α and β chains. In either case, $\gamma\delta$ or $\alpha\beta$, there is co-expression of the CD3 family of molecules which are thought to be involved in transducing signals from the T cell receptor into the cell. The functions of the $\alpha\beta$CD3 complex are best understood. These molecules are expressed on a majority of peripheral T lymphocytes and are concerned with the recognition of foreign antigens (probably in the form of processed peptides) in association with major histocompatibility molecules.[8] Thus, $\alpha\beta$CD3 molecules are of major importance in the role of T lymphocytes in immune responses. The role of $\gamma\delta$CD3 expressing T lymphocytes is poorly understood, although it is known that they can participate in cytotoxic reactions.

Within the thymus, rearrangements of the genes which code for the γ and δ molecules pre-date those of the α and β chains genes. However, it is also known that many of these rearrangements are not productive in the sense that they do not lead to the expression of the appropriate proteins. In fact the proportion of cells which express $\gamma\delta$CD3 receptors within the thymus is very low (no more than a few percent) but these cells are evident some days before the appearance of $\alpha\beta$CD3 expressing cells. The $\gamma\delta$CD3 cells are probably a separate lineage to the $\alpha\beta$CD3 cells[9] (see Fig. 2).

There is little doubt that initiation of rearrangements of $\alpha\beta$ chain genes occurs within the thymus. For example, a single stem cell taken from the early embryo thymus can generate multiple $\alpha\beta$ T cell receptors when it is grown within an epithelial thymic primordium.[10] The rearrangement of β chain genes precedes that of α chain genes. Of the three β chain gene segments which code for the variable part of the molecule rearrangements occur between the D and J segments prior to the production of full V-D-J rearrangements (Fig. 2). In both cases, rearrangements also involve constant region (C) genes producing, in the case of D-J-C rearrangements 1.0 kb mRNA transcripts and in the case of V-D-J-C rearrangements 1.3 kb mRNA transcripts.[11] The rearrangement and expression of β chain genes prior to α chain genes results in the presence of detectable cytoplasmic β chains within proliferating cells of the thymus prior to the expression of $\alpha\beta$CD3 molecules on cell surfaces.[12] CD3 expression occurs earlier in the lineage and again CD3 expression can be detected within the cytoplasm of cells prior to expression on cell surfaces.

The signals involved in these growth and differentiation steps are under active investigation. In terms of growth signals, it has been shown that both IL-2 and IL-4 can independently stimulate the proliferation of early thymic precursors removed from the thymic environment and grown in vitro.[13,14] However, the progeny of the stimulated cells do not undergo an ordered progression of T cell receptor gene rearrangements and phenotypic changes as observed in the intact thymus.[15] In fact, to date full rearrangements of the β chain genes and expression of αβCD3 receptors has not been observed in these cell cultures and so the physiological significance of the results is open to question. However, IL-2 receptors have been demonstrated on a majority of developing lymphocytes within the intact thymus during at least part of the proliferative phase. There is some debate about the significance of this observation because of reports that the receptors detected are of low affinity for IL-2 and therefore may not be functional.[16] In a further study antibodies to IL-2 receptors have been shown to reduce cell proliferation within thymus organ cultures—an effect that can be reversed by the addition of recombinant IL-2.[17] However, growth inhibition was not observed in another study.[18] Further support for the role of growth factors in thymus lymphocyte proliferation has come from *in situ* hybridization studies where low levels of interleukin IL-4 mRNA has been detected in a majority of developing thymus lymphocytes just prior to the stage when αβ T cell receptors are expressed.[19] At earlier stages of development, a role for IL-1 in lymphocyte maturation has been suggested from studies demonstrating the importance of IL-1 derived from phagocytic cells of the thymus on the induction of proliferation in precursor populations.[20]

The signalling systems which initiate these growth factor mechanisms are poorly understood. It has been suggested that the CD2 molecule on immature thymocytes might by interacting with its complementary molecule LFA-3 on thymic epithelium cells lead to the activation of the IL-2 growth system.[21] Further work is needed in this area. The ability of T cell precursors to proliferate outside the thymus without full receptor gene rearrangement suggests that these growth systems are not by themselves sufficient to induce the process of T cell receptor gene rearrangements described earlier. Recently, we have shown that antibodies to CD3 molecules will inhibit the full rearrangement of β chain genes so that D-J but not V-D-J rearrangements are produced.[22] These experiments have been carried out in organ cultures where the

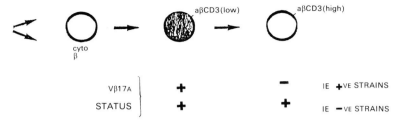

Fig. 3 Expression of the Vβ17a product by T cells confers reactivity to the MHC class II antigen IE. In IE$^+$ mouse strains (but not in IE$^-$ strains), Vβ17a$^+$ cells are clonally deleted before they can proceed to the αβCD3 (high) stage.

treated thymus lobes support normal levels of proliferation and indeed show evidence of phenotypic maturation but lack expression of αβCD receptors. How this effect is mediated is presently unknown but we have suggested the possibility that the antibodies react with γδCD3 cells in the early thymus and perhaps inhibit a signalling effect they have on αβ precursor cells.

Selection of the T lymphocyte repertoire within the thymus

The majority of newly formed thymus lymphocytes expressing αβCD3 receptors are unable to respond to antigens and must undergo further maturation before they can function as peripheral mature T lymphocytes. These CD4$^+$CD8$^+$ thymocytes express low levels of αβ receptors and although they have been shown to be capable of mobilising calcium in response to various cell stimuli[23] they invariably undergo cell death when separated from the thymus and placed in vitro. Indeed, the latter result has given rise to the notion that these cells may normally undergo cell death and are therefore not the precursors of mature peripheral T cells. However, recent studies provide an alternative explanation, namely that these cells may be subjected to considerable negative selection as a means of removing autoreactive cells. The V segments of some of the β chain genes have been shown to produce receptors with affinity for histocompatibility molecules. For example, the product of the Vβ17 gene in the mouse produces αβ receptors which have affinity for IE molecules and using a monoclonal antibody which recognises the Vβ17 product, it has been shown that cells expressing this product are deleted from the peripheral T cell repertoire in those strains of mice that express IE.[24] However, Vβ17 positive cells are present within the cortex of the IE$^+$ thymus and so the supposition is that the deletion process occurs during the maturational phase when the cells convert from an immature to a mature phenotype (Fig. 3). Further support for this idea has come from recent studies on the reactivity of products of the Vβ6 and Vβ8 genes for the minor histocompatibility antigen Mls.[25] Perhaps most dramatically, the concept of negative selection as a means of removing autoreactive cells has been obtained in transgenic mice in which the transgene is an αβ T cell receptor for the male H-Y antigen. In both male and female mice the transgene is expressed at the expense of endogenous T cell receptor genes so that the repertoire in each case is heavily biased to reactivity to the H-Y antigen.[26] In female mice no gross effect is seen on thymus size or the peripheral T cell pool but in male mice the thymus is small and cells expressing receptors coded by the transgene in association with CD4 and CD8 appear to be eliminated because of their potential autoreactivity.

The mechanisms involved in the deletion of autoreactive cells are not known but we have recently found that antibodies directed to the CD3 component of the αβCD3 receptor induce a process of apoptosis in immature thymus cells within thymus organ cultures. Apoptosis is characterized by the activation of endogenous endonucleases which cleave DNA into small fragments as a result of which nuclei become condensed and affected cells are phagocytosed by macrophages. The activation of this mechanism when the receptors of immature cells bind self antigens might be the means by which autoreactive cells are removed.

It is well known that the T cells of an individual respond best to peptides derived from foreign antigens when associated with the major histocompatibility antigens possessed by the particular individual. This major histocompatibility restriction of immune responsiveness is determined by the thymus[27] and so presumably a mechanism of positive selection must occur at some stage of T lymphocyte development which favours the survival of those T cells which have receptors which will recognize foreign peptides in association with self MHC. The way in which this positive selection is achieved is presently unknown and there has been controversy as to whether it is determined by interaction of developing T lymphocytes with thymic epithelial cells or with antigen presenting cells. These are important matters requiring further investigation.

SIGNALS IN B LYMPHOCYTE ONTOGENY

Introduction

B lymphocytes are known to be generated from haemopoietic stem cells within the fetal liver and later the bone marrow.[28] The rate of production of B lymphocytes is very high[29] and rivals that of the production of T lymphocytes within the thymus. The cell kinetics of B lymphocyte development have been extensively studied and it is clear that within a proliferating pre-B cell population rearrangements of the genes coding for the immunoglobulin heavy and light chains are proceeding. In fact heavy chain rearrangements precedes that of the light chains and a proportion of pre B cells are characterized by the presence of cytoplasmic μ chains in the absence of light chain expression.[30] Only later are μ and light chains co-expressed on the surface of newly formed B lymphocytes which then leave the cell cycle. Because of the difficulty of studying this process in organs such as fetal liver and bone marrow where there is a complex mixture of cells, many of the investigations have been carried out on immature B lymphocytes transformed by the Abelson virus.[31] These lines not only express an immature phenotype but some of them continue to differentiate in vitro.

Stromal cell requirements in B lymphocyte ontogeny

Early attempts to generate B lymphocytes from stem cells in colony type assays in either liquid or semi-solid culture conditions were unsuccessful. However, B lymphocytes could be generated in organ cultures of fetal liver[32] suggesting that cell interactions within the organ are important. Later, stromal cells derived from bone marrow were shown to be capable of supporting B lymphopoiesis under certain defined conditions.[33] By producing cell clones derived from these stromal cultures, it has become clear that not all stromal cell types are capable of supporting lymphopoiesis.[34] One clonal cell line (designated 1xN/A6) has been shown to secrete a growth factor which will support the proliferation of factor-dependent B cell precursors obtained from long term bone marrow cultures.[35] This factor has been purified to a single 25-Kd species and is distinct from previously described haemopoietic factors. Using direct expression in mammalian cells, a complementary DNA clone encoding this factor, designated IL-7, has been isolated.[36] The variety of cells capable of responding to

IL-7 is unknown but both pre-B cells (identified by the B220 antigen) and their B220⁻ precursors respond.

Clearly, considerable progress is now being made in understanding the factors which regulate B lymphopoiesis. Various membrane glycoproteins are known to be expressed on pre B cells: their possible functional importance and other aspects of B lymphopoiesis are discussed fully in a recent review.[37]

REFERENCES

1 Miller JFAP, Osoba D. Current concepts of the immunological function of the thymus. Physiol Rev 1967; 47: 437–487
2 MacDonald HR, Lees RK, Bron C, Sordat B, Miescher G. T cell antigen receptor expression in athymic (Nu/Nu) mice. J Exp Med 1987; 166: 195–209
3 Ben Spimane S, Houllier F, Tucker G, Thierry JP. In vitro migration of avian hemopoietic cells to the thymus. Preliminary characterization of a chemoattractive mechanism. Cell Differentiation 1983; 13: 1–24
4 Moore MAS, Owen JJT. Experimental studies on the development of the thymus. J Exp Med 1967; 126: 715–726
5 Spangrude GJ, Heinfeld S, Weissman IL. Purification and characterization of mouse hemopoietic stem cells. Science 1988; 241: 58–62
6 Moore MAS, Owen JJT. Stem cell migration in the developing myeloid and lymphoid system. Lancet 1967; ii: 658
7 MacDonald HR, Budd RC, Howe RC. A CD3-subset of CD4⁻8⁺ thymocytes: a rapidly cycling intermediate in the generation of CD4⁺CD8⁺ cells. Eur J Immunol 1988; 18: 519–523
8 Dembic Z, Haas W, Weiss S et al. Transfer of specificity of murine α and β T cell receptor genes. Nature 1986; 320: 232
9 Pardoll DM, Fowlkes BJ, Bluestone JA et al. Differential expression of two distinct T cell receptors during thymocyte development. Nature 1987; 326: 79–81
10 Williams GT, Kingston R, Owen MJ, Jenkinson EJ, Owen JJT. A single micromanipulated stem cell gives rise to multiple T cell receptor gene rearrangements in the thymus in vitro. Nature 1986; 324: 63–64
11 Snodgrass HR, Kisielow P, Kiefer M, Steinmetz M, von Boehmer H. Ontogeny of the T cell antigen receptor within the thymus. Nature 1985; 313: 592–595
12 Owen JJT, Kingston R, Jenkinson EJ. Generation of cells expressing cytoplasmic and/or surface T cell receptor β chains during the development of mouse fetal thymus. Immunology 1986; 59: 23–27
13 Ceredig R. Proliferation in vitro and interleukin production by 14 day fetal and adult Lyt2⁻/L3T4⁻ mouse thymocytes. J Immunol 1986; 137: 2260–2267
14 Palacios R, Sideras P, von Boehmer H. Recombinant interleukin 4/BSF.1 promotes growth and differentiation of intrathymic T cell precursors from fetal mice in vitro. EMBO J 1987; 6: 91–95
15 Pelkonen J, Sideras P, Rammensee H-G, Karjalainen K, Palacios R. Thymocyte clones from 14 day mouse embryos. J Exp Med 1987; 166: 1245–1258
16 Lowenthal JW, Howe RC, Ceredig R, MacDonald HR. Functional status of interleukin 2 receptors expressed by immature Ly2⁻L3T4⁻ thymocytes. J Immunol 1986; 137: 2579–2582
17 Jenkinson EJ, Kingston R, Owen JJT. Importance of IL-2 receptors in mitrathymic generation of cells expressing T cell receptors. Nature 1987; 329: 160–162

18 Plum J, De Smedt M. Differentiation of thymocytes in fetal organ cultures: lack of evidence for the functional role of the interleukin 2 receptor expressed by prothymocytes. Eur J Immunol; 18: 795–799
19 Sideras P, Funa K, Zalcberg-Quintana I et al. Analysis by in situ hybridisation of cells expressing mRNA for interleukin 4 in the developing thymus and in peripheral lymphocytes from mice. Proc Natl Acad Sci 1988; 85: 218–221
20 Papiernik M, Penit C, El Rouby S. Control of prothymocyte proliferation by thymic accessory cells. Eur J Immunol 1987; 17: 1303–1310
21 Alcoten A, Ramarli D, Richardson NE, Chang H-C, Reinherz EL. Functional and molecular aspects of human T lymphocyte activation via T3-Ti and T11 pathways. Immunol Rev 1987; 95: 5–36
22 Owen JJT, Owen MJ, Williams GT, Kingston R, Jenkinson EJ. The effects of anti-CD3 antibodies on the development of T cell receptor $\alpha\beta$ + lymphocytes in embryonic thymus organ cultures. Immunology 1988; 63: 639–642
23 Havran WL, Poenic M, Kimma J, Tsien R, Weiss A, Allison JP. Expression and function of the CD3-antigen receptor on murine CD4 + 8 + thymocytes. Nature 1987; 300: 70–173
24 Kappler J, Roehm N, Marrack P. T cell tolerance by clonal elimination in the thymus. Cell 1987; 49: 273–280
25 MacDonald HR, Schneider R, Lees RK et al. T cell receptor Vβ use predicts reactiority and tolerance to Mls^a-encoded antigens. Nature 1988; 322: 40–5
26 Kisielow P, Bluthmann H, Staerz UD, Steinmetz M, von Boehmer H. Tolerance in T cell receptor transgenic mice involves deletion of non mature CD4 + 8 + thymocytes. Nature 1988; 333: 742–746
27 Zinkernagel RM. Thymus and lymphohaemopoietic cells: their role in T cell maturation in selection of T cells H-2 restriction specificity and in H-2 linked gene control. Immunol Rev 1978; 42: 224–270
28 Owen JJT, Wright DE, Habu S, Raff MC, Cooper MD. Studies on the generation of B lymphocytes in fetal liver and bone marrow. J Immunol 1977; 118: 2067–2072
29 Osmond DG, Nossal GJV. Differentiation of lymphocytes in mouse bone marrow II Kinetics of maturation and renewal of anti-globulin binding cells studied by double labelling. Cell Immunol 1974; 13: 132–136
30 Raff MC, Megson M, Owen JJT, Cooper MD. Early production of intracellular IgM by B lymphocyte precursors in the mouse. Nature 1976; 259: 224–225
31 Alt FW, Blackwell TK, Depinho RA, Reth MG, Yancopoulos GD. Regulation of genome rearrangement events during lymphocyte differentiation. Immunol Rev 1986; 89: 5
32 Owen JJT, Cooper MD, Raff MC. In vitro generation of B lymphocytes in mouse fetal liver, a mammalian bursa equivalent. Nature 1974; 249: 361–362
33 Whitlock CA, Witte ON. Long term culture of B lymphocytes and their precursors from murine bone marrow. Proc Natl Acad Sci USA 1982; 79: 3608–3611
34 Whitlock CA, Tidmarsh GF, Muller-Sieburg C, Weissman IL. Bone marrow stromal cell lines with lymphopoietic activity express high levels of a pre B neoplasia-associated molecule. Cell 1987; 48: 1009–1014
35 Namen AE, Schmierer AE, March CJ et al. B Cell precursor growth-promoting activity. J Exp Med 1988; 167: 988–1002
36 Namen AE, Luptor S, Hjenilk K et al. Stimulation of B-cell progenitors by cloned murine interleukin-7. Nature 1988; 333: 571–573
37 Kincade PW. Experimental models for understanding B lymphocyte formation. Adv Immunol 1987; 41: 181–267

T cells and lymphokines

M Feldmann
M Londei
Charing Cross Sunley Research Centre, Hammersmith, London

C Haworth
Department of Haematology, Charing Cross and Westminster Medical School, Hammersmith, London

> T lymphocytes are one of the richest sources of protein mediators. Many of their effects, such as T cell help, growth stimulation, macrophage activation or suppression are caused by the release of these molecular mediators, which include the interleukins IL-2, IL-3, IL-4, IL-5, IL-6, interferons α and β (IFNα and β), tumour necrosis factor (TNF), lymphotoxin (LT), granulocyte macrophage colony stimulating factor (GM-CSF) and transforming growth factor β (TGFβ). These molecules are only produced transiently after activation of the cells, and the CD4 (cluster differentiation antigen 4) cells are the richest sources of cytokines.

T lymphocytes are considered to be the most important immune regulatory cells, influencing the function of all other components of the immune system.[1] This includes B cells, in the phenomenon known as 'T cell help' of the antibody production, activation and stimulation of T and natural killer (NK) cells, and activation of macrophages. However T cells can also affect virtually all other cells in the body.

There are two ways in which T cells can influence the activities of other cells. One involves cell contact, recognition and the subsequent destruction by T cells with cytotoxic properties. These chiefly have the CD8 (cluster differentiation antigen 8) marker, but some CD4 cells, appropriately triggered are also cytotoxic. The other, much more versatile way in which T cells communicate and influence other cells is by the production and secretion of a variety of potent mediator molecules, termed lymphokines or more generically 'cytokines'.

T cells are a particularly rich sources of cytokines. At last count they are able to produce over 10 cloned products, e.g. IL-1α, IL-2, IL-3, IL-4, IL-5, IL-6, TNF, LT, IFNα, IFNγ, GM-CSF, TGFβ; as well as a number of products identified but still to be cloned. It thus appears that the majority of T cell effects are mediated by the production of lymphokines.

The production of lymphokines by T cells is typically transient, and only occurs for 24 to 48 hours after activation of the cells before ceasing.[2] This highly regulated synthesis and secretion places a major emphasis on the specific activation of T cells by their stimulus, the antigen presenting cells expressing HLA (human leucocyte antigen) molecules and antigen.

Until recently it was considered that CD4 cells were the major T cell producers of lymphokines. Deeper analysis of CD8 T cells has shown that they can also produce a number of lymphokines, including IL-2. It is of interest that the potent immunosuppressive agent, cyclosporin A, which has made such an impact on clinical transplantation is a potent inhibitor of T cell cytokine production.[3]

One of the important aspects of T cell derived cytokines is that many act in synergy with others, and thus the net effect may be considerably greater than that of the individual components. Well known synergies are those of INF_γ and TNF in cytostasis, cytotoxicity, inflammation and HLA induction,[4] and of IL-2 and IL-4 in T cell growth.[5]

LYMPHOKINES AND T CELL GROWTH

Until about 1986, the current dogma was that T cell growth was dependent on IL-2, and IL-2 alone,[6] and the capacity to clone T cells in IL-2 supported that concept. However, with the cloning and expression of IL-4 it became clear that other molecules also regulated T cell growth.[5] Currently it is known that various cytokines can influence T cell growth but none with anywhere near the effect of IL-2. These include IL-4, IL-1, IL-6, TNF, LT, GM-CSF and for a rare subset of T cells, IL-3.[5,7-9] It is likely but not known yet whether various T cell subpopulations differ in their requirements for T cell growth.

T CELL FUNCTIONS AND LYMPHOKINE PRODUCTION

CD4 T cells are often termed 'helper cells' because of their capacity to assist antibody production by B cells. This activity is now known to be mediated in large part by a variety of T cell produced lymphokines, such as IL-2, IL-4, IL-5 (in mouse), IL-6, TNF and lymphotoxin acting in concert at different states of the B cell activation process. IL-4, IL-5 and IFN are of importance in Ig (immunoglobulin) class regulation.

CD8 cells are often termed 'cytotoxic/suppressor' cells as these functions are considered to be mediated by these cells. CD8 cell mediated cytotoxicity is chiefly not mediated by lymphokines but perforin and proteases, however TNF, LT and IFNα and γ may be involved, and may be especially important in cytotoxicity mediated by CD4 cells. IL-2, IL-4, IFNγ and perhaps IL-6 can regulate the cytolytic process in T cells, and IFNα also for NK cells.

The mechanism of immune suppression by 'suppressor T cells' is currently controversial. However, T cells make TGFβ which is a potent immunosuppressive entity.[10]

INTERLEUKIN-2 (IL-2)

Interleukin-2 first termed T cell growth factor, is much more than a T cell growth factor. It acts on T cells, NK cells, B cells and activated monocytes[11] after binding to a complex receptor, comprised of 2 chains. The p55 chain which is recognized by the anti Tac monoclonal antibody, and the p75 chain each have a low affinity for IL-2, but together combine to yield a high affinity receptor.[12] On all these cells, IL-2 acts as an activating factor and a growth factor for T, B and NK cells. The activation of T cells leads to cytolytic function and secretion of lymphokines. IL-2 is a simple polypeptide chain of 146 amino acids, the natural form of which is glycosylated, but recombinant *Escherichia coli* produced non-glycosylated IL-2 functions as efficiently in vitro and in vivo.

The discovery of IL-2 has had a profound influence on immunology, as it has permitted the culture and propagation of T cells and their cloning, and the subsequent surge in information about T cells. Clinically there has already been use of IL-2 in cancer therapy. IL-2 is used both in vivo and in vitro, to stimulate cells with properties resembling activated NK cells, which are termed lymphokine activated killer cells. Certain types of cancer, e.g. renal cell cancer and melanomas tend to respond to this therapy, but the side effects are severe, and it is too early to establish whether it will have a long term role in cancer therapy.[13]

INTERLEUKIN-4 (IL-4)

Like many other cytokines, this entity has had a number of previous names, e.g. B cell stimulatory factor-1. IL-4 is produced by T cells, NK and mast cells. Since all haemopoietic cells (and many others) express receptors for IL-4, it is apparent that IL-4 has a plethora of effects. Most studies have been on B cells where it acts as an early stimulating and growth factor, induces HLA Class II molecules, and at a later stage favours the production of IgG_1 and IgE antibodies. On T cells it is both stimulatory and a growth factor, rather less potent on most T cells than IL-2, on macrophages it is an activating factor and induces HLA Class II molecules, on mouse mast cells it induces proliferation especially in synergy with IL-3 (see Ref. 14 for review).

INTERLEUKIN-5 (IL-5)
(synonyms: eosinophil-CSF, BCDF2)

The gene for this cytokine is located on the q arm of chromosome 5 in humans together with other haemopoietic growth factor genes. The purified recombinant protein has two main target cell populations in mouse (1) B cells; and (2) eosinophils and their progenitor cells. In man the B cell differentiating properties of IL-5 (increased IgM and IgA production and enhanced IL-4 induced IgE production) have not yet been observed. Mouse and human IL-5 cDNAs are 77% homologous. Currently only T cells are known to produce IL-5.[15,16]

IL-5 activates mature peripheral blood eosinophils—as demonstrated by chemiluminescence, superoxide generation and C3bi expression, and prolongs their half life. It also stimulates eosinophil production from progenitor cells, with the eosinophil promyelocyte being the most sensitive target cell. Thus in the mouse, at least, T cell activation can result in both eosinophilia and enhanced IgE production. However, eosinophilia is not a common consequence of cell mediated immune responses and the regulation of IL-5 gene expression is still poorly understood, especially in humans. In studies using tumor T cell clones it has been found that IL-5 mRNA is expressed at lower levels than GM-CSF in phorbol ester and anti CD3 activated T cells. Further knowledge in this field is important as it would lead to understanding of hypereosinophilic syndrome.

IL-6—INTERLEUKIN-6

(Synonyms: Interferon B2, hepatocyte stimulating factor, plasmacytoma growth factor, BSF-2)
This cytokine (as can be seen from its number of 'aliases') has a wide variety of activities on numerous target cells. It shows homology with G-CSF[17] and the two cytokines developed after duplication of a group of genes. G-CSF is located on chromosome 17q and IL-6 on chromosome 6 in humans.

IL-6 is constitutively expressed in a number of tumour lines and may be induced in mitogen stimulated lymphocytes, and cytokine stimulated fibroblasts. The IL-6 receptor is also widely expressed—including mature B cells and resting T cells. The latter observation implicates IL-6 as an autocrine growth regulator.[18]

Even within the lymphohaemopoietic system IL-6 has numerous activities. It stimulates mature B cells to produce IgG and may be involved in Ig class switching. Like IL-1, it is active in the thymocyte proliferation assays, is an autocrine T-cell stimulator, and is a potentiator of haemopoietic stem cell growth. In addition, it stimulates hepatocytes to release acute phase proteins.[19] The interferon properties of IL-6 are still highly controversial.

Increased production of IL-6 is associated with autoimmunity. In particular constitutive production of IL-6 by certain tumours (cardiac myxomas, cervical carcinomas and bladder tumours) has been associated with co-existing autoimmune phenomena in these diseases which remit with adequate control of the underlying tumour. High levels of IL-6 have also been detected in the synovial fluid of rheumatoid joints.[20] The control of expression of the IL-6 gene is thus likely to receive a great deal of attention in view of its therapeutic potential.[21]

HAEMOPOIETIC GROWTH FACTORS IL-3 AND GM-CSF

Activated T cells produce two multilineage haemopoietic growth factors, IL-3 and GM-CSF, both of which are discussed in this Issue (*see* Dexter). It is interesting to note that activated T cells do not produce the mono-lineage growth factors G-CSF and M-CSF (CSF-1).

In vitro IL-3 and GM-CSF have overlapping activities.[22] However, GM-CSF has a more pronounced effect on stimulated mature granulocyte, macrophage and eosinophil function, whereas IL-3 has a more pronounced effect on stimulating early erythroid and megakaryocyte progenitor cell growth and in the mouse it stimulates mast cell growth and differentiation together with IL-4.

The genes for both growth factors lie in a haemopoietic growth factor 'hot spot' on chromosome 5q in humans (C 11 in mice) and although the two cytokines are not significantly related at the genomic or protein level there is significant sequence homology of the 5' regions controlling gene transcription similar to the common regulations sequence of IL-2 and IFN_γ. However IL-3 and GM-CSF are variably expressed suggesting other control mechanisms operate.[23]

In addition, although human and mouse GM-CSF are 70% homologous at the DNA level, for IL-3 the degree of homology is reduced to 43%. It has been estimated that in human T cells IL-3 and GM-CSF mRNA is less than in mouse.[24] It is important to establish whether the IL-3 in mouse and humans have similar physiological relevance. As IL-3 action in vitro is important for its capacity to stimulate early progenitor cell growth, its physiological effect in the context of the human immune response has to be fully assessed as haemopoietic progenitor cells are infrequent in the circulation of active haemopoiesis is not prominant at the site of inflammation. The short serum half life (2 min) of IL-3 and GM-CSF rule out the possibility that T cell producing IL-3 and GM-CSF act as long range stimulators of bone marrow function.

TNFα AND LYMPHOTOXIN (TNFβ)

These two cytokines are genetically linked, separated by 1.2kb and located within the HLA complex of Chromosome 6 in man (17 in mouse). There is some evidence that a polycistronic mRNA is transcribed which is later cleaved (M Turner, personal communication). Although the two lymphokines are only 28% homologous at the amino acid level they act through a common receptor and thus have overlapping activities. These activities are often enhanced by Interferon-γ. Control of TNFα production occurs mainly at the post-transcriptional level, though TNFα mRNA levels increase following stimulation, e.g. by endotoxin.[25] TNFα was initially thought to be produced by macrophages but is now known to be also produced by T and NK cells. LT is produced by T, NK and B cells.

TNFα has a variety of physiological properties, stimulation of fibroblast growth and neutrophil function, the induction of procoagulant activity and haemopoietic growth factor expression by endothelial cells. In addition it enhances IL-2 receptor expression in T cells and HLA class II expression in many T cells, and is an autocrine T cell growth factor. These roles of the molecule, together with the fact that some mRNA exists in unstimulated T cells supports the concept that TNFα is one of the first lymphokines released by T cells when stimulated and is hence critical to the immune response. AntiTNF antibodies inhibit the mixed lymphocyte response.

Other properties of TNF include direct cytotoxicity on some tumour cells[26]—the property which defined the molecule originally and to which it owes its name, and the inhibition of haemopoietic progenitor cell growth. TNF has profound pro-inflammatory effect inducing PGE_2 and Interleukin-1 production, and most of its activities are shared with IL-1.

TNFα is clinically important. It has been demonstrated to be identical with 'cachexin' and hence implicated in the pathology of the wasting associated with chronic diseases—chronic parasitic, viral and bacterial infections, and malignancy. The use of anti TNFα antibodies to protect against lethal septic shock has identified TNFα as important early in the pathogenesis of septic shock. For maximal effect the antibodies should be given prior to induction of septicaemia, which supports the concept that TNFα release is important early in the process.[27] Augmented TNFα gene expression is also detected in the graft versus host disease, and has been implicated in the chronicity of rheumatoid arthritis.[28]

Initial results suggest that the modification of the toxicity of TNF through anti-TNFα antibodies will be therapeutically important, e.g. meningococcal septicaemia and septic shock. However, the direct anti-tumour effect of TNFα does not appear to have important therapeutic applications,[29] as in vivo, in mice, anti-tumour effects are most likely to be necrosis induced by thrombosis. For a more detailed review of the TNFs *see* Balkwill, this Issue.

TRANSFORMING GROWTH FACTOR β

TGFβ mRNA is transcribed within 2 hours of stimulation of T cells. However, the release of the protein is delayed and can occur between 2 and 4 days later (D Chantry, personal communication). This suggests that T cell produced TGFβ is physiologically important late in the immune response. In contrast, however, platelets and granules contain preformed TGFβ, which is released on activation and therefore has an immediate importance in wound healing. A wide variety of other cells also produce TGFβ.

The molecule has a broad spectrum of activities (see Hsuan, this Issue) and exists in at least 2 forms. $TGFβ_1$ has 99% amino acid homology between mouse and man, confirming its importance as a critical molecule. A wide variety of tissues are targets for TGFβ activity. It is stimulatory, e.g. for synthesis of collagen, fibronectin and differentiation of epithelial cells, and hence is important in wound healing—as implied by platelet release of TGFβ on activation. Within the lymphoid system, however, TGFβ is mainly inhibitory. It blocks NK function, reduces T cell cytotoxicity, reduces IL-2 induced IL-2 receptor expression, inhibits Ig synthesis, and inhibits IL-1 synthesis and release.[10]

Thus the kinetics of TGFβ transcription and protein release together with observation of the properties of the recombinant molecule in vitro may be (overly?) simply interpreted as showing that the activating T cells result in a programmed release of initially immune stimulating molecules and, later, down regulatory molecules of which $TGFβ_1$ is an important example.

CONCLUSION

T lymphocytes are major producers of cytokines, and respond to a number of cytokines, especially IL-2 by growth and activation. Many of these T cell derived molecules mediate inflammation, and so inhibiting their production may be beneficial. In some pathological states, e.g. septic shock antibodies to TNFα may be beneficial whereas in others, the presence of increased amounts of cytokine, e.g. TGFβ may be of therapeutic benefit.

REFERENCES

1 Feldmann M, Owen MJ, Lamb JR. In: T Cells. Wiley, New York: 1989 (In press)

2 Buchan GS, Barrett K, Fujita T et al. Detection of activated T cell products in the rheumatoid joint using cDNA probes to interleukin 2, IL-2 receptor and interferon γ. Clin Exp Immunol 1988; 71: 295–301
3 Shevach EM. The effects of cyclosporin A on the immune system. Annu Rev Immunol 1985; 3: 397–423
4 Lee SH, Aggarwal BB, Rinderknecht E, Assisi F, Chiu H. The synergistic antiproliferative effect of γ-interferon and human lymphotoxin. J Immunol 1984; 133: 1083–1086
5 Spits H, Yssel H, Takebe Y et al. Recombinant IL-4 promotes growth of human T cells. J Immunol 1987; 139: 1142–1147
6 Poiez BJ, Ruscetti FW, Mier JW, Woods AM, Gallo RC. T cell lines established from human T lymphocytic neoplasias by direct response to T cell growth factors. Proc Natl Acad Sci USA 1980; 77: 6815–6819
7 Woods A, West J, Rasmussen R, Bottomley K. Granulocyte macrophage colony stimulation factor produced by cloned L3T4a[+], class II restricted T cells induce HT-2 cells to proliferate. J Immunol 1987; 138: 4298–4302
8 Yokota S, Geppert, TD, Lipsky PE. Enhancement of antigen and mitogen induced human T lymphocyte proliferation by tumour necrosis factor-α^1. J Immunol 1988; 140: 531–536
9 Londei M, Verhoef A, De Berardinis P et al. Definition of a population of CD4$^-$8$^-$ T cells expressing the αβ T cell receptor responsive to IL-2, IL-3 and IL-4. (Submitted)
10 Kehrl JA, Wakefield LM, Roberts AB et al. Production of transforming growth factor β by human T lymphocytes and its potential role in the regulation of T cell growth. J Exp Med 1986; 163: 1037–1050
11 Smith KA. Interleukin-2. Ann Rev Immunol 1984; 2: 319–333
12 Tsudo M, Kozak RW, Goldman CK, Waldmann T. Demonstration of a new non-Tac polypeptide that binds Interleukin-2: a potential participant in a multichain Interleukin-2 receptor complex. Proc Natl Acad Sci USA 1986; 83: 9694–9698
13 Rosenberg SA, Lotze MT, Muul LM et al. A progress report on the treatment of 157 patients with advanced cancer using lymphokine-activated killer cells and interleukin-2 or high-dose interleukin-2 alone. New Engl J Med 1987; 316: 889–897
14 Paul WE. B cell stimulatory factor 1/IL-4. Ann Rev Immunol 1987; 5: 429–459
15 Warren DJ, Sanderson CJ. Production of a T cell hybrid producing a lymphokine stimulating eosinophil differentiation. Immunology 1985; 54: 615–623
16 Azuma C, Tanabe T, Konishi M et al. Cloning of cDNA for human T-cell replacing factor (interleukin-5) and comparison with the murine homologue. Nucleic Acids Res 1986; 14: 9149–9158
17 Hirano T, Taga T, Nakano N et al. Purification to homogeneity and characterization of human B cell differentiation factor (BCDF or BSFp.2). Proc Natl Acad Sci USA 1985; 82: 5490–5494
18 Taga T, Kawanishi Y, Hardy RH, Hirano T, Kishimoto T. Receptors for B cell stimulatory factor 2 (BSF2): Quantitation, specificity, distribution and regulation of the expression. J Exp Med 1988; 166: 967–987
19 Gauldie J, Richards C, Harnish D, Landsdorp ?, Baumann H. Interferon β2/B cell stimulatory factor type 2 shares identity with monocyte derived hepatocyte stimulatory factor and regulates the major acute phase protein response in liver cells. Proc Natl Acad Sci USA 1987; 84: 7251–7255
20 Hirano T, Matsuda T, Turner M et al. Excessive production of B cell stimulatory factor 2 (BSF2/IL-6) in rheumatoid arthritis. Eur J Immunol 1988; (In press)
21 Yasukawa K, Hirano T, Watanabe Y et al. Structure and expression of human B cell stimulatory factor-2 (BSF-2/IL-6). EMBO J 1987; 6: 2939–2945

22 Sieff CA, Emerson SG, Donahue RE, Nathan DG. Human recombinant granulocyte-macrophage colony stimulating factor: A multilineage hematopoietin. Science 1985; 230: 1171–1173
23 Kelso A, Gough N. Expression of haemopoietic growth factor genesis murine T lymphocytes. In: Webb DR, Goeddel DU, eds. Lymphokines, Vol. 13, 1987, pp.209–238
24 Otsuka T, Miyajma A, Brown N et al. Isolation and characterisation of an expressible cDNA encoding human IL-3. J Immunol 1988; 140: 2288–2295
25 Old LJ. Tumour necrosis factor. Science 1985; 230: 630–632
26 Helson L, Green S, Calswell EA, Old LJ. Effect of tumour necrosis factor on cultured human melanoma cells. Nature 258: 731–732
27 Tracey KJ, Fong Y, Hesse DG et al. Anti-cachexin/TNF monoclonal antibodies prevent septic shock during lethal bacteriaemia. Nature 1987; 330: 662–664
28 Brennan FM, Chantry D, Jackson A, Maini R, Feldmann M. Anti-TNF antibody down regulates IL-1 production in rheumatoid synovial cell cultures. (Submitted)
29 Selby P, Hobbs S, Viner C et al. Tumour necrosis factor in man: clinical and biological observations. Br J Cancer 1987; 56: 803–808.

Cytokine regulation of B-cell growth and differentiation

Robin E. Callard
Department of Immunology, Institute of Child Health, London

> In the last few years, more than ten soluble factors (cytokines) important for regulating B cell growth and differentiation have been identified and their genes cloned. These factors are now known to influence each separate stage of normal B cell responses, namely the activation of quiescent B cells, their proliferation and differentiation into antibody secreting cells and the regulation of immunoglobulin class and subclass production. An important feature of all of these factors is their lack of target cell specificity. Each one has multiple activities both on B cells and on a range of other cell types, often in synergy with other factors. How their multiple functions are controlled in vivo is only now beginning to be understood, opening the way to the use of factors—or more probably, specific inhibitors—for the treatment of a variety of immunological diseases including allergy, autoimmunity, and possibly some forms of B cell malignancies.

Optimal antibody production to the majority of antigens depends on complex interactions between B cells, regulatory (helper) T cells (Th), and antigen presenting cells. Communication between these cells is known to involve cell contact and conjugate formation through specific receptor ligand binding at the surface membrane.[1-4] In addition, intercellular signalling between B cells, T cells and monocytes can be mediated at a distance by soluble factors (cytokines). A role for soluble factors in Th-B cell interactions was first indicated by experiments in which supernatants from activated T cells were found to replace Th in specific antibody responses.[5,6] Since then, a large number of B cell growth and differentiation factors (BCGF & BCDF) have been described, including some derived from non-T cells.[7] Many of these have now been cloned and the use of recombinant factors has considerably enhanced our understanding of how B cell responses are controlled. To avoid some of the confusion which has arisen previously from experimentation with poorly defined and/or partially purified factors, only cloned factors known to regulate B cell growth and differentiation will be discussed in this chapter.

RECOMBINANT FACTORS WHICH REGULATE B-CELL ACTIVATION, PROLIFERATION AND DIFFERENTIATION

Terminology

The various cloned factors known to regulate B cell function are listed in Table 1. Six are interleukins (IL-1, 2, 4–7) and these are listed with their common synonyms (BCGF$_1$, TRF, BCDF, etc). The term interleukin was originally coined to describe factors involved in signalling between leukocytes. This definition is no longer appropriate since some (especially IL-1 and IL-6) are also produced by, and act on, cells other than leukocytes. Nonetheless, this terminology has proved valuable for the unequivocal identification of a particular factor since it has only ever been applied to cloned factors with a published cDNA sequence. This is particularly important in instances where different factors have been given the same name—e.g. both IL-5 and IL-6 are known as T cell replacing factors (TRF). The other factors (IFN, TNF, C3, sCD23) were all named before they were found to have activity on B cells and have not been assigned an interleukin number. Low molecular weight BCGF[8] has not been included in Table 1. Although this factor has been cloned,[9] recombinant material is not generally available, and the vast majority of experiments have been carried out with a commercial preparation which contains significant amounts of IL-2, IFN$_\gamma$, TNF$_\alpha$, and GMCSF as impurities[7] (Callard et al., unpublished observations).

Properties

All of the factors listed in Table 1 have been identified in humans and mice and (except for CD23) cloned in both species. Their cellular origin, molecular weight, human chromosomal gene loca-

Table 1 Cloned factors which control B cell growth and differentiation

Factor (synonyms)	Source[2]	$M_r(\times 10^{-3})$[3]	Human chromosome	Activation	Proliferation	Differentiation
IL-1	TBMF	15	2	+?	+?	+?
IL-2	T	15	4	?	+	+
IL-4 (BSF1, BCGF1, BCGF$_\gamma$)	T	15	5	+	+	+
IL-5 (BCGF$_{II}$, BCGF$_\mu$, TRF, EDF)	T	15(22)	5	+(m)	+(m)	+(m)
IL-6 (BSF2, TRF, BCDF, IFN$_{\beta 2}$)	TMEF	21(26)	7	?	+	+
IL-7	S	15(25)	?	?	+(pre-B)	?
s-CD23	B	25	?	?	+	+
C3	M	190(115+75)	19	?	+	+
IFN$_\alpha$	L	17–23	9	?	+/−	+/−
IFN$_\gamma$	T	20–24	12	?	+/−	+/−
TNF$_\alpha$	M	17(X3)	6	?	−	−
TGFβ	TBP	12·5(×2)	19	?	−	+/− (isotype)

[1] m = mouse, ? = unknown, + = positive response, − = inhibition, +/− = both enhancement and inhibition have been reported
[2] T = T cells, B = B cells, M = monocytes, E = endothelial cells, F = fibroblasts, S = bone marrow stromal cells, L = leukocytes, P = placenta
[3] Molecular weight of human IL's (except for IL-7 which is mouse) is that of the core peptide with the Mr for glycosylated factor in parenthesis. Note that C3 is a heterodimer, TNF is a homotrimer, and TGFβ a homodimer
[4] Abbreviations: IL = interleukin; IFN = interferon; TNF = tumour Necrosis factor; TGFβ = transforming growth factor; CD = cluster differentiation antigen

lization, and activities on B cells are summarised in Table 1. IL-7 stimulates proliferation of B cell progenitors[10] with no reported activity on mature B cells. Of interest is the location of human IL-4 and IL-5 together with IL-3, GMCSF, CSFl and the CSFl receptor (c-fms) on Chromosome 5. The genomic organisation of IL-3, IL-4, IL-5 and GMCSF is similar suggesting that they may be derived from a common ancestral gene.

Source

Most of the factors in Table 1 are produced by T cells and are likely to be important in Th-B cell interactions. Some of them (IL-1, IL-6, IFN_γ) are also secreted by non-lymphoid cells. Of the rest, sCD23 is produced by B cells[11] IL-7 by bone marrow stromal cells, and TNF, C3 and IFN_α by monocytic cells.

REGULATION OF B CELL RESPONSES

The various factors listed in Table 1 will be discussed in the context of their role in B cell regulation. Normal B cell responses can be conveniently divided into three distinct stages—activation from resting cells, proliferation, and differentiation into antibody secreting cells (Fig. 1). Although this scheme takes no account either of B cell subpopulations, or of diverging differentiation pathways, it is a useful model for understanding the importance of B cell growth and differentiation factors for regulating B cell responses.

B cell activation

Antigen or anti-Ig binding to surface membrane Ig (smIg) sets off a cascade of biochemical reactions which primes (activates) the cell to respond to other signals without inducing cell division (Fig.2). To begin with, phospholipase C activated through a smIg linked G-binding protein cleaves phosphatidyl inositol bisphosphate (PIP2) releasing inositol triphosphate (IP3) and diacylglycerol (DAG). IP3 then induces a rapid increase in cytosolic calcium released from intracellular stores, and DAG activates protein kinase C (PKC). Phorbol esters (e.g. TPA) directly activate PKC without increasing intracellular calcium. Measurements of membrane phospholipid turnover, protein phosphorylation and intracellular calcium can therefore be used to detect B-cell activation by

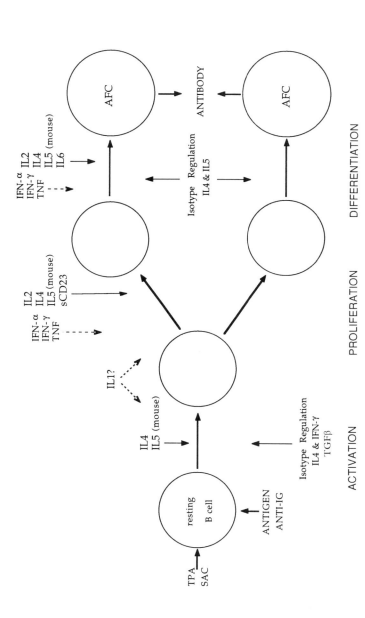

Fig. 1 Lymphokine regulation of B-cell activation, proliferation and differentiation. Small resting B cells are activated by antigen (or anti-Ig) binding to smIg, by IL-4 and (in mice) IL-5. Other ligands such as the phorbol ester TPA binding directly to PKC or *Staphylococcus aureus* cowan 1 (SAC) also activate B cells. Cell division results from costimulation with two independent activation signals (e.g. IL-4 and anti-IgM) or from an activation signal (anti-IgM) followed by a progression (growth factor) signal. At least five different factors are important for differentiation into antibody forming cells (AFC). Isotype regulation may involve heavy chain switching (IL-4 and IFNγ) or selection of precommitted cells (IL-5). This scheme does not consider any role for B cell subpopulations or divergent paths of differentiation and should be considered only as a convenient model for the function of B cell growth and differentiation factors in B cell responses.

this pathway, usually within minutes. Later events, such as increases in cell volume and expression of activation antigens—notably MHC class II and CD23, are also important indicators of B cell activation.

Both IL-4 and IL-5 are also able to activate resting B cells.

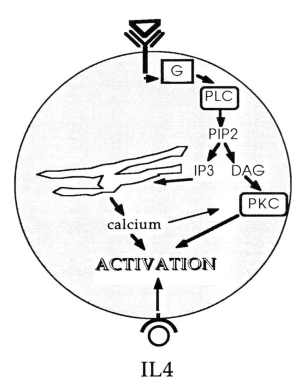

Fig. 2 B cell activation. Binding of antigen or anti-Ig to smIg results in cleavage of phosphatidyl inositolbisphosphate (PIP2) by phospholipase C into inositol triphosphate (IP3) and diacylglycerol (DAG). IP3 induces calcium release from the endoplasmic reticulum and DAG activates protein kinase C. Together these two signals initiate a chain of biochemical reactions from the surface membrane to the nucleus. IL-4 also activates B cells but through a different pathway without calcium release or activation of PKC. B cell activation results in increases in size and expression of activation antigens such as MHC Class II and CD23, but not DNA synthesis.

Table 2 Activation of human B cells

	IL-4	Anti-IgM
Calcium flux	−	+
PKC activation	−	+
Protein phosphorylation	+	+
Increase in size	+	+
Increase in Class II	+	+
Increase in CD23	+	±
Increase in IL2R (CD25)	−	+
Increase in surface IgM	+	−

Activation with IL-4 results in protein phosphorylation,[12] changes in cell volume[13] and expression of activation antigens including MHC class II,[13,14] CD23,[15] and surface IgM,[16] but not PKC activation or calcium mobilization[12] (Table 2). B cell activation with IL-4 is inhibited with IFN$_\gamma$.[17] IL-5 has been shown to induce expression of the IL-2 receptor on resting B cells in mice but not humans.[18] Whether protein phosphorylation or calcium mobilisation occurs with IL-5 is not known.

It is important to recognise that IL-4, IL-5, and anti-IgM do not activate B cells by the same transmembrane signalling pathway (Table 2). Moreover, each activation signal alone induces transition from G_0 to G_1 in the cell cycle, but does not result in cell division (DNA synthesis).

B cell proliferation

Under appropriate experimental conditions, costimulation with two independent signals (e.g. IL-4 and anti-IgM, IL-5 and dextran sulphate) will result in B cell proliferation whereas either signal alone will not (Table 3.). IL-2, IL-4, IL-5, TNF and IFN$_\gamma$ have all been shown to be growth factors in costimulation assays.

Table 3 Costimulation with IL-4 and anti-IgM[1]

Signal 1	Signal 2	Proliferation (^{3}HTdR dpm)
−	−	4273 ± 1068
anti-IgM	−	9753 ± 1124
−	IL-4	3548 ± 968
anti-IgM	IL-4	64632 ± 3692

[1]Human tonsillar B cells stimulated for 72 hours with anti-IgM and IL-4. ^{3}HTdR uptake was measured over the final eight hours

In the case of IL-4, cell division results from two activation signals rather than an initial activation step with anti-IgM followed by a growth (progression) signal provided by IL-4. Since high affinity IL-2 receptors are not detectable on resting B cells, but are induced on activation, IL-2 is more likely to be a progression factor.[19,20] IL-5 is a growth factor in costimulation assays only in mice and has no such activity in humans.[21] TNF and IFN (α and γ) have been reported as growth factors in costimulation assays[22-25] but whether these act directly on B cells, or indirectly through other cell types, is not entirely clear. C3 also seems to be important for B cell proliferation.[26] Most mature B cells carry both types of C3 receptor (CR1 and CR2) and antibodies to the receptor have been shown to enhance proliferation. In addition, cross linked C3d and C3b promote cell division by murine B cells.[27]

Some B cell growth factors also induce proliferation of B cell lines.[28] Of particular interest are those known to be derived from B cells.[29] These 'autocrine' factors may be important for regulating normal B cell responses as well as promoting cell division by transformed B cells.[29] Monocyte derived IL1 has been shown to support growth of EBV-transformed B-LCL[30] but these preparations also contain other factors including IL-6 and an autocrine role for IL-1 is now in doubt. More recently, a soluble Mr 25K fragment of CD23 (sCD23) released spontaneously from the surface of EBV-transformed B-LCL and activated normal B cells has been shown to be an autocrine B cell growth factor for normal and transformed B cells.[11,31] IL-6 has been identified as an autocrine growth factor for human myeloma cells,[32] but this factor is a BCDF not a BCGF for normal B cells in costimulation assays[33] suggesting that it may have different activities on subpopulations of B cells, or B cells in different states of activation. None of the other factors (IL-2, IL-4, IL-5, TNF or IFN α/γ) have yet been identified as autocrine growth factors, nor do they promote growth of indicator human B cell lines[28] although IL-2 enhances proliferation by the murine BCL1 line.[34]

B cell differentiation

B cell differentiation factors promote Ig secretion in costimulation assays and/or B cell lines. Of the factors listed in Table 1, IL-2, IL-5 (in mice only) and IL-6 (in humans) will induce Ig secretion by normal B cells in costimulation assays with various activation signals (anti-IgM, SAC, dextran sulphate etc.) and will enhance Ig secretion by selected indicator B cell lines.[28,33–38] Blocking IL-6 antibodies inhibit PWM induced antibody secretion but not proliferation indicating that IL-6 is an essential BCDF for T dependent (polyclonal) Ig secretion.[39] IFN_γ and IFN_α have both been shown to enhance Ig secretion by normal B cells and some B cell lines.[40–42] IFNs may act directly on B cells,[43] but indirect action through non-B cells or synergy with other factors cannot always be ruled out.[35,44] Neither IL-1 nor TNF have been unequivocally identified as differentiation factors, but each has been shown to augment differentiation in response to other factors.[25,45] Antibodies to C3 receptors will enhance B cell differentiation to PWM[46] and C3 may be important for differentiation of memory B cells in germinal centres.[26]

T cell replacing factors

The requirement for T helper cells in specific antibody responses to some antigens (usually polyvalent or TI Type 2) can be replaced by T cell replacing factors (TRF).[5,47] In mice, IL-5 is a TRF for responses to sheep red cells and haptenated protein antigens.[48–50] In contrast, IL-5 is entirely without TRF activity in man.[21] IFN_γ may also be a TRF in mice[52] although it is not in man[53] (Smith & Callard, unpublished observations). On the other hand, IL-2 is a TRF in man[53] but not in mice, although it may enhance Ig secretion in synergy with other factors.[54] None of the other factors listed in Table 1 has TRF activity in either species. Whether TRFs function simply as differentiation factors or must also activate B cells and/or promote cell division is not known. It is also not known whether resting B cells will respond to TRF. In humans, small dense (resting?) B cells will respond to antigen in the presence of T cells but not to TRF[55] suggesting that an initial T cell dependent activation step may be required.

Immunoglobulin isotype selection

Three lymphokines (IL-4, IL-5, and IFN_γ) have been implicated in Ig class switching. Secretion of both IgG1 and IgE by lipopoly saccharide (LPS) stimulated mouse B cells is enhanced with IL-4.[56] IFN_γ inhibits this response and increases secretion of

IgG2a.[51,56] In vivo administration of a monoclonal antibody to IL-4 profoundly inhibits IgE but not IgG1 production in response to anti-IgD or the nematode parasite *Nippostrongylus brasiliensis*.[57] Both isotypes are inhibited with IFN_γ.[58] Both IgM and IgA production by LPS stimulated mouse spleen cells are increased with IL-5.[59-63] This effect is enhanced with IL-4 but it is not inhibited with IFN_γ.

It is important to distinguish between factors which control switch region recombination and those which select subpopulations of already committed B cells. When resting B cells are preincubated with IL-4, IgG1 but not IgE, production is increased on subsequent stimulation with the LPS.[64] Moreover, IL-4 enhances IgG1 production by surface $IgM^+/IgG1^-$ B cells.[56,65] Similar findings have also been reported for IgG2a secretion with IFN_γ.[56] Both IL-4 and IFN_γ therefore seem to act as true switch factors, probably by opening DNA switch regions for efficient recombination.[66,67] In contrast to the effect of IL-4 on IgG1 responses, optimal IgE production requires the presence of IL-4 at much higher doses (10 000 u/ml vs 600 u/ml) more than 48 hours after activation (exposure to LPS),[56,68] i.e. during proliferation and/or differentiation. Although IL-4 may function by selective expansion of B cells precommitted to the production of IgE, recent evidence showing synthesis of sterile 1gECH transcripts by B cells stimulated with LPS and IL-4 is consistent with a switch mechanism. Induction of IgA secretion by Peyer's patch B cells with IL-5 occurs only with surface IgA^+ and not IgA^- cells. Moreover, surface IgA expression was not induced on $smIgM^+/IgA^-$ cells.[63] IL-5 therefore seems to be a differentiation factor on B cells which have already undergone isotype switching. In contrast, induction of IgA secretion by TGF_β is found only on $smIgA^-$ cells.

In man, IgE and IgA secretion in response to IL-4 and/or IL-5 requires the presence of T cells.[66,69-70] This is particularly important for IL-5 which has no detectable effect at all on purified (T depleted) human B cells.[21] A requirement for T cells is also suggested by the findings that IL-4 is essential for IgE secretion induced with T cell clones,[70] and that IgE secretion can be induced in human B cells by T cells activated with antibody to CD3.[71] Apparently IL-4 and IL-5 act in quite different ways on murine and human B cells.

There is no evidence for IgG subclass regulation by lymphokines in man, and in our experience neither IL-4, IL-5 or IL-6 have any effect on Ig subclasses in specific antibody responses by human lymphocytes (Callard & Smith unpublished observations). As IgG subclasses in man and mouse have probably evolved independently,[72] this is not altogether surprising.

Factors which inhibit B cell responses

Inhibition of B cell responses has been reported for several factors. As discussed above, IFN_γ inhibits B cell activation and IgG1 secretion induced with IL-4.[17,73] In addition, TNF has been shown to inhibit B cell responses to pokeweed mitogen.[74] Recently, IL-4 has been shown to inhibit IL-2 dependent B cell proliferation and differentiation in costimulation assays with SAC.[75] In our own work, IL-4 was found to profoundly inhibit TRF activity of IL-2 (Table 4.). The mechanism of this inhibition is unknown, but it serves to emphasize the important point that a single factor may promote or suppress B cell responses depending on the particular function being measured.

Table 4 Effect of IL-4 on specific antibody responses by E^- cells cultured with antigen and TRF (IL-2)

TRF	rhIL-4 Units/ml	Antibody response (ng/ml)
none	0	<1
IL-2	0	83±64
IL-2	0.1	2±1
IL-2	1[1]	14±9
IL-2	10	<1

[1]Optimal dose of IL-4 for B cell proliferation in costimulation assays with anti-IgM

B CELL GROWTH AND DIFFERENTIATION FACTORS HAVE MULTIPLE ACTIVITIES

From the discussion so far, it is not only evident that each step of B cell activation, proliferation and differentiation is regulated by more than one factor (Fig. 1) but that each factor may have several distinct activities. Why this should be so is not known. It may reflect a requirement for independent control of antibody (isotype) responses to different types of antigen (e.g. protein and carbohydrate), and/or in different microenvironments (e.g. IgA production in the gut).[76] Factors may also be important for control of antigen presentation by B cells. A related question is that of B cell subpopulations. Human B cell subsets can be identified by surface markers such as IgD,[77,78] FMC7[79] and CD5,[80,81] but little is known of their individual responses to B cell growth and differentiation factors or their importance for isotype regulation.

Even more notable than the diverse actions of B cell growth and differentiation factors on B cells is their extraordinary range of target cells. No factor has yet been identified with specificity only for B cells. This lack of target specificity is exemplified by IL-4 which has receptors on a wide range of cell types.[82-84] Target cells for IL-2, IL-4, IL-5 and IL-6 are listed in Table 5. How such diverse activities are controlled in vivo is a vital question, especially if these factors are to be exploited therapeutically. From our present understanding there seem to be two possibilities. Synergistic combinations of factors may be required for a particular cellular response. There are many examples of this type of control for B cells. For example, anti-IgM and IL-4,[56] IL-4 and IL-5;[76] IL-2 and IFN_γ[35] etc. In principle, synergistic combinations of two factors would permit independent control of ten cell functions with five factors, 45 cell functions with 10 factors and so on.

Control could also be provided by local microenvironments. The action of factors may be restricted to short distances in vivo by local degradation mechanisms or the production of inhibitors (IFN_γ for example). It is also likely that some factors are involved in membrane interactions. For example, the secretory apparatus of T cells is orientated towards antigen presenting B cells[2] and secretion of IL-4 is known to be concentrated towards the site of membrane stimulation.[85] In addition, IL-4 has been shown to enhance conjugate formation between Th and B cells.[3] Gap junctions between antigen specific T and B cells have been

Table 5 B-cell growth and differentiation factors are not tissue specific

Factor	Target cells
IL-2	T-cells, B-cells, Macrophages
IL-4	T-cells, B-cells, Macrophages, Mast cells Haemopoietic progenitors (Erythroid, Megakaryocyte, Granulocyte, Monocyte)
IL-5	B-cells (mice), T-cells, Eosinophils
IL-6 (BSF-2)	B-cells, T-cells, Thymocytes, Hepatocytes, other non-lymphoid cells

described raising the possibility of direct cytoplasmic transfer.[1] This may be the mechanism of cognate T cell help. Other factors, however, clearly function at a distance. IL-6 can be detected in serum and urine, and is greatly elevated during rejection of renal transplants.[86] Secretion of IL-6 by monocytes and endothelial cells during inflammation may be important locally for activation of T cells as well as B cells,[87] and systematically to enhance haeomopoiesis (in synergy with IL-3)[88] and induce acute phase reactant secretion by the liver.[89] In this way, soluble factors may cordinate complex responses to infection.

FACTORS IN THE FUTURE

Several important areas of future work can be identified. There is no doubt that more B cell growth and differentiation factors have yet to be identified and cloned. These may be important not just for B cell growth and differentiation. B cell ontogeny is likely to be under the control of different factors of which IL-7 is only the first. In addition, factors may be involved in B cell trafficking and migration to the appropriate areas in lymphoid tissues. How the different factors combine to control B cell responses in vivo is a crucial question. Staining of tissue sections with monoclonal antibodies together with *in situ* hybridization using specific gene probes for the different factors and their receptors will enable these questions to be answered. Independent lymphokine regulation of B cell subpopulations responding to different antigenic signals should also be a profitable area of future research, especially with regards to isotype regulation and/or switching. In the long term, selective control of B cell functions with lymphokines (or more probably with specific inhibitors) should permit therapeutic intervention in a number of diseases including allergy, autoimmunity, and possibly some forms of B cell malignancy.

REFERENCES

1 Sanders VM, Snyder JM, Uhr JW, Vitetta ES. Characterization of the physical interaction between antigen-specific B and T cells. J Immunol 1986; 137: 2395–2404
2 Kupfer A, Swain SL, Janeway CA, Singer SL. The specific direct interaction of helper T cells and antigen presenting B cells. Proc Natl Acad Sci USA 1986; 83: 6080–6083
3 Sanders VM, Fernandez-Botran R, Uhr JW, Vitetta ES. Interleukin 4 enhances

the ability of antigen-specific B cells to form conjugates with T cells. J Immunol 1987; 139: 2349–2354
4 Mitchison NA. The carrier effect in the secondary response to hapten carrier conjugates. II. Cellular co-operation. Eur J Immunol 1971; 1: 18–27
5 Schimpl A, Wecker E. Replacement of T-cell function by a T-cell product. Nature New Biol 1972; 237: 15–17
6 Dutton RW. Separate signals for the initiation of proliferation and differentiation in the B cell response to antigen. Transplant Rev 1975; 23: 66–77
7 O'Garra A, Umland S, Defrance T, Christiansen J. B-cell factors are pleiotropic. Immunology Today 1987; 9: 45–54
8 Mehta SR, Conrad D, Sandler R, Morgan J, Montagna R, Maizel AL. Purification of human B cell growth factor. J Immunol 1985; 135: 3298–3302
9 Sharma S, Mehta S, Morgan J, Maizel A. Molecular cloning and expression of a human B-cell growth factor gene in Escherichia coli. Science 1987; 235: 1489–1492
10 Namen AE, Lupton S, Hjerrild K et al. Stimulation of B-cell progenitors by cloned murine interleukin-7. Nature 1988; 333: 571–573
11 Swendeman S, Thorley-Lawson DA. The activation antigen BLAST-2, when shed, is an autocrine BCGF for normal and transformed B cells. EMBO J 1987; 6: 1637–1642
12 Justement L, Chen Z, Harris L et al. BSF1 induces membrane protein phosphorylation but not phosphoinositide metabolism, calcium mobilization, protein kinase C translocation, or membrane depolarisation in resting murine B lymphocytes. J Immunol 1986; 137: 3664–3670
13 Rabin EM, Ohara J, Paul WE. B-cell stimulatory factor 1 activates resting B cells. Proc Natl Acad Sci USA 1985; 82: 2935–2939
14 Noelle R, Krammer PH, Ohara J, Uhr JW, Vitetta ES. Increased expression of Ia antigens on resting B cells: an additional role for B-cell growth factor. Proc Natl Acad Sci USA 1984; 81: 6149–6153
15 Defrance T, Aubry JP, Rousset F et al. Human recombinant interleukin 4 induces Fcε receptors (CD23) on normal human B lymphocytes. J Exp Med 1987; 165: 1459–1467
16 Shields JG, Armitage RJ, Jamieson BN, Beverley PCL, Callard RE. Increased expression of surface IgM but not IgD or IgG on human B cells in response to interleukin 4. 1988 Immunology (In press).
17 Mond JJ, Carman J, Sarma C, Ohara J, Finkelman FD. Interferon-gamma suppresses B cell stimulation factor (BSF-1) induction of Class II MHC determinants on B cells. J Immunol 1986; 137: 3534–3537
18 Loughnan MS, Takatsu K, Harada N, Nossal GJV. T-cell replacing factor (interleukin 5) induces expression of interleukin 2 receptors on murine splenic B cells. Proc Natl Acad Sci USA 1987; 84: 5399–5403
19 Prakash S, Robb RJ, Stout RD, Parker DC. Induction of high affinity IL-2 receptors on B cells responding to anti-Ig and T cell-derived helper factors. J Immunol 1985; 135: 117–122
20 Mittler R, Rao P, Olini G et al. Activated human B cells display a functional IL-2 receptor. J Immunol 1985; 134: 2392–2399
21 Clutterbuck E, Shields JG, Gordon J et al. Recombinant human interleukin-5 is an eosinophil differentiation factor but has no activity in standard human B cell growth factor assays. Eur J Immunol 1987; 17: 1743–1750
22 Harada H, Shioiri-nakano K, Mayumi M, Kawai T. Distinction of two subtypes of human leukocyte interferon (IFN-alpha) on B cell activation. J Immunol 1983; 131: 238–243
23 Defrance T, Aubry J-P, Vanbervliet B, Banchereau J. Human interferon-gamma acts as a B cell growth factor in the anti-IgM antibody co-stimulatory assay but has no direct B cell differentiation activity. J Immunol 1986; 137: 3861–3867

24 Morikawa K, Kubagawa H, Suzuki T, Cooper MD. Recombinant interferon-alpha, -beta, and -gamma enhance the proliferative response of human B cells. J Immunol 1987; 139: 761–766
25 Kehrl JH, Miller A, Fauci AS. Effect of tumor necrosis factor alpha on mitogen-activated human B cells. J Exp Med 1987; 166: 786–791
26 Klaus GGB, Humphrey JH. A re-evaluation of the role of C3 in B-cell activation. Immunology Today 1986; 7: 163–165
27 Melchers F, Erdei A, Schulz T, Dierich MP. Growth control of activated, synchronized murine B cells by the C3d fragment of human complement. Nature 1985; 317: 264–267
28 Shields JG, Smith SH, Levinsky RJ, Defrance T, De Vries JE, Banchereau J, Callard RE. The response of selected human B cell lines to B cell growth and differentiation factors. Eur J Immunol 1987; 17: 535–540
29 Gordon J, Ley SC, Melamed MD, Aman P, Hughes-Jones NC. Soluble factor requirements for the autostimulatory growth of B lymphoblasts immortalised by Epstein-Barr virus. J Exp Med 1984; 159: 1554–1559
30 Gordon J, Guy G, Walker L. Autocrine models of B-lymphocyte growth. II. Interleukin-1 supports the proliferation of transformed lymphoblasts but not the stimulation of resting B cells triggered through their receptors for antigen. Immunology 1986; 57: 419–423
31 Cairns J, Flores-Romo L, Millsum MJ, Guy GR, Gillis S, Ledbetter JA, Gordon J. Soluble CD23 is released by B lymphocytes cycling in response to interleukin 4 and anti-Bp50 (CDw40). Eur J Immunol 1988; 349–353
32 Kawano M, Hirano T, Matsuda T et al. Autocrine generation and requirement of BSF-2/IL-6 for human multiple myelomas. Nature 1988; 332: 83–85
33 Hirano T, Yasukawa K, Harada H et al. Complementary DNA for a novel human interleukin (BSF-2) that induces B lymphocytes to produce immunoglobulin. Nature 1986; 324: 73–76
34 Brooks KH, Vitetta ES. Recombinant IL-2 but not recombinant interferon-gamma stimulates both proliferation and IgM secretion in a Ly-1[+] clone of neoplastic murine B cells (BCL1). J Immunol 1986; 137: 3205–3210
35 Nakagawa T, Nakagawa N, Volkman DJ, Fauci AS. Sequential synergistic effect of interleukin 2 and interferon-gamma on the differentiation of a tac-antigen-positive B cell line. J Immunol 1986; 136: 164–168
36 Swain SL, Dutton RW. Production of a B cell growth promoting activity (DL)BCGF, from a cloned T cell line and its assay on the BCLI B cell tumour. J Exp Med 1982; 156: 1821–1834
37 Muraguchi A, Kishimoto T, Miki Y et al. T-cell-replacing factor- (TRF) induced IgG secretion in a human B blastoid cell line and demonstration of acceptors for TRF. J Immunol 1981; 127: 412–416
38 Ralph P, Jeong G, Welte K et al. Stimulation of immunoglobulin secretion in human B lymphocytes as a direct effect of high concentrations of IL-2. J Immunol 1984; 133: 2442–2445
39 Muraguchi A, Hirano T, Tang B et al. The essential role of B cell stimulatory factor 2 (BSF-2/IL-6) for the terminal differentiation of B cells. J Exp Med 1988; 167: 332–344
40 Sidman CL, Marshall JD, Shultz LD, Gray PW, Johnson HM. Gamma-interferon is one of several direct B-cell-maturing lymphokines. Nature 1984; 309: 801–804
41 Leibson HJ, Gefter M, Zlotnik A, Marrack P, Kappler JW. Role of gamma-interferon in antibody-producing responses. Nature 1984; 309: 799–801
42 Peters M, Ambrus JL, Zheleznyak A, Walling D, Hoofnagle JH. Effect of interferon-alpha on immunoglobulin synthesis by human B cells. J Immunol 1986; 137: 3153–3157
43 Harfast B, Huddlestone JR, Casali P, Merigan TC, Oldstone MBA. Interferon

acts directly on human B-lymphocytes to modulate immunoglobulin synthesis. J Immunol 1981; 127: 2146–2150
44 Nakagawa T, Hirano T, Nakagawa N, Yoshizaki K, Kishimoto T. Effect of recombinant IL 2 and gamma-IFN on proliferation and differentiation of human B cells. J Immunol 1985; 134: 959–966
45 Jelinek DF, Lipsky PE. Enhancement of human B cell proliferation and differentiation by tumor necrosis factor-alpha and interleukin 1. J Immunol 1987; 139: 2970–2976
46 Weiss L, Delfraissy J-F, Vazquez A, Wallon C, Galanaud P, Kazatchkine MD. Monoclonal antibodies to the human C3b/C4b receptor (CR1) enhance specific B cell differentiation. J Immunol 1987; 138: 2988–2993
47 Singer A, Hodes RJ. Mechanisms of T cell-B cell interaction. Annu Rev Immunol 1983; 1: 211–241
48 Takatsu K, Harada N, Hara Y et al. Purification and physicochemical characterization of murine T cell replacing factor (TRF). J Immunol 1985; 134: 382–389
49 Kinashi T, Harada N, Severinson E et al. Cloning of complementary DNA encoding T-cell replacing factor and identity with B-cell growth factor II. Nature 1986; 324: 70–73
50 Alderson MR, Pike BL, Harada N, Tominaga A, Takatsu K, Nossal GJV. Recombinant T cell replacing factor (interleukin 5) acts with antigen to promote the growth and differentiation of single hapten-specific B lymphocytes. J Immunol 1987; 139: 2656–2660
51 Snapper CM, Paul W. Interferon-gamma and B cell stimulatory factor-1 reciprocally regulate Ig isotype production. Science 1987; 236: 944–947
52 Brunswick M, Lake P. Obligatory role of gamma interferon in T cell-replacing factor-dependent, antigen-specific murine B cell responses. J Exp Med 1985; 161: 953–971
53 Callard RE, Smith SH, Shields JG, Levinsky RJ. T cell help in human antigen specific antibody responses can be replaced by interleukin 2 (IL-2). Eur J Immunol 1986; 16: 1037–1042
54 Swain SL. Role of BCGFII in the differentiation to antibody secretion of normal and tumor B cells. J Immunol 1985; 134: 3934–3943
55 Callard RE, Tiernan SL. Specific antibody responses by high and low density human peripheral blood B cells: T helper cells and T cell replacing factor (TRF) act on different B cell subpopulations. Immunology 1987; 62: 451–456
56 Snapper CM, Finkelman FD, Paul WE. Regulation of IgG1 and IgE production by interleukin 4. Immunol Rev 1988; 102: 51–75
57 Finkelman FD, Katona IM, Urban JF, Snapper CM, Ohara J, Paul WE. Suppression of in vivo polyclonal IgE response by a monoclonal antibody to the lymphokine B-cell stimulatory factor 1. Proc Natl Acad Sci USA 1986; 83: 9675–9678
58 Finkelman FD, Katona IM, Mosmann TR, Coffman RL. IFN-gamma regulates the isotypes of Ig secreted during in vivo humoral immune responses. J Immunol 1988; 140: 1022–1027
59 Takatsu K, Tominaga A, Harada N. T cell-replacing factor (TRF)/interleukin 5 (IL-5): molecular and functional properties. Immunol Rev 1988; 102: 107–135
60 Yokota T, Coffman RL, Hagiwara H et al. Isolation and characterization of lymphokine cDNA clones encoding mouse and human IgA-enhancing factor and eosinophil colony-stimulating factor activities: Relationship to interleukin 5. Proc Natl Acad Sci USA 1987; 84: 7388–7392
61 Coffman RL, Shrader B, Carty J, Mosmann TR, Bond MW. A mouse T cell product that preferentially enhances IgA production. I. biologic characterization. J Immunol 1987; 139: 3685–3690
62 Bond MW, Shrader B, Mosmann TR, Coffman RL. A mouse T cell product

that preferentially enhances IgA production. II. physicochemical characterization. J Immunol 1987; 139: 3691–3696
63 Harriman GR, Kunimoto DY, Elliott JF, Paetkau V, Strober W. The role of IL-5 in IgA B cell differentiation. J Immunol 1988; 140: 3033–3039
64 Snapper CM, Paul WE. B cell stimulatory factor-1 (interleukin 4) prepares resting murine B cells to secrete IgG1 upon subsequent stimulation with bacterial lipopolysaccharide. J Immunol 1987; 139: 10–17
65 Isakson PC, Pure E, Vitetta ES, Krammer PH. T cell derived B cell differentiation factor(s). Effect on the isotype switch of murine B cells. J Exp Med 1982; 155: 734–748
66 Lutzkar S, Rothman P, Pollock R, Coffman R, Alt FW. Mitogen- and IL-4-regulated expression of germ-line Ig-gamma-2b transcripts: evidence for directed heavy chain class switching. Cell 1988; 53: 177–184
67 Winter E, Krawinkel U, Radbruch A. Directed Ig class switch recombination in activated murine B cells. EMBO J 1987; 6: 1663–1671
68 Snapper CM, Finkelman FD, Paul WE. Differential regulation of IgG1 and IgE synthesis by interleukin 4. J Exp Med 1988; 167: 183–196
69 Pene J, Rousset F, Briere F, Chretien I, Wideman J, Bonnefoy JY, De Vries JE. Interleukin 5 enhances interleukin 4-induced IgE production by normal human B cells. The role of soluble CD23 antigen. Eur J Immunol 1988; 18: 929–935
70 Del Prete G, Maggi E, Parronchi P et al. IL-4 is an essential factor for the IgE synthesis induced in vitro by human T cell clones and their supernatants. J Immunol 1988; 140: 4193–4198
71 Yang X-D, De Weck AL, Stadler BM. Induction of human in vitro IgE synthesis via stimulation by anti-CD3 antibody. Eur J Immunol 1988; 18: 467–471
72 Wang A-C, Tung E, Fudenberg HH. The primary structure of a human IgG2 heavy chain: genetic, evolutionary, and functional implications. J Immunol 1980; 125: 1048–1054
73 Rabin EM, Mond JJ, Ohara J, Paul WE. Interferon-gamma inhibits the action of B cell stimulatory factor (BSF)-1 on resting B cells. J Immunol 1986; 137: 1573–1576
74 Kashiwa H, Wright SC, Bonavida B. Regulation of B cell maturation and differentiation I. Suppression of pokeweed mitogen-induced B cell differentiation by tumor necrosis factor (TNF). J Immunol 1987; 138: 1383–1390
75 Jelinek DF, Lipsky PE. Inhibitory influence of IL-4 on human B cell responsiveness. J Immunol 1988; 141: 164–173
76 Murray PD, McKenzie DT, Swain SL, Kagnoff MF. Interleukin 5 and interleukin 4 produced by Peyer's patch T cells selectively enhance immunoglobulin A expression. J Immunol 1987; 139: 2669–2674
77 Jelinek DF, Splawski JB, Lipsky PE. Human peripheral blood B lymphocyte subpopulations: functional and phenotypic analysis of surface IgD positive and negative subsets. J Immunol 1986; 136: 83–92
78 Mosier DE, Zitron IM, Mond JJ, Ahmed A, Scher I, Paul WE. Surface immunoglobulin D as a functional receptor for a subclass of B lymphocytes. Immunol Rev 1977; 37: 89–104
79 Bloem AC, Chand MA, Dollekamp I, Rijkers GT. Functional properties of human B cell subpopulations defined by monoclonal antibodies HB4 and FMC7. J Immunol 1988; 140: 768–773
80 Antin JH, Emerson SG, Martin , Gadol N, Ault KA. Leu-1+ (CD5+) B cells. A major lymphoid subpopulation in human fetal spleen: Phenotypic and functional studies. J Immunol 1986; 136: 505–510
81 Richard Y, Leprince C, Dugas B, Treton D, Galanaud P. Reactivity of Leu-1+ tonsillar B cells to a high molecular weight B cell growth factor. J Immunol 1987; 139: 1563–1567
82 Lowenthal JW, Castle BE, Christiansen J. Expression of high affinity receptors

for murine interleukin 4 (BSF-1) on hemopoietic and nonhemopoietic cells. J Immunol 1988; 140: 456–464
83 Park LS, Friend D, Sassenfeld HM, Urdal DL. Characterisation of the human B cell stimulatory factor 1 receptor. J Exp Med 1987; 166: 476–488
84 Ohara J, Paul WE. Receptors for B-cell stimulatory factor-1 expressed on cells of haematopoietic lineage. Nature 1987; 325: 537–540
85 Poo W-J, Conrad L, Janeway CA. Receptor-directed focussing of lymphokine release by helper T cells. Nature 1988; 332: 378–380
86 Van Oers MHJ, Van Der Heyden AAPAM, Aarden LA. A novel interleukin in serum and urine of renal transplant recipients. Clin Exp Med 1988; 71: 314–319
87 Garman RD, Jacobs KA, Clark SC, Raulet DH. B-cell-stimulatory factor 2 (beta 2 interferon) functions as a second signal for interleukin 2 production by mature murine T cells. Proc Natl Acad Sci USA 1987; 84: 7629–7633
88 Wong GG, Witek-Giannotti JS, Temple PA et al. Stimulation of murine hemopoietic colony formation by human IL-6. J Immunol 1988; 140: 3040–3044
89 Gauldie J, Richards C, Harnish D, Lansdorp P, Baumann H. Interferon beta-2/ B-cell stimulatory factor type 2 shares identity with monocyte-derived hepatocyte-stimulating factor and regulates the major acute phase protein response in liver cells. Proc Natl Acad Sci USA 1987; 84: 7251–7255

Tumour necrosis factor

F R Balkwill
Imperial Cancer Research Fund, Lincoln's Inn Fields, London

Tumour necrosis factor, TNF, possesses the attributes of a typical cytokine, being a pleiotropic cell regulatory protein whose activity is largely determined by the cell type to which it binds and the presence of other protein regulators. Thus TNF can be a growth factor, cytotoxin, cytostatic agent or inducer of differentiation. This cytokine is also an important inflammatory mediator regulating the activity of neutrophils, eosinophils, T and B lymphocytes and modulating the properties of the vascular endothelium. All of these actions may play a role in the ability of TNF to induce necrosis of experimental animal tumours, but the potential of this cytokine in therapy of human cancer is uncertain. The increasing evidence for a role for TNF in the pathophysiology of acute and chronic disease makes the use of specific TNF antagonists an equally interesting therapeutic possibility.

Tumour necrosis factor (TNF) is a cytokine.[1] Until 1985 it was known as a macrophage factor that would cause necrosis of experimental animal tumours, but with the availability of the purified recombinant product,[2] other (and probably more important) properties were discovered. TNF is a typical cytokine because it possesses a wide range of cell regulatory, immune and inflammatory properties that overlap with other members of the cytokine network such as interleukin-1 (IL-1) and interferon-γ (IFN-γ).[3] TNF also interacts with other members of the cytokine network, inducing them, and enhancing or inhibiting their action. Local and transient production of TNF is of benefit to the host in controlling immunity, inflammation and repair but sustained and systemic production can be harmful.

HISTORY

Tumour necrosis factor is named after one of its properties that has been observed by clinicians for several centuries—anecdotal cases of tumour regression, and even cure, in some cancer patients with concomitant infections. At the turn of the century these observations led a New York surgeon, William Coley, to derive a systemic cancer therapy that undoubtedly cured a minority of patients with inoperable and metastatic carcinoma and sarcoma.[4] 'Coleys mixed toxins', a crude filtrate of bacterial broths of erysipelas bacteria and *Bacillus prodigiosus* were used as a systemic cancer therapy until the 1930s when they were replaced by the more quantifiable techniques of chemotherapy and radiotherapy. Research on the ability of bacterial products to induce tumour necrosis and regression continued in animal models and a lipopolysaccharide constituent of bacterial cell walls, endotoxin, was found to cause this phenomenon.[5] In 1962, O'Malley et al.[6] reported that this 'tumour necrosis activity' could be transferred in the serum of endotoxin treated animals and then, in 1975, the first evidence was provided that the 'tumour necrosis factor' was actually made by host cells (probably monocytes) in response to the bacterial toxin.[7] Apart from causing necrosis of animal tumours, this factor was cytotoxic for some tumour cells in vitro. Nine years later the TNF gene was successfully cloned and expressed in *Escherichia coli*[2] providing sufficient quantities of homogeneous product to fully investigate its molecular and biologic properties.

THE TNF MOLECULE AND ITS RELATIONSHIP WITH LYMPHOTOXIN, LT

The TNF gene is closely linked to that of another cytokine, with almost identical properties, lymphotoxin, and both genes map within the major histocompatability complex region on the short arm of chromosome 6.[8] In solution, the biologically active TNF molecule exists as a trimer with 17 kD subunits,[9] but TNF is first produced in the cell as a 26 kD propeptide. It appears that this 26 kD molecule is found within the cell membrane and is, in fact, biologically active at this site. The structure of this 26 kD molecule resembles other transmembrane proteins with hydrophilic, hydrophobic and then hydrophilic regions, and is cleaved to form the 17 kD extracellular molecule.[10] In contrast LT does not appear to code for a transmembrane protein. Lymphotoxin and TNF are antigenically distinct but show 30% amino acid homology and share the same cell surface receptor.

TNF and LT are not only induced by endotoxin, but a variety of other stimuli including tumour promoters, viruses and mitogens. Moreover, as members of the cytokine network, their production can be stimulated by other cytokines notably IFN-γ, IL-1 and the Colony stimulating factors (CSFs).[1,3]

At first monocytes and macrophages were thought to be the sole producers of TNF, and T lymphocytes the producers of LT, but now there is evidence that lymphocytes and transformed cell lines of haemopoietic and nonhaemopoietic origin can produce TNF.[1]

CELL SURFACE RECEPTORS FOR TNF

TNF exerts its cytotoxic and cell regulatory activities by interacting with a specific cell surface receptor which it shares with LT.[1,11] This receptor exists on a variety of normal and malignant cells with numbers ranging from 10^3 to 10^4 receptors per cell. Recent evidence indicates that some cells, particularly human monocytes, possess two binding sites of different affinity, low affinity binding sites outnumbering high affinity sites by more than 10 to 1.[12] High and low affinity sites have recently been described for other cytokine receptors for instance interleukin-2.

One of the ways cytokines interact and influence each other's action is by transmodulation of receptor expression.[3] In this respect, it is of interest that TNF receptor RNA and cell surface expression can be upregulated by interferons α, β and γ, particularly as these two classes of cytokine can have synergistic activities.[3,11]

There is, as yet, little information on the signals transduced after the binding of TNF to its receptor, although one study has indicated an involvement of protein kinase C, possibly via direct phosphorylation of specific receptor proteins.[13] Whatever the 'second messengers', the binding of TNF to its receptor results in a rapid change in transcription and translation resulting in an altered profile of cellular protein synthesis, and thus changes in cell function. The affinity and density of receptors for TNF does not appear to account for its diversity of action.

TNF AS A GROWTH FACTOR

TNF will stimulate the growth of various human diploid fibroblasts and some tumour cell lines (reviewed in 1 & 14). This mitogenic action is synergistic with Epidemal growth factor (EGF), Platelet derived growth factor (PDGF) and insulin.[14] Synergy with EGF may be attributed, at least in part, to a TNF-induced increase in EGF receptor expression. TNF is also able to induce some of the 'competence' genes e.g. c-fos and c-myc, which are thought to play a role in transition from G_0 to G_1 phase of the cell cycle, but this induction is weak and more transient than that seen with other growth factors.[14] TNF may also stimulate cells to produce other growth factors, e.g. PDGF.

CYTOTOXIC ACTIVITIES OF TNF

Paradoxically, TNF is a potent cytotoxin for some cells particularly when they have been metabolically compromised by inhibitors of RNA or protein synthesis or viruses, (see Ref. 1 for review). TNF is also toxic for some transformed cells and will suppress normal human and murine haemopoietic cell colony formation in vitro. The cytotoxic action of TNF is protein synthesis independent and may involve several different mechanisms (see Ref. 15 for review). TNF can activate phospholipases, which break down phospholipids to arachidonic acid from which toxic leukotrienes and free oxygen radicals can be generated. Phospholipase activation can be inhibited by corticosteroids and these will protect susceptible cells from the toxicity of TNF. The cytotoxic activity of TNF can also be blocked to protease inhibitors, although the actual target of such inhibitors is unknown. As TNF can be cytocidal for normal cells when protein or RNA synthesis is inhibited, it may be that cells are protected from TNF toxicity by proteins that need to be continuously synthesized. Such proteins may prevent the activation of a nuclease. A characteristic breakdown and release of DNA occurs in cells susceptible to TNF prior to cytolysis. This could be caused by free oxygen radicals, or could be due to activation of an endonuclease. The basis of the susceptibility/resistance of cells to the cytotoxic action of TNF is unknown. One small study has linked the ability of TNF to induce the cytokine interleukin-6 with resistance to cytotoxicity.[16] In some cases resistance to the cytotoxic action of TNF may be due to autocrine production of small amounts of TNF or LT. For instance, some human epithelial cell lines resistant to TNFs cytotoxic action continuously expressed TNF message and protein.[17] Susceptibility to the TNF cytokine may also be dependent on other cytokines or growth factors to which a cell is exposed. For instance, EGF and transforming growth factor α (TGF-α) interfere with the antiproliferative effects of TNF in some cell lines.[18] The ability of TNF to be mitogenic, cytostatic or cytotoxic is therefore dependent on a complex series of extracellular and intracellular events.

THE ROLE OF TNF IN IMMUNE CELL KILLING

Activated macrophages destroy cancer cells more effectively than normal cells. TNF is a cytotoxic agent and agents that stimulate macrophage cytotoxicity also stimulate TNF production. There are now three lines of evidence suggesting that TNF can be directly involved in the killing mechanisms of macrophages (for review see Ref. 1): first, there is a strong correlation between susceptibility of cell lines to direct killing by TNF and activated macrophages; second, preincubation of target cells with inhibitors of RNA synthesis increases their susceptibility to monocyte mediated cytotoxicity; and third, killing of tumour cells by activated macrophages can be inhibited by monoclonal antibodies to TNF. However, macrophage mediated cytotoxicity is unlikely to be the result of extracellular release of TNF. Little, if any TNF can be found in culture fluids and it is more likely that the membrane bound form of TNF is the effector molecule.[10] This would provide effective local concentrations of the cytokine and prevent more generalized cell damage. There are other recognized ways by which cells kill, notably the generation of pore-forming molecules that assemble in the cell membrane, but the finding that monoclonal antibodies to TNF can, in some experimental systems, totally inhibit killing by activated macrophages, indicates a central role for this cytokine. TNF and LT may also be involved in the cytotoxic action of lymphocytes and natural killer cells.

TNF INDUCES A CELLULAR ANTIVIRAL STATE

Another contribution to host defence that may be made by TNF is the induction of a cellular antiviral state.[19] This action was originally thought to be the exclusive property of the interferons, but now it appears that both TNF and LT have intrinsic antiviral activity without inducing an interferon-like intermediate cytokine. TNF and LT can protect cells from infection by both DNA and RNA viruses, but do not act on such a broad spectrum of cells as the alpha and beta interferons.

EFFECTS OF TNF ON CELLS INVOLVED IN IMMUNITY AND INFLAMMATION

TNF is a powerful neutrophil activator promoting adherence to endothelial cells or particulate matter—stimulating phagocytosis, respiratory burst activity, and degranulation.[20] TNF also activates eosinophils, particularly stimulating their toxicity for *Schistosoma mansoni* larvae.[21] TNF also has immunoregulatory activity on T cells.[22] Normal resting T cells do not bind TNF, but upon activation TNF receptors are induced, and, at least in vitro, TNF will increase Class I MHC and IL-2 dependent T cell proliferation and IFN-γ production. TNF may also be involved in the control of B cell function particularly as a co-stimulator of B cell proliferation and Ig secretion.[23]

Vascular endothelial cells are important targets for TNF and this cytokine exerts a variety of different effects which collectively promote coagulation, inflammation and immunity (*see* Ref. 24 for review).

TNF inhibits the activity of thrombomodulin, augments the secretion of inhibitors of plasminogen activators, and induces the synthesis and transient cell surface expression of tissue factor procoagulant activity. TNF greatly increases the expression of endothelial leucocyte adhesion molecules and Class I MHC antigens, and can alter the morphology of endothelial cells in vitro changing their typical 'cobblestone' morphology to a more elongated form. Surprisingly however, TNF is a very powerful stimulator of neovascularisation in vivo.[25]

EFFECTS OF TNF ON BONE AND CARTILAGE

When leucocytes are exposed to mitogens or antigens in vitro, they release bone resorbing activity which can be reproduced by purified TNF or LT.[26] The potency of these cytokines in stimulating bone resorption is comparable to that of parathyroid hormone. TNF will also stimulate chrondrocytes to degrade proteoglycans[27] and will elicit the secretion of proteolytic enzymes, such as collagenase, from synovial cells and fibroblasts surrounding bone and cartilage.[28]

THE ROLE OF TNF IN DISEASE

Localized and transient production of cytokines such as TNF would therefore appear to be an important component of host defence systems. There is, however, increasing evidence that sustained and/or systemic cytokine production may contribute to the signs and symptoms of disease.

Infectious disease

Three observations suggest that excess production of TNF has a central involvement in endotoxic shock (*see* Ref. 29 for review): First, administration of purified recombinant TNF to rats can reproduce the signs associated with endotoxic shock such as hypotension, cardiomyopathy and diarrhoea. This is followed by an overwhelming metabolic acidosis, respiratory arrest and death; second, antibodies against TNF will protect animals against the lethality of some bacterial infections. For instance if baboons were passively immunized with murine monoclonal antibodies to human TNF, they could survive an LD100 dose of live *E. coli*; and third, experiments using a highly sensitive biological assay to TNF showed that 10 of 11 patients with meningococcal meningitis who had circulating levels of TNF in serum, died of their disease, as compared to only 8 of 68 who survived.[30]

TNF is also one of the host factors involved in inducing acute phase responses in infection and injury. When administered to mice, TNF induces the acute phase reactants serum amyloid P-component (homologous to human C-reactive protein), C3 and fibrinogen, although its activity is not as strong as the cytokine IL-1.[31] The same reactants can be induced in isolated hepatocytes.

High levels of TNF can be found in the blood of animals and humans with malaria and recent experiments suggest that TNF may be involved in the pathogenesis of this disease.[32] Injection of mice with *Plasmodium berghei* produces acute neurological manifestations and lesions similar to those seen in human cerebral malaria, a severe complication of *Plasmodium falciparum* infection. One injection of a neutralizing rabbit antibody to TNF, 4–7 days after infection, completely protected mice from the cerebral complications without modifying the parasitaemia.

The contribution of TNF to the cachectic state

Progressive weight loss is a common sign of certain chronic diseases. In 1985 Beutler et al. purified a host produced protein they called cachectin from rabbits infected with *Trypanosoma brucei* which interfered with a key enzyme in lipid biosynthesis.[29] They subsequently found that pure cachectin was identical to tumour necrosis factor. It has, however, proved difficult to reproduce signs and symptoms of cachexia with the purified recombinant cytokine, particularly as animals appear to develop a tolerance to its action. However, if increasing twice daily doses of TNF are given cachexia is sustained and weight loss occurs mainly as a result of anorexia. Unlike partially starved pair-fed animals, TNF injected mice showed depletion of whole body protein and lipid stores.[33] Chronic production of TNF during disease was mimicked when the human TNF gene (human TNF will act on murine tissues) was transfected into rodent tumour cells and a tumourigenic cell line was obtained which constitutively secreted TNF. Nude mice injected intramuscularly with such cells developed severe cachexia and weight loss before tumours became substantial. Raised serum levels of TNF have been detected in a number of chronic diseases (reviewed in 1). Moreover, RNA purified from a proportion of human bowel cancers contained high levels of TNF when compared to adjacent normal tissues (Naylor et al. unpublished observations) and several human tumour cell lines can produce TNF.[1,17]

Although TNF was first discovered due to its ability to make some animal tumours regress, sustained production of this cytokine by a cancer, or as part of a host response to a malignancy could actually promote disease progression as well as contributing to cachexia. The ability of TNF to promote lysis of bone and cartilage could facilitate tumour spread, and tumour growth could be enhanced by the mitogenic activity of TNF and its ability to stimulate angiogenesis.

TNF and immune disorders

Recent evidence has suggested that TNF is involved in the aetiology of skin and gut lesions seen in acute graft versus host disease (GVHD).[34] Systemic administration of antibodies to TNF prevented skin epidermal cell necrosis, foci of lichenoid hyperplastic reactions and the loss of hypodermic fat in mice with GVHD. In the gut, therapy with anti-TNF antibody prevented gut dilatation and crypt cell necrosis.

ANTICANCER ACTIVITY OF TNF IN ANIMAL MODELS

Tumour necrosis factor was first identified as one of the host produced factors capable of mediating tumour necrosis and regression after bacterial infection or endotoxin injection. When the protein was purified, the gene cloned, and homogeneous recombinant product made available, tumour necrosis activity against the Meth A murine sarcoma was readily demonstrated.[2] Further experiments over the past four years have shown that TNF and LT have anticancer activity in other murine transplantable tumours, murine experimental metastasis models, and human tumour xenografts in nude mice inducing necrosis, regression, and occasionally cure (see Ref. 1 for review). The most effective route of administration is local, in or near the tumour, or i.v., although some responses have been achieved with i.p. therapy.

As might be expected from its pleiotropic cell regulatory activities, there is evidence that TNF exerts anticancer activity in these models by a variety of mechanisms which are dependent largely on tumour type, tumour site, the stage of tumour development, and route of cytokine administration. There is almost certainly a host component to the anti-cancer activity and two studies have recently shown that T cells may be an important component of this (at least in murine syngeneic tumours which may be more immunogenic than human tumours[35,36]). A generalized inflammation may also play a role when TNF acts on peritoneal xenograft tumours in nude mice.[37] In some models modulation of the vascular endothelium is important, with TNF only acting on established and well vascularized tumours, and anticoagulant therapy being able to abrogate the anti-tumour action of TNF.[38] Toxicity, with the signs and symptoms of septicaemic shock, was a major problem in some animal studies, particularly when murine TNF was used. This toxicity did however vary from laboratory to laboratory and may have been, in part, due to host factors such as subclinical infection. Ibuprofen or indomethacin protected against the lethal toxicity of high doses of TNF in rats,[39] but it is not yet clear whether cyclo-oxygenase inhibitors will also abrogate the antitumour activity of TNF.

ANTICANCER ACTIVITY OF TNF IN HUMANS

Phase I clinical trials with recombinant human TNF from 4 different commercial sources are currently being carried out worldwide (see Ref. 1 for review). A review of clinical trials in which 219 patients were treated for four weeks or less, revealed 2 partial responses (a greater than 50% reduction in measurable tumours) in 193 patients receiving systemic therapy (i.m. or i.v.).[1] However, when TNF could be given directly into the tumour 10 of 22 patients were partial responders and 3 of 4 patients who received intrapleural therapy responded likewise. Side effects of this therapy were similar to those recorded for the interferons—a 'flu-like' syndrome with reversible fever, rigors, headaches and other 'flu-like' symptoms. At higher doses hypotension became dose limiting and bone marrow toxicity was observed.

These initial results, although in a Phase I setting in patients with advanced disease, are disappointing. Certainly Coley's toxins gave a complete response (total disappearance of tumour) in a minority of patients with very advanced metastatic disease, presumably by inducing TNF and other cytokines.[4]

Thus at this point in time, TNF antagonists appear to have more therapeutic potential in human disease than the cytokine itself. However, further understanding of the way TNF induces tumour necrosis, optimization of its delivery, and the combination of TNF with other cytokines such as interferon-γ, may lead to improved prospects for the use of this powerful cytokine in human cancer.

REFERENCES

1 Balkwill FR. Tumour necrosis factor and lymphotoxin. In: Balkwill FR, Cytokines in Cancer Therapy. Oxford: Qxford University Press, 1988 (In press).
2 Pennica D, Nedwin GE, Hayflick JS et al. Human tumour necrosis factor: precursor structure, expression and homology to lymphotoxin. Nature 1984; 312: 724–729.
3 Balkwill FR. Understanding and exploiting the cytokine network. In: Balkwill FR, Cytokines in Cancer Therapy. Oxford: Oxford University Press, 1988 (In press).
4 Coley Nauts H, Fowler GA, Bogatko FH. A review of the influence of bacterial infection and of bacterial products (Coley's toxins) on malignant tumors in man. Acta Med Scand 1953; (Supplement); 274–277: 29–97
5 Shear MF, Perrault A. Chemical Treatment of tumors. IX reactions of mice with primary subcutaneous tumors to injection of a hemorrhage-producing bacterial polysaccharide. JNCI 1944; 44: 461–476.
6 O'Malley WE, Achinstein B, Shear MH. Action of bacterial polysaccharide on tumours II. Damage of sarcoma 37 by serum of mice treated with Serratia marcescens polysaccharide, and induced tolerance. JNCI 1962; 29: 1169–1175.

7 Carswell EA, Old LJ, Kassel RJ, Green S, Fiore N, Williamson B. An endotoxin-induced serum factor that causes necrosis of tumours. Proc Natl Acad Sci USA 1975; 72: 366–3670.
8 Spies T, Morton CC, Nedospasov SA, Fiers W, Pious D, Strominger JL. Genes for the tumor necrosis factors alpha and beta are linked to the human major histocompatibility complex. Proc Natl Acad Sci USA 1986; 83: 8699–8702.
9 Wingfield P, Pain RH, Craig S. Tumor necrosis factor is a compact trimer. FEBS Lett 1987; 211: 179–184.
10 Kriegler M, Perez C, DeFay K, Albert I, Lu SD. A novel form of TNF/cachectin is a cell surface cytotoxic transmembrane protein: Ramifications for the complex physiology of TNF. Cell 1988; 53: 43–53.
11 Aggarwal BB, Eessalu TE, Hass PE. Characterization of receptors for human tumour necrosis factor and their regulation by gamma interferon. Nature 1985; 318: 665–667.
12 Imamura K, Spriggs D, Kufe D. Expression of tumor necrosis factor receptors on human monocytes and internalization of receptor bound ligand. J Immunol 1987; 139: 2989–2992.
13 Scheurich P, Unglab R, Maxeiner B, Tinoma B, Zugmaier G, Pfizenmaier K. Rapid modulation of tumor necrosis factor membrane receptors by activators of protein kinase C. Biochem Biophys Commun 1986; 141: 855–860.
14 Vilcek J, Palombella VJ, Zhang Y Lin JX, Feinman R, Reis LFL, Le J. Mechanisms and significance of the miotogenic and antiviral actions of TNF. Ann Inst Pasteur/Immunol 1988; 139: 307–311.
15 Fiers W, Brouckaert P, Goldberg AL et al. Structure-function relationship of tumour necrosis factor and its mechanism of action. In: Tumour necrosis factor and related cytokines. (Ciba Foundation Symposium 131). Chichester: Wiley, 1987; pp. 109–123.
16 Defilippi P, Poupart P, Tavernier, J, Fiers W, Content J. Induction and regulation of mRNA encoding 26-kDA protein in human cells lines treated with recombinant human tumor necrosis factor. Proc Natl Acad Sci USA 987; 84: 4557–4561.
17 Spriggs D, Imamura K, Rodriguez C, Horiguchi J, Kufe DW. Induction of tumor necrosis factor expression and resistance in a human breast tumor cell line. Proc Natl Acad Sci USA 1987; 84: 6563–6566.
18 Sugarman BJ, Lewis GD, Eessalu TE, Aggarwal BB, Shepard HM. Effects of growth factors on the antiproliferative activity of tumor necrosis factor. Cancer Res 1987; 47: 780–786.
19 Mestan J, Digel W, Mittnacht S et al. Antiviral effects of recombinant tumour necrosis factor in vitro. Nature 1986; 323: 816–819.
20 Shalaby MR, Aggarwal BB, Rinderknect E, Svedersky LP, Finkle BS, Palladino MA. Activation of human polymorphonuclear neutrophil functions by interferon gamma and tumor necrosis factor. J Immunol 1985; 135: 2069–2073.
21 Silberstein DS, David JR. Tumor necrosis factor enhances eosinophil toxicity to Schistosoma mansoni larvae. Proc Natl Acad Sci USA 1986; 83: 1055–1059.
22 Scheurich P, Thoma B, Ucer U, Pfizenmaier K. Immunoregulatory activity of recombinant human tumour necrosis factor (TNF) alpha: Induction of TNF receptors of human T cells and TNF alpha mediated enhancement of T cell responses. J Immunol 1987; 138: 1786–1790.
23 Kehrl JH, Miller A, Fauci AS. Effect of tumour necrosis factor alpha on mitogen-activated human B cells. J Exp Med 1987; 166: 786–791.
24 Pober JS. Effect of tumour necrosis factor and related cytokines on vascular endothelial cells. In: Tumour necrosis factor and related cytokines. Ciba Foundation Symposium 131. Chichester: Wiley, 1987: pp. 170–184.

25 Leibovich SJ, Polverini PJ, Shepard HM, Wiseman DM, Shively V, Nuseir N. Macrophage-induced antiogenesis is mediated by tumour necrosis factor alpha. Nature 1987; 329: 630–632.
26 Bertolini DR, Nedwin GE, Bringman RS, Smith DD, Mundy GR. Stimulation of bone resorption and inhibition of bone formation in vitro by human tumour necrosis factors. Nature 1986; 319: 516–518.
27 Saklatvaia J. Tumour necrosis factor alpha stimulates resorption and inhibits synthesis of proteoglycan in cartilage. Nature 1986; 322: 547–549.
28 Dayer JM, Beutler B, Cerami A. Cachetin/tumour necrosis factor stimulates collagenase and prostaglandin E2 production by human synovial cells and dermal fibroblasts. J Exp Med 1985; 162: 2163–2168.
29 Cerami A, Beutler B. The role of cachetin /TNF in endotoxic shock and cachexia. Immunol Today 1988; 9: 28–31.
30 Waage A, Halstensen A, Espevik T. Association between tumour necrosis factor in serum and fatal outcome in patients with meningococcal disease. Lancet 1987; 355–357.
31 Mortensen RF, Shapiro J, Lin BF, Douches S, Neta N. Interaction of recombinant Il-1 and recombinant tumour necrosis factor in induction of mouse acute phase proteins. J Immunol 1988; 140: 2260–2266.
32 Grau GE, Fajardo LF, Piguet PF, Allet B, Lambert PH, Vassalli P. Tumor necrosis factor (cachetin) as an essential mediator in murine cerebral malaria. Science 1987; 237: 1210–1212.
33 Tracey KJ, Lowry SF, Cerami A. The pathophysiologic role of cachetin/TNF in septic shock and cachexia. Ann Inst Pasteur Immunol 1988; 139: 311–316.
34 Piguet PF, Grau GE, Allet B, Vassalli P. Tumor necrosis factor/cachetin is an effector of skin and gut lesions of the acute phase of graft-vs-host disease. J Exp Med 1987; 166: 1280–1289.
35 Palladino JR, Refaat Shalaby M, Kramer SM et al. Characterization of the antitumour activities of human tumor necrosis factor alpha and the comparison with other cytokines: induction of tumor specific immunity. J Immunol. 1987; 138: 4023–4032.
36 Havell EA, Fiers W, North RJ. The antitumor function of tumor necrosis factor (TNF). J Exp Med 1988; 167: 1067–1085.
37 Balkwill FR, Ward BG, Moodie E, Fiers W. Therapeutic potential of tumor necrosis factor alpha and gamma interferon in experimental human ovarian cancer. Cancer Res 1987; 47: 4755–4758.
38 Shimomura K, Manda T, Mukomoto S, Katsumasa K, Nakano K, Mori J. Recombinant human tumor necrosis factor-alpha: thrombus formation is a cause of anti-tumour activity. Int J Cancer 1988; 41: 243–247.
39 Kettlehut K, Fiers W, Goldberg AL. The toxic effects of tumour necrosis factor in vivo and their prevention by cyclooxygenase inhibitors. Proc Natl Acad Sci USA 1987; 84: 4273–4277.

Epidermal growth factor and transforming growth factor α

Antony W Burgess
Melbourne Tumour Biology Branch, Ludwig Institute for Cancer Research, Victoria 3050, Australia

> This review describes the discovery and initial characterization of the epidermal growth factors (EGFs) and transforming growth factors α (TGFα), the biosynthesis and tissue distribution of these molecules and a brief description of the effects of these molecules in culture and animals. An analysis of the similarities between the EGFs and TGFαs from different organisms is used to describe the features of the molecules which appear to be critical for their function. The review concludes with a discussion of the relationship between the production of the EGF or TGFα to cancer induction and/or metastasis.

DISCOVERY AND CHARACTERIZATION

It is almost thirty years since Stanley Cohen discovered epidermal growth factor (EGF)[1] as a contaminant of nerve growth factor. EGF was recognized by its ability to accelerate the eruption of mouse teeth and the opening of eyelids of new-born mice. The abundance of EGF in mouse salivary glands facilitated its purification and by 1972 the full amino acid sequence of mouse EGF had been determined.[2] Although no human equivalent of EGF had been purified at that time, it was known that a similar protein was present in concentrates of human urine.[3] As is wont to happen in science, just as these observations were being reported, another purification project was coming to completion after more than 35 years. The human urinary protein responsible for the inhibition of gastric acid secretion (β-urogastrone) was finally purified and analyzed.[4] Harry Gregory recognized that the amino acid composition of murine EGF, human urinary EGF and β-urogastrone were closely related. The biology of urogastrone indicated that it might also promote the proliferation and epithelialization of gastric mucosa, so Gregory concluded, 'that urogastrone and human epidermal growth factor are one and the same'.

Joseph De Larco and George Todaro discovered that the retroviral transformation of murine fibroblastic cells was associated with the secretion of a molecule they termed sarcoma growth factor (SGF).[5] Subsequently, purification studies revealed that SGF consisted of two active components termed the transforming growth factors TGFα and TGFβ.[6,7] TGFα was characterized by its ability to bind to the EGF receptor, while TGFβ potentiated the clonal effects of TGFα on growth of normal rat kidney cells. The biological properties of TGFα can be explained by its ability to activate the EGF receptor. The amino acid sequence similarity between EGFs and TGFαs are displayed in Figure 1.

There is no structural relationship between TGFα and TGFβ (for more information about TGFβ see Hsuan, this issue) however, TGFβ can modulate the availability of the EGF/TGFα receptor.[8] Consequently, any consideration of the biology of EGF or TGFα should include the possible effects of TGFβ.

BIOSYNTHESIS AND TISSUE DISTRIBUTION

EGF is synthesized as a precursor of 1217 amino acids which includes at least seven repeat amino acid sequences homologous to the original 53 amino acid EGF mitogen.[9,10] The physiological role(s) of EGF is still subject to considerable speculation (see below) and very few tissues contain significant amounts of either immunoreactive EGF or EGF mRNA. The male submaxillary gland is the only concentrated source of EGF in the mouse.[11] The female mouse salivary gland has less than 1/10th the levels of the male gland, but it still contains more than 100 times as much EGF as any other tissue in a female mouse. The next highest levels of EGF (69 ng/ml and 65 ng/ml respectively) occur in urine and milk. Whilst some EGF can be detected in association with the oesophagus, stomach and duodenum, most of this is likely to be adsorbed from the secretions from the submaxillary gland.[12]

Both prepro EGF and mature EGF have been detected in mouse kidney.[13,14] Neither the EGF protein nor mRNA are detectable

Fig. 1 Similarities of 'EGF-like' peptides known to interact with the EGF receptor

GROWTH FACTOR	AMINO ACID SEQUENCE
	6 14 20 31 33 42
rat EGF	N S N T G C P P S Y D G Y C L N G G V C M Y V E S V D - - - - R Y V C N C V I G Y I G E R C Q H R D L R
mouse EGF	N S Y P G C P S S Y D G Y C L N G G V C M H I E S L D - - - - S Y T C N C V I G Y S G D R C Q T R D L R W W E L R
guinea pig EGF	Q D A P G C P P S H D G Y C L H G G V C M H I E S L N - - - - T Y A C N C V I G Y V G E R C E H Q D L D D W E
human EGF	N S D S E C P L S H D G Y C L H D G V C M Y I E A L D - - - - K Y A C N C V V G Y I G E R C Q Y R D L K W W E L R
rat TGFα	V V S H F N K C P D S H T Q Y C F H - G T C R F L V Q E E - - - - K P A C V C H S G Y V G V R C E H A D L L A
human TGFα	V V S H F N D C P D S H T Q F C F H - G T C R F L V Q E D - - - - K P A C V C H S G Y V G A R C E H A D L L A
VVP	D I P A I R L C G P E G D G Y C L H - G D C I H A R D I D - - - - G M Y C R C S H G Y T G I R C Q H V V L V D Y Q R S
SFGF	I V K H V K V C N H D Y E N Y C L N N G T C F T I - A L D N V S I T P F C V C R I N Y E G S R C Q F I N L V T Y
MGF	I I K R I K L C N D D Y K N Y C L N N G T C F T V - A L N N V S L N P F Q A C H I N Y V V G S R C Q F I N L I T I K

Alignment of 'EGF/TGFα'-like sequences known to bind to the EGF receptor: VVP = vaccinia virus protein; SFGF = Shope fibroma growth factor; and MGF = Myxoma growth factor.

during fetal development or in early mouse neonates and the first prepro EGF mRNA only appears in the kidney two weeks after birth.[15] No EGF mRNA appears in the salivary gland until after weaning. Urine and milk contain EGF so it is tempting to suggest that the major function of salivary gland EGF is a replacement of the lumenal activity of the EGF in milk.

Although the detectable levels of ECG in other tissues are low, there are several suggestions that even these levels are significant. For example, EGF-immunoreactive molecules have been identified within neuronal fibres of the telencephalon area of the adult rat brain.[16] It has been suggested that this EGF-like peptide may serve as a trophic factor for particular neurons within the brain.

The prepro EGF molecule has not been studied in detail and there is still no indication of the biological function of the EGF precursor molecule detected in the kidney. High molecular weight forms of human EGF can be purified by immunoaffinity chromatography, but these molecules appear to be precursors of biologically active human EGF (also called urogastrone).

TGFs were first detected in the conditioned medium of murine 3T3 fibroblasts transformed with the Moloney murine sarcoma virus.[5] Originally the molecule(s) responsible for the EGF-like activity in this conditioned medium was referred to as sarcoma growth factor. A considerable effort was made to purify SGF and gradually it became clear that its ability to bind to the EGF receptor (TGFα) could be separated from its stimulatory activity on the clonal growth of normal rat kidney cells (TGFβ).[6,7]

Initially, it was thought that the SGF was uniquely associated with transformed cells; however, at the same time as the distinction between TGFα and TGFβ was discovered, it was also realized that both TGFα and TGFβ could also be extracted from normal tissues.[6,17] The levels of TGFα in many tissues were thought to be quite low, however, recent observations on self-renewing epithelial tissues (e.g. skin and gastrointestinal tract) have detected significant concentrations of TGFα and TGFα mRNA.[18,19] EGF-like activity has been detected during fetal development and it was generally assumed that this activity was due to TGFα synthesized by the embryo. Careful analyses have shown that no TGFα is synthesized by the embryo; rather the TGFα mRNA is expressed in the maternal decidua.[20] The level of TGFα mRNA expressed in the decidua reaches a maximum at day 8 but is present until day 15. It appears that the embryo may induce TGFα production in the decidua as the mRNA levels are highest in the region adjacent to the embryo. There is no detectable synthesis in the uterus, placenta or other maternal tissues. Since many cells of the decidua and the embryo have TGFα receptors, it has been suggested that TGFα may have an autocrine function on decidual growth and a paracrine influence on embryonic development.

In situ hybridization has been used to investigate the biosynthesis of TGFα in the skin.[18] TGFα mRNA and protein are present throughout the stratified epidermis. In vitro keratinocytes[21] and other 'untransformed' epithelial cells in culture (e.g. pituitary cells[22]) produce even higher amounts of TGFα. Interestingly, the production of TGFα by keratinocytes is enhanced by the presence of exogenous EGF or TGFα. Thus at sites of wound healing the initial release of TGFα or EGF-like peptides by platelets could induce the autocrine production of TGFα to amplify the healing process.

Our understanding of the processing of the prepro EGF molecule is still very limited. In the mouse salivary gland the precursor is broken down to the 53 amino acid mitogen which is associated with several binding proteins in cytoplasmic granules.[23] It is proposed that in other tissues (e.g. kidney) the EGF precursor is expressed as a transmembrane protein. However, there is no indication of the biological activity for the EGF precursor.

The secretion of biologically active TGFα occurs via a membrane-associated intermediate.[24,25] The 50 amino acid form of TGFα is derived from a 160 amino acid precursor which is anchored to the cell surface via its C-terminus. As well as the 50 amino acid TGFα mitogen, higher molecular weight forms are released from the N-glycosylated 160 amino acid precursor. The portion of the TGFα sequence anchored in the cell membrane is palmitoylated (presumably at a cysteine residue) and it has been suggested that the palmitoylation could slow the passage of the TGFα precursor through the golgi and cell surface membranes, thus allowing more efficient cleavage of the precursor and thus TGFα production. Again no biological activity has yet been attributed to the surface associated TGFα precursor, but unprocessed membrane-bound TGFα could still be available for interaction with the EGF receptor, thus permitting a role for TGFα in direct contact cell-to-cell signalling processes.

BIOLOGICAL EFFECTS IN VITRO AND IN VIVO

EGF and TGFα have been observed to have many biological actions both in vitro and in vivo. Initial observations have centred around the proliferative effects of these molecules on fibroblasts, keratinocytes and epithelial cells. However, the proliferation of some squamous cell carcinomas (with elevated EGF receptor levels) and the production of wool fibres from hair follicles are inhibited by EGF.[26] Thus, apart from modulating proliferation, it is important to note that EGF can have profound effects on the production of specialized cellular products involved in the localization, mobility and function of the target cells. It is now recognized that many growth factors act on both the proliferative phase of cell development as well as the differentiated phase. The physiological effects of growth factors such as EGF or TGFα will depend on the mode of delivery and the status of the target cells. Low levels of EGF may stimulate the proliferation of keratinocytes and thus induce skin hyperplasia, but at pharmacological levels the function of other epithelia e.g. ovary, thyroid, thymus and hair follicle can be inhibited.

A particularly interesting observation relates to the effects of EGF on tooth development. As mentioned earlier, EGF was discovered as the contaminant in nerve growth which was responsible for the premature opening of mouse neonate eyes and accelerated tooth eruption. The obvious conclusion from this effect of EGF on tooth eruption is that EGF induces the teeth to grow faster. Indeed, the conclusion was substantiated by the mitogenic action of EGF on ondontogenic cells in vitro. Actually, the injection of EGF into neonatal mice decreases the size of incizors.[27] The early eruption is associated with the effects of EGF on the properties of the overlying epidermis.

Considerable care is required when attempting to extrapolate from in vitro observations to the likely physiological roles of EGF or TGFα. Firstly, it is essential to establish which of these two molecules (and which form) is present in the tissue of interest. In many respects the pharmacological actions of EGF and TGFα are remarkably similar. The potency of both in the eyelid opening assay is identical.[28] Experiments describing the action of EGF pellets on mammary duct development demonstrated that EGF induced the formation of new ductal end buds, replaced the requirement for oestrogen and prolactin for the normal histomorphology of the mammary stem cell layer, and stimulated mammary ductal diameter.[29] The authors concluded that EGF 'must be considered a strong candidate for a naturally occurring mammary tissue mitogen.' Immunohistochemical localization of either EGF or TGFα would help to substantiate this conclusion. It is important to determine the roles of TGFα and EGF in different epithelia and which form of the molecule (membrane bound, high molecular weight or processed mitogen) is present in the tissue. Some evidence is accumulating that there is a strong interaction between the action of EGF/TGFα receptor and steroid hormones,[30] but this needs to be investigated in more detail.

In vitro

The range of mesenchymal and epithelial cells influenced in vitro by EGF and/or TGFα is astonishing. In many respects these observations serve to emphasize the need to understand the availability of these molecules during development and tissue homeostasis. In many situations the effects of EGF have been shown to be dependent on other molecules and in some situations the effects are almost certainly indirect, as the apparent target cells do not even display detectable EGF receptors. One example of the indirect actions of EGF is its apparent effects on lymphoid cells. EGF decreases the blastogenic response of spleen and thymus cells to lymphoid mitogens.[31] It has been established that whilst large thymus epithelial cells lack EGF receptors, the small thymic epithelial cells produce prostaglandin PGE_2 in response to EGF. Presumably it is the PGE_2 which suppresses lymphoid blastogenesis. Keratinocytes respond to both EGF and TGFα but as mentioned earlier, TGFα is likely to be the physiological stimulus for these cells. Several interesting murine keratinocyte cell lines have been derived which are dependent on EGF for their survival and proliferation in vitro.[32] When these cells are transformed by tumourigenic retroviruses they become independent of an exogenous source of EGF.[33] These experiments demonstrate the close association between the availability of EGF (or TGFα) and one of the important steps in the development of carcinomas.

TGFα biosynthesis occurs in many self-renewing tissues and its role in neoplastic development is still unclear. Although retroviruses induce the production of TGFα in various cell lines, the cells of some tissues subject to epithelial transformation are already stimulated by TGFα. In these situations the initial neoplastic events presumably involve the production of aberrant proteins or overproduction of proteins involved in the cellular responses to growth factors such as TGFα.

The biological effects of EGF on fundic epithelia are dependent on the EGF concentration.[34] At high concentrations (2–10 nM) EGF stimulates mucin production but has no apparent effect on the rate of proliferation of these cells. However, at low concentrations 20–200 pM EGF has no effect on mucin production but stimulates proliferation significantly. The molecular basis for the differential effects of EGF on fundic cells is not yet understood in detail, but it is interesting to note that only the high affinity EGF receptors would be occupied in the low concentration range, whereas all of the cell surface EGF receptors would be occupied in the experiments using higher concentrations of EGF.

The actions of EGF and TGFα are modulated by several other growth factors.[35] In particular, bombesin, platelet derived growth factor (PDGF) and transforming growth factor β are known to act in synergy with either EGF or TGFα. Cells pretreated with PDGF are more sensitive to the action of EGF.[36] Interestingly, even though the PDGF treatment downmodulates almost all of the high affinity EGF receptors the cells are still able to respond more effectively to exogenous EGF. The synergy between TGFα and TGFβ is most striking. TGFα stimulates the growth of small clusters of NRK cells in soft agar culture, but in the presence of TGFβ, large colonies of NRK cells are produced by TGFα (or EGF). The action of TGFβ on NRK cells in the presence of EGF or TGFα presumably leads to the induction of an extracellular matrix protein[37] which allows the non-adherent NRK cells to proliferate more effectively in response to TGFα.

Even the effects of a single growth factor acting on a particular cell line can be difficult to interpret. The effects of TGFα on an endometrial carcinoma cell line have been studied in detail.[38] When seeded at low densities (5×10^3 cells/cm^2), high concentrations of TGFα (830 pM–5 nM) inhibit the growth of these cells: mitogenic stimulation was only detected at lower concentrations of TGFα (~ 16 pM). When the endometrial cells are seeded at 2.5×10^4 cells/cm^2 and then treated with TGFα (>830 pM), the cells are stimulated to proliferate. Presumably, at higher densities the endothelial cells stimulated by TGFα (1 nM) produce molecule(s) capable of synergizing with the TGFα to allow proliferation rather than differentiation. Although the nature of the synergistic molecules is still obscure, it must be recognized that these types of synergistic interactions are likely to occur in steady-state or regenerating tissues. The modulating molecules and their biological properties must be identified before we can hope to approach the physiological properties of TGFα or EGF. There are already specific candidates such as interleukin-1 and fibroblast growth factor, but now that sufficient quantities of the highly purified recombinant modulators are available, it will soon be possible to study the physiological effects of combinations of several growth factors.

The pleiotrophic action of EGF and TGFα in vitro suggests a myriad of functions for these molecules in vivo. Almost all fibroblast, epithelial and muscle cells respond to EGF or TGFα. However, the tissue location of these molecules may restrict their major effects. Physiologically, the action of either growth factor might be limited by the sites of biosynthesis. If we are to understand the roles of EGF or TGFα in the development of specific tissues, we must design techniques for the accurate delivery of the growth factors. Small hydrostatic pumps or pellet delivery systems are being designed at present.[39] Even though the in vivo actions of EGF were amongst the earliest observations of growth factor action we still have an extremely limited understanding of the pharmacokinetics or delivery systems for these molecules.

In vivo

The discovery of both human and murine EGFs was closely associated with their physiological effects. Human EGF (urogastrone) was detected in the urine of pregnant women by its ability to cure experimental stomach ulcers in dogs.[40] Subsequent work shows that human EGF inhibited the release of acid from the gastric mucosa. This aspect of EGF action has had intriguing possibilities for many years, but the rapid destruction of EGF in the stomach necessitates large and frequent doses. Since EGF can bind to highly charged polymers, even at low pH, it has been suggested that molecular carriers such as sucralfate could increase the concentration of EGF in the stomach.[41]

When EGF and TGFα are administered at pharmacological levels there are effects on many tissues: skin thickening, retardation of hair production by follicles, cell production and function in the gastrointestinal tract, cranio-facial morphogenesis, blood vessel development, neonatal growth, the immune and endocrine systems. Indeed, the effects of EGF are so widely distributed it is difficult to distinguish between the direct and referred responses. For example, EGF modulates the release of luteinizing hormone and thyroid hormone and it is difficult to distinguish the EGF responses from the responses to reduced levels of these hormones.[42] EGF and triiodothyronine (T3) induce some similar physiological responses, however, the potency of each can be quite different. T3 is more potent in the tooth eruption assay whereas EGF is a better stimulator of palpebral morphogenesis.[43] In some tissues T3 and EGF actually have the opposite effects: EGF retards external ear development whereas T3 accelerates this process. Both EGF and thyroid hormone retard hair follicle development in sheep.[26] Since EGF is known to reduce the secretion of thyroid hormone in mice and to lower the plasma levels of thyroid hormone in sheep, it is still not clear whether the effects of EGF on hair follicle development are directly controlled by EGF (or TGFα). A similar situation pertains to our understanding of the decrease in reproductive functions in sheep treated with EGF.[44] Whilst EGF has no effect on the sensitivity of the pituitary to luteinizing hormone releasing hormone, it does inhibit the hypothalamic pulse generator, thus preventing the release of luteinizing hormone. However, EGF has a direct effect on the ovaries, impairing the response to gonadotrophins. The relative importance of these effects on the reproductive system is yet to be established.

The effects of TGFα and EGF are not always equivalent. Whilst these two molecules are equipotent in the new-born eyelid opening assay, for example, TGFα is a more potent promoter of calcium release from fetal rat long bones[45,46] and there is a distinct difference between their actions on blood vessels.[47] EGF and TGFα both inhibit smooth muscle contraction in response to prostaglandin F2 and in vivo both stimulate arterial blood flow.[47] However, TGFα is considerably more potent than EGF in eliciting the changes in blood flow.[47] Interestingly, pretreatment of mice with either EGF or TGFα desensitizes the vasculature responses to EGF; pretreatment with TGFα does not impair subsequent treatments with TGFα.

Several studies recently have indicated that EGF may play a role in the central nervous system.[16] Rabbit antibodies to murine EGF detect the EGF epitope within rodent brain neuronal fibres and terminals. Furthermore, EGF supports the survival and outgrowth of processes from telencephalic neurons of the rat brain.[48] The molecular characteristics of this immunoreactive EGF have not been identified as yet, so some caution is needed when interpreting these results.

When administered to neonatal mice the effects of EGF can have a long latency. Daily treatment of neonatal mice for 30 days with EGF stimulated an increase in body weight and accelerated the opening of the eyes and vagina.[49] Accelerated vaginal opening did not require daily treatment. EGF administered between 14 and 18 days after parturition was sufficient to cause this effect and subsequently for inducing premature oestrous.

There are now many studies which indicate that EGF stimulates the proliferation of cells in the gastrointestinal tract. The EGF needs to be administered intravenously.[50] EGF delivered intragastrically does not alter intestinal cell production. The largest effects of EGF are seen in the colon where EGF stimulates increased DNA synthesis (and also mitosis). Neither thyroxine nor cortisol appear to modulate cell production in the intestine.

The in vitro responses of keratinocytes to EGF (and TGFα) are reflected in the enhanced rate of wound epithelialization. Wound healing actually requires both proliferation and migration of keratinocytes.[51] TGFα stimulates both of these processes. Whilst EGF is not as potent as TGFα, it is still able to stimulate wound-healing. EGF has already been used to increase the strength of corneal grafts and the improved rate of epithelialization means that the wounds heal more quickly.

What then are the physiological roles of EGF and TGFα? Of course the answer is unknown, however, some speculation is in order. The distribution of EGF is limited to a few organs, such as the male mouse salivary gland, Brunner's gland, breast milk and the kidney (albeit in the precursor form). EGF is difficult to detect in self-renewing epithelia, but TGFα is present in significant levels. The extraordinary difference in the level of EGF in the male and female salivary gland and the strong synergistic action between EGF and oestradiol may provide a clue to the action of EGF. Given the presence of high concentrations of androgens in male mice, perhaps the oesophageal mucosa is sensitive to these hormones and requires protection from the EGF in the salivary secretions.

GENES, HOMOLOGIES AND STRUCTURE

The EGF mitogens isolated from mouse salivary glands and human urine are both 53 amino acids long. Whilst other EGF mitogens can be slightly smaller than this, the active forms are all between 48 and 53 residues. Precursor forms with molecular weights of 9000, 28 000 and 30 000 have been detected in the mouse salivary gland[52] and human urine.[53] However, it was most unexpected when molecular cloning indicated that the mRNA for murine EGF contained more than 4800 nucleotides. Further analysis of the EGF mRNA revealed that a prepro EGF protein of 1217 amino acids (MW ~133 000) was encoded and that there were eight repeating EGF-like segments, only the last of which corresponded to the 53 amino acid mitogenic EGF peptide.[9,10] It is still not clear why the EGF precursor is so large or why it is apparently over redundant. The biosynthetic processing of prepro EGF has not been determined in detail and the fate of the EGF-like proteins encoded by the homologous repeats is unknown. These peptides could represent a family of proteins with similar but distinct biological properties. There is one report of prepro EGF being present in murine kidneys, but there is no data on the biological activity of this precursor.[13,14]

The mRNA encoding TGFα is also 4800 bases long, however, most of this is associated with a long 3′ untranslated region.[54] The coding sequence implies that a precursor of 160 amino acids is translated from this message. The residues between 8 and 18 correspond to a typical signal sequence involved in protein secretion. The Val.Val.Ser.His.Phe N-terminal sequence of the 50 amino acid TGFα polypeptide starts at position 39 of the translated sequence, so some proteolytic cleavage of the precursor must occur after the signal sequence is removed. The protein sequence in the TGFα precursor immediately following the C-terminus of the secreted protein consists of 23 hydrophobic amino acids characteristic of a transmembrane domain. The TGFα precursor appears to be inserted into the plasma membrane and the mature mitogen released by a specific membrane associated protease.[24,25] If cells producing TGFα lacked this protease the TGFα would remain as a transmembrane protein capable of participating in direct contact intercellular signalling. Similar functions have been proposed for prepro EGF, but as yet there is no evidence to support these notions.

Similarities to the EGF/TGFα mitogenic amino acid sequence

motif have been identified in a diverse range of molecules: hormone receptors, plasminogen activators and extracellular matrix proteins to name a few.[55,56] The function of this motif in these other molecules is unknown. In most cases whilst the proteins are similar, there are changes which would almost certainly abolish the ability of these molecules to bind with high affinity to the EGF/TGFα receptor. If we consider all of the EGF or TGFα molecules known to bind to and activate the EGF receptor, all have six cysteine residues which are presumably arranged as identical disulphide bonds; and residues G_{18}, G_{36}, Y_{37}, G_{39}; R_{41} and L_{47} are **invariant**. Structure function studies have demonstrated the importance of Leucine 47 and any non-conservative substitutions at this position might be expected to reduce the affinity of homologues for the EGF/TGFα receptor.[57] Most of the seven repeat sequences in prepro EGF have at least two substitutions at the invariant positions. In all of these repeats, the positions of the cysteine residues are also altered. If these peptides were produced they are unlikely to interact with the EGF receptor. There are a number of possibilities for the function of these sequences. They could represent a protein framework motif which is used to generate similar structures for a number of proteins, vestigial copies from an ancient gene amplification with no function at present or precursors for growth factors with unknown specificity. The repeats observed in mammalian prepro EGF are not an isolated phenomenon. At least two genes (Notch and Delta) or *Drosophila* and the lin-12 gene in *C. elegans* contain multiple copies of the EGF-like motif.[58,59] The third repetitive element of the Notch locus has all of the cysteines and the invariant residues are also preserved.[58] This segment would be an excellent candidate EGF-like molecule. The other 35 EGF-like Notch repeats have at least two substitutions at the EGF invariant positions. The lin-12 locus of *C. elegans* encodes 11 peptide units which are similar to each other and to the EGF mitogen motif.[59] However, all of the 'repeats' have at least two substitutions at the invariant positions.

Interesting similarities have been noted between the early regions of prepro EGF and the light density lipoprotein (LDL) receptor.[56] This relationship together with the C-terminal 'transmembrane' sequence in the prepro EGF has led to the notion that the prepro EGF protein could act as a cell surface receptor. It is suggested that the N-terminal region of prepro EGF could act as a ligand binding domain. The subcellular location and function of prepro EGF requires further investigation and the presence of this protein in the kidney[13] affords an opportunity to improve our understanding of its function. The molecular nature of the EGF-like cross-reactivity in the brain will also be interesting.

Although antibodies can be of immense importance for defining the tissue distribution of particular epitopes, some care is necessary before making a direct association between the epitope and the presence of the native molecule. Cross-reacting epitopes might be expected from some of the similarities described earlier. Either definitive molecular analyses or bioassays of the immunoreactive protein are important adjuncts to immunofluorescent data. One interesting example has been described using monoclonal antibodies generated against peptide sequences derived from rat or human TGFα. The antibody raised against the C-terminal region of human TGFα recognizes native molecules and can be used to measure the levels of TGFα in conditioned media.[60] When this antibody is used to analyze cell lysates a 21 000 dalton protein is detected. This protein was concentrated in a perinuclear region, however, small amounts were still detectable in the cytoplasm. Biosynthetic studies on TGFα have detected cell-associated precursors with high molecular weight, but these are on the plasma membrane. The perinuclear location of the 21 000 dalton epitope suggests an immunological cross-reaction between similar molecules, but it is important to establish that the molecule detected in the perinuclear region is actually TGFα. In this context, it should be noted that the anti-TGFα peptide antibodies used in these studies do not recognize native TGFα as efficiently as TGFα peptides or denatured TGFα.

Another class of molecules share homologies with the EGF/TGFα family. These are proteins from three viruses capable of transforming fibroblasts or epithelial cells. The vaccinia virus encodes a protein with all of the EGF cysteine and invariant residues intact.[61] Indeed, this molecule has been shown to bind to the EGF receptor and to initiate cell division. It appears that this virus uses the EGF receptor to attach to its target cell. The Shope fibrosarcoma virus and the myxomatosis virus encode related proteins which have conserved all of the EGF disulphides and all but one of the invariant residues (glycine$_{36}$).[62,63] In both viruses this residue 36 is asparagine. Initial data indicate that these proteins bind to the EGF receptor but do *not stimulate* a mitogenic response.[64] However, the EGF region of the Shope protein has been synthesized using solid phase peptide chemistry and this analogue bound to the EGF receptor and stimulated a mitogenic response in NRK cells.[65] It is possible that other regions of the Shope protein are involved in modulating the cellular response. It will be interesting when the present conundrum surrounding the activity of the EGF-like proteins in these two viruses is resolved.

EGF is only a small protein but the elucidation of its three dimensional structure has proved difficult. Attempts to crystallize EGF have not been successful, however, two-dimensional NMR analyses have yielded detailed models for the structures of human,[66,67] mouse[68] and rat EGF.[69] Similar data will soon be available for human TGFα. The first residue and last six residues of mouse EGF appear to be in motion with respect to the remainder of the molecule. However, the relative positions of residues 2–47 have been determined in sufficient detail to identify the hydrogen bonding pattern and the folding of the polypeptide backbone.[68] The dominant feature of the molecule is a central antiparallel β-sheet between residues 19 and 32. The C-terminal region from residue 34 to 48 forms a separate domain and has a short anti-parallel β-sheet and a left-handed alphabetical loop. The surface containing the side chains for leucine 47, glycine 36 and leucine 47 is quite hydrophobic and has a distinct cleft. This opposite surface is acidic and contains several polar side-chains. It is likely that the leucine residue positions 26 and 47 form hydrophobic interactions with the receptor. The enzymatic removal of the leucine 47 side chain essentially destroys the activity of murine EGF.[57] Since this side chain is a central feature of the proposed binding surface this is not all that surprising. Cleavage of the murine EGF backbone at position 21 would be expected to disrupt the binding surface and experimentally this is associated with a reduction in the ability of EGF to bind to its receptor. Neither tyrosine 37 nor arginine 41 (two of the invariant residues) appear to be associated with the proposed binding surface, however, these residues are in close juxtaposition together with the side chain of valine 34. The role of these residues is not yet clear but these may be required for directing the appropriate processing of prepro EGF or there may be further interactions between EGF and other closely associated molecules.

At the time of this review, there were no reliable reports of peptide analogues of EGF or TGFα which could act as EGF antagonists. Fragments of the EGF or TGFα molecule are essentially inactive in either the receptor or mitogenic assay. Since the binding surface appears to contain residues from the

N-terminus, the central β-sheet and the C-terminus, it is quite probable that high affinity ligands will require analogous residues from the cysteine at position six to the arginine at position 48.

EGF, TGFα AND CANCER

There is no evidence to suggest that EGF *per se* is associated with either the induction, promotion or invasiveness of tumour cells. The EGF biosynthesis is restricted to a few tissues. Neither the EGF precursor nor the EGF mitogen are produced by transformed cells. In contrast, TGFα is often associated with proliferating epithelia and tumour cells.[70] Whilst many in vitro and in vivo experiments have used EGF to modulate cellular proliferation or to maintain the transformed state, most of these EGF experiments should be interpreted to reflect the likely action(s) of TGFα. In some cases (e.g. angiogenesis) TGFα appears to be more potent than EGF; in other experiments TGFα appears to act for longer. However, the biological outcome of most experiments with EGF can be expected to reflect the likely action(s) of TGFα.

There are several aspects of TGFα biology which are relevant to tumourigenesis: the inappropriate or over-expression of TGFα,[71,72] the amplification of the EGF receptor on some tumour cells[73] and the increased responsiveness of cells to TGFα caused by disturbances to the biochemical pathways normally stimulated by the activated EGF receptor TGFα complex.[74]

The discovery of TGFα was associated with the effects of mouse and feline sarcoma viruses on the receptors for EGF.[5] Retroviral infection of murine 3T3 fibroblast normal rat kidney cells, mice lung cells and cat embryo fibroblasts caused a profound and permanent loss of detectable membrane receptors for EGF. This phenomenon did not occur when the same cells were transformed by DNA tumour viruses. These observations were followed quickly by evidence that the virally transformed cells secreted a polypeptide growth factor capable of binding to the EGF receptor.[75] This molecule was eventually purified and named transforming growth factor α (TGFα). TGFα is capable of inducing the growth of fibroblasts in soft agar—a property usually associated with tumour cells, however, the role of TGFα in the initiation or maintenance of naturally occurring tumours is still far from clear. TGFα mRNA and protein are associated with normal self-renewing, proliferative epithelia.[18] Both normal epithelial progenitor cells and carcinomas may require TGFα for survival and proliferation, but TGFα secretion may not always be caused by the tumorigenic event. It would be interesting to follow the cause of TGFα secretion in virally induced sarcomas where there is reason to believe that the induction of TGFα may be closely associated with the transformation process. Experimentally, artificial viruses encoding the synthesis of EGF or TGFα are sufficient to transform non-tumorigenic cells to malignant cells.[76,77]

Epidermal keratinocytes produce TGFα both in vivo and in vitro,[18] however, tumour promoters such as 12-0-tetradecanoyl-phorbol-13-acetate enhance (2-3-fold) the secretion of TGFα.[78] Since phorbol esters are strong hyperplastic agents for epidermis, it is likely that TGFα underlies the perturbed growth and differentiation associated with agents such as these. Chronic elevation of TGFα secretion may allow a sufficient increase in the rate of cell turnover to increase the risk of a complementary mutational event which leads to self-renewal rather than differentiation. In the presence of excess TGFα, this class of mutations would be expected to lead to the accumulation at a local site of immature cells, i.e. a primary tumour.

Other tumorigenic events are associated with an increased production of TGFα. When a non-tumorigenic mouse mammary epithelial cell line (NMuMG) is transformed by an activated Harvey *ras* gene or the polyoma middle T antigen (pyt), the cells will form tumours in nude mice. Conditioned media from the *ras* and pyt transformed cells appear to contain more TGFα than the conditioned medium from the NMuMG cells. Interestingly, the EGF receptors were down regulated on NMuMG-*ras* cells, but not on NMuMG-pyt cells. It is possible that the 'EGF-like', 'TGF-like' activity detected in the CM from the NMuMG-pyt cells contains other mitogenic substances (e.g. transforming growth factor β and fibroblast growth factor) relevant to the proliferation of breast epithelial cells. Primary malignant gliomas have a high incidence of amplified copies of the EGF receptor gene.[79] More than 30% of gliomas have multiple copies of the EGF receptor gene and this is invariably associated with high levels of expression of the EGF receptor[79] or its cytoplasmic domain.[80] Many gliomas and epithelial tumours are associated with the production of TGFα. Presumably the excess level of activated receptor in the cells with amplified genes coupled with the availability of TGFα is sufficient to convert these receptor-rich cells to tumourigenic cells.

In the urine of some brain tumour patients there is an elevated level of high molecular weight urinary TGFα. When the tumour is removed surgically, the levels of urinary high molecular weight TGFα are reduced.[81]

POTENTIAL CLINICAL AND INDUSTRIAL USES OF EGF/TGFα

Although EGF has been available in large quantities for more than ten years, relatively few clinical studies have been published. EGF has been used to accelerate the in vitro growth of keratinocytes for applications to burns patients.[82] Animal tests indicated that EGF accelerates wound healing[51] and some limited experience with the use of EGF to accelerate the healing of surgical wounds from corneal grafts appears to be quite promising.[83] The wounds treated with EGF achieve a higher tensile strength several days earlier than the untreated grafts. There are similar indications for the use of TGFα and model studies with partial thickness wounds have shown that EGF accelerates healing. Several studies are underway on the use of EGF or TGFα for assisting the healing of full thickness wounds in diabetic patients. Many of these patients have suffered with chronic ulceration for several years but various growth factor preparations (including platelet extracts which contain EGF-like molecules) seem to improve the rate of healing of the wounds.

The large-scale experiments on the use of EGF to defleece sheep have been undertaken in Australia.[44] When administered at pharmacological doses, EGF inhibits the proliferation of hair follicle cells and the formation of the mature wool fibre.[84] The wool fibre thins but is extruded from the follicle and after a few days the wool lifts easily from the skin. A number of logistic problems are associated with this technique, namely premature and inconvenient shedding of the wool. Furthermore, the lack of sufficient wool stubble leaves the sheep susceptible to sunburn and cold.

Although EGF retards the initial growth of neonatal mice over a longer term, in controlled doses it can promote growth and possibly increase the efficiency of food utilization. These properties could be a valuable adjunct to other growth modulators in the production of poultry and fish. However, before wide-scale applications are attempted, it will be important to understand the role and properties of both EGF and TGFα in different animal species, in particular, the effects of long-term administration of EGF or TGFα on the reproductive systems of these animals.

There are some indications that high levels of EGF can act as a tumour promoter in animals treated with carcinogens.[85] The use of EGF for the treatment of gastric ulcers has been considered since its initial discovery. However, the in vivo half-life of EGF is quite short and extended effects require high doses or frequent applications. Until recently the availability of EGF or TGFα restricted its possible uses in this area. The production of recombinant EGF or synthetic TGFα can now be accomplished on a larger scale and the use of polymer delivery systems to extend the bioavailability could make EGF a useful agent for the treatment of gastrointestinal ulcers or mucositis.[41] Cancer patients can develop severe mucositis during chemotherapy and mouth ulcers are often a serious side-effect. Treatment of the patient with combinations of haemopoietic and epithelial growth factors to increase mucous production and/or neutrophil levels could ameliorate some of these difficulties.[86]

Since quite a number of squamous cell carcinomas and gliomas have elevated levels of EGF receptors, consideration has been given to the preparation of cytotoxic conjugates of EGF for killing cancers which display more than 100 000 surface EGF receptors per cell. A pseudomonas toxin-EGF fusion protein has been prepared and is known to be capable of killing cells with elevated levels of EGF receptors.[87] Daunomycin or ^{131}I-EGF or TGFα conjugates should be capable of similar killing and might penetrate tumour tissue more effectively than monoclonal antibodies or large toxin conjugates.

There is a considerable interest in the angiogenic effects of TGFα.[47] Many tumours secrete TGFα and as well as being involved as an autocrine (or paracrine) stimulator, TGFα could also be responsible for the 'invasion' of these tumours by blood vessels. Antagonists to TGFα might be able to compete with the autocrine actions of TGFα (although this might be thwarted by the intracellular association of the autocrine TGFα and the EGF receptor) and to decrease the vascularization of the tumour mass. The destruction of tumour blood vessels can lead to the complete destruction of a primary cancerous lesion. EGF or TGFα antagonists have been difficult to synthesize, however, neutralizing antibodies may be effective angiogenesis antagonists. If we could improve our understanding of the factors controlling the biosynthesis of TGFα it might even be possible to shut down its autocrine production at tumour sites.

REFERENCES

1 Cohen S. Isolation of a mouse submaxillary gland protein accelerating incisor eruption and eyelid opening in the new born animal. J Biol Chem 1962; 237: 1555-1562
2 Savage CR, Inagami T, Cohen S. The primary structure of epidermal growth factor. J Biol Chem 1972; 247: 7612-7621
3 Starkey RH, Cohen S, Orth DN. Epidermal growth factor: Identification of a new hormone in human urine. Science 1975; 189: 800-802
4 Gregory H. Isolation and structure of urogastrone and its relationship to epidermal growth factor. Nature 1975; 257: 325-327
5 De Larco JE, Todaro GJ. Growth factors from murine sarcoma virus-transformed cells. Proc Natl Acad Sci USA 1978; 75: 4001-4005
6 Roberts AB, Anzano MA, Lam LC, Smith JM, Sporn MB. New class of transforming growth factors potentiated by epidermal growth factor: Isolation from non-neoplastic tissues. Proc Natl Acad Sci USA 1981; 78: 5339-5343
7 Holley RW, Armour R, Baldwin JH. Density-dependent regulation of growth of BSC-1 cells in cell culture: growth inhibitors formed by the cells. Proc Natl Acad Sci USA 1978; 75: 1864-1866
8 Massague J. Transforming growth factor β modulates the high affinity receptors for epidermal growth factor and transforming growth factor. J Cell Biol 1985; 100: 1508-1514
9 Scott J, Urdea M, Quiroga M, et al. Structure of a mouse submaxillary messenger RNA encoding epidermal growth factor and seven related proteins. Science 1983; 221: 236-240
10 Gray A, Dull TJ, Ullrich A. Nucleotide sequence of epidermal growth factor cDNA predicts a 128,000-molecular weight protein precursor. Nature 1983; 303: 722-725
11 Byyny RL, Orth DN, Cohen S. Radio-immunoassay of epidermal growth factor. Endocrinology 1972; 90: 1261-1266
12 Joh T, Itoh M, Katsumi K, et al. Immunoreactive epidermal growth factor in mouse digestive organs. Use of a sensitive enzyme immunoassay. Acta Endocrinol 1987; 115: 203-210
13 Rall LB, Scott J, Bell GI, Grawford RJ, Penschow JD, Niall HD, Coghlan JP. Mouse prepro-epidermal growth factor synthesis by the kidney and other tissues. Nature 1985; 313: 228-231
14 Kashimata M, Hiramatsu M, Minami N, Minami N. Biochemical properties of epidermal growth factor in the mouse kidney. Comp Biochem Physiol 1987; 86: 651-653
15 Popliker M, Shatz A, Avivi A, Ullrich A, Schlessinger J, Webb CG. Onset of endogenous synthesis of epidermal growth factor in neonatal mice. Dev Biol 1987; 119: 38-44
16 Fallon JH, Seroogy KB, Loughlin SE, Morrison RS, Bradshaw RA, Knauer DJ, Cunningham DD. Epidermal growth factor immunoreactive material in the central nervous system: location and development. Science 1984; 224: 1107-1109
17 Sporn MB, Roberts AB, Wakefield LM, Assoian RK. Transforming growth factor-β: Biological function and chemical structure. Science 1986; 233: 532-534
18 Derynck R, Roberts AB, Winkler ME, Chen EY, Goeddel D. Human transforming growth factor-α: precursor structure and expression in *E. coli*. Cell 1984; 38: 287-297
19 Malden LT, Novak U, Burgess AW. Expression of transforming growth factor alpha messenger RNA in the normal and neoplastic gastrointestinal tract. Int J Cancer 1989, In press
20 Han VK, Hunter ES 3d, Pratt RM, Zendegui JG, Lee DC. Expression of rat

transforming growth factor α mRNA during development occurs predominantly in the maternal decidua. Mol Cell Biol 1987; 7: 2335–2343
21 Coffey RJ Jr, Derynck R, Wilcox JN, et al. Production and autoinduction of transforming growth factor-alpha in human keratinocytes. Nature 1987; 328: 817–820
22 Kobrin MS, Samsoondar J, Kudlow JE. α-Transforming growth factor secreted by untransformed bovine anterior pituitary cells in culture. J Biol Chem 1986; 261: 14414–14419
23 Kasselberg AG, Orth DN, Gray ME, Stahlman MT. Immunocytochemical localization of human epidermal growth factor/urogastrone in several human tissues. J Histochem Cytochem 1985; 33: 315–322
24 Bringman TS, Lindquist PB, Derynck R. Different transforming growth factor-alpha species are derived from a glycosylated and palmitoylated transmembrane precursor. Cell 1987; 48: 429–440
25 Teixido J, Gilmore R, Lee DC, Massague J. Integral membrane glycoprotein properties of the prohormone pro-transforming growth factor-alpha. Nature 1987; 326: 883–885
26 Thorburn GD, Waters MJ, Dolling M, Young IR. Fetal maturation and epidermal growth factor. Proc Aust Phys Pharmacol Soc 1981; 12: 11–15
27 Rhodes JA, Fitzgibbon DH, Macchiarulo PA, Murphy RA. Epidermal growth factor-induced precocious incisor eruption is associated with decreased tooth size. Dev Biol 1987; 121: 247
28 Smith JM, Sporn MB, Roberts AB, Derynck R, Winkler ME, Gregory H. Human transforming growth factor-α causes precocious eyelid opening in new born mice. Nature 1985; 315: 515–516
29 Coleman S, Silberstein GB, Daniel CW. Ductal morphogenesis in the mouse mammary gland: evidence supporting a role for epidermal growth factor. Dev Biol 1988; 127: 304–315
30 Traish AM, Wotiz HH. Prostatic epidermal growth factor receptors and their regulation by androgens. Endocrinology 1987; 121: 1461–1467
31 Nieburgs AC, Korn JH, Picciano PT, Cohen S. Thymic epithelium in vitro. IV. Regulation of growth and mediator production by epidermal growth factor. Cell Immunol 1987; 108: 396–404
32 Weissman BE, Aaronson SA. Balb and Kirsten murine sarcoma viruses alter growth and differentiation of EGF-dependent Balb/c mouse epidermal keratinocyte lines. Cell 1983; 32: 599–606
33 Weissman BE, Aaronson SA. Members of the src and ras oncogene families supplant the epidermal growth factor requirement of Balb/MK-2 keratinocytes and induce distinct alterations in their terminal differentiation program. Mol Cell Biol 1985; 5: 3386–3396
34 Yoshida S, Kasuga S, Hirao Y, Fuwa T, Nakagawa S. Effect of biosynthetic human epidermal growth factor on the synthesis and secretion of mucin glycoprotein from primary culture of rabbit fundal mucosa cells. In Vitro Cell Dev Biol 1987; 23: 460–464
35 Rozengurt E. Early signals in the mitogenic response. Science 1986; 234: 161–166
36 Stiles CD. The molecular biology of platelet-derived growth factor. Cell 1983; 33: 653–655
37 Thorne HJ, Jose DG, Zhang HY, Dempsey PJ, Whitehead RH. Epidermal growth factor stimulates the synthesis of cell-attachment proteins in the human breast cancer cell line PMC42. Int J Cancer 1987; 40: 207–212
38 Korc M, Haussler CA, Trookman NS. Divergent effects of epidermal growth factor and transforming growth factors on a human endometrial carcinoma cell line. Cancer Res 1987; 47: 4909–4914
39 Murray JB, Brown L, Langer R, Kalgsbrun M. A microsustained release system for epidermal growth factor. In Vitro Cell Dev Biol 1983; 19: 743–748

40 Sandweiss DJ. The immunizing effect of the anti-ulcer factor in normal human urine (anthelone) against the experimental gastrojejunal (peptic) ulcer in dogs. Gastroenterology 1943; 1: 965–969
41 Nexo E, Poulsen SS. Does epidermal growth factor play a role in the action of sucralfate? Scand J Gastroenterol Suppl 1987; 127: 45–49
42 Ahren B. Epidermal growth factor (EGF) inhibits stimulated thyroid hormone secretion in the mouse. Peptides 1987; 8: 743–745
43 Hoath SB, Pickens WL. Effect of thyroid hormone and epidermal growth factor on tactile hair development and craniofacial morphogenesis in the postnatal rat. J Craniofac Genet Dev Biol 1987; 7: 161–167
44 Radford HM, Avenell JA, Panaretto BA. Some effects of epidermal growth factor on reproductive function in Merino sheep. J Reprod Fertil 1987; 80: 113–118
45 Stern PH, Krieger NS, Nissenson RA, Williams RD, Winkler ME, Derynck R, Strewler GJ. Human transforming growth factorα stimulates bone resorption in vitro. J Clin Invest 1985; 76: 2016–2019
46 Ibbotson KJ, Harrod J, Gowen M, D'Souza S, Smith DD, Winkler ME, Derynck R, Mundy GR. Human recombinant tranforming growth factor alpha stimulates bone resorption and inhibits formation in vitro. Proc Natl Acad Sci USA 1986; 83: 2228–2232
47 Gan BS, Hollenberg MD, MacCannell KL, Lederis K, Winkler MW, Derynck R. Distinct vascular actions of epidermal growth factor-urogastrone and transforming growth factor-alpha. J Pharmacol Exp Ther 1987; 242: 331–337
48 Morrison RS, Kornblum HI, Leslie FM, Bradshaw RA. Trophic stimulation of cultured neurons fron neonatal rat brain by epidermal growth factor. Science 1987; 238: 72–75
49 Imada O, Hayashi N, Masamoto K, Kasuga S, Fuwa T, Nakagawa S. Long-latency growth-promoting activity of EGF when administered to mice at the neonatal stage. Am J Physiol 1987; 253: E251–E254
50 Goodlad RA, Wilson TJ, Lenton W, Gregory H, McCullagh KG, Wright NA. Intravenous but not intragastric urogastrone-EGF in trophic to the intestine of parenterally fed rats. Gut 1987; 28: 573–582
51 Schultz GS, White M, Mitchell R, et al. Epithelial wound healing enhanced by transforming growth factor-alpha and vaccinia growth factor. Science 1987; 235: 350–352
52 Frey P, Forand R, Maciag T, Shooter EM. The biosynthetic precursor of epidermal growth factor and the mechanism of its processing. Proc Natl Acad Sci USA 1979; 76: 6294–6298
53 Tsukumo K, Nakamura H, Sakamoto S. Purification and characterization of high molecular weight human epidermal growth factor from human urine. Biochem Biophys Res Commun 1987; 145: 126–133
54 Derynck R, Roberts AB, Winkler ME, Chen EY, Goeddel DV. Human transforming growth factor-α: Precursor structure and expression in E. coli. Cell 1984; 38: 287–297
55 Sasaki M, Kato S, Kohno K, Martin GR, Yamada Y. Sequence of the cDNA encoding the laminin B1 chain reveals a multidomain protein containing cysteine-rich repeats. Proc Natl Acad Sci USA 1987; 84: 935–939
56 Russell DW, Schneider WJ, Yamamoto T, Luskey KL, Brown MS, Goldstein JL. Domain map of the LDL receptor: sequence homology with the epidermal growth factor precursor. Cell 1984; 37: 577–585
57 Burgess AW, Lloyd CJ, Smith S, et al. Murine epidermal growth factor: Structure and function. Biochemistry 1988; 27: 4977–4985
58 Wharton KA, Johansen KM, Xu T, Artavanis-Tsakonas S. Nucleotide sequence from the neurogenic locus notch implies a gene product that shares homology with proteins containing EGF-like repeats. Cell 1985; 43: 567–581
59 Greenwald I. *lin*-12, a nematode homeotic gene, is homologous to a set of

mammalian proteins that include epidermal growth factor. Cell 1985; 43: 583–590
60 Hazarika P, Pardue RL, Earls R, Dedman JR. Identification and subcellular localization of a 21-kilodalton molecule using affinity-purified antibodies against alpha-transforming growth factor. Biochemistry 1987; 26: 2067–2070
61 Reisner AH. Similarity between the vaccina virus 19K early protein and epidermal growth factor. Nature 1985; 313: 801–803
62 Chang W, Upton C, Hu S-L, Purchio AF, McFadden G. The genome of Shope fibroma virus, a tumorigenic poxvirus, contains a growth factor gene with sequence similarity to those encoding epidermal growth factor and transforming growth factor alpha. Mol Cell Biol 1987; 7: 535–540
63 Upton C, Macen JL, McFadden G. Mapping and sequencing of a gene from myxoma virus that is related to those encoding epiderml growth factor and transforming growth factor α. J Virol 1987; 61: 1271–1275
64 Strayer DS, Leibowitz JL. Inhibition of epidermal growth factor-induced cellular proliferation. Am J Pathol 1987; 128: 203–209
65 Lin YZ, Caporaso G, Chang PY, Ke XH, Tam JP. Synthesis of a biological active tumor growth factor from the predicted DNA sequence of Shope Fibroma virus. Biochemistry 1988; 27: 5640–5645
66 Cooke RM, Wilkinson AJ, Baron M, et al. The solution structure of human epidermal growth factor. Nature 1987; 327: 339–341
67 Makino K, Morimoto M, Nishi M, et al. Proton nuclear magnetic resonance study on the solution conformation of human epidermal growth factor. Proc Natl Acad Sci USA 1987; 84: 7841–7845
68 Montelione GT, Wüthrich K, Nice EC, Burgess AW, Scheraga HA. Solution structure of murine epidermal growth factor: determination of the polypeptide backbone chain-fold by nuclear magnetic resonance and distance geometry. Proc Natl Acad Sci USA 1987; 84: 5226–5230
69 Mayo KH, Schaudies P, Savage CR, De Marco A, Kapstein R. Structural characterization and exposure of aromatic residues in epidermal growth factor from the rat. Biochem J 1986; 239: 13–18
70 Derynck R. Transforming growth factor-α. In: Kahn P, Graf T, eds. Oncogenes and Growth Control. Berlin: Springer-Verlag, 1986; pp. 58–64
71 Finzi E, Fleming T, Segatto O, et al. The human transforming growth factor type alpha coding sequence is not a direct-acting oncogene when overexpressed in NIH 3T3 cells. Proc Natl Aca Sci USA 1987; 84: 3733–3737
72 Yeh YC, Tsai JF, Chuang LY, et al. Elevation of transforming growth factor alpha and its relationship to the epidermal growth factor and alpha-fetoprotein levels in patients with hepatocellular carcinoma. Cancer Res 1987; 47: 896–901
73 Ullrich A, Crussens L, Hayflick JS, et al. Human epidermal growth factor receptor DNA sequence and aberrant expression of the amplified gene in A431 epidermoid carcinoma cells. Nature 1984; 309: 418–425
74 Di Fiore PP, Pierce JH, Fleming TP et al. Overexpression of the human EGF receptor confers an EGF-dependent transformed phenotype to NIH 3T3 cells. Cell 1987; 51: 1063–1070
75 Roberts AB, Lamb LC, Newton DL, Sporn MB, De Larco JE, Todaro GJ. Transforming growth factors: Isolation of polypeptides from virally and chemically transformed cells by acid/ethanol extraction. Proc Natl Acad Sci USA 1980; 77: 3494–3498
76 Rosenthal A, Lindquist PB, Bringman TS, Goeddel DV, Derynck R. Expression in rat fibroblasts of a human transforming growth factor-α cDNA results in transformation. Cell 1986; 46: 301–309
77 Stern DF, Hare DL, Cecchini MA, Weinberg RA. Construction of a novel oncogene based on synthetic sequences encoding epidermal growth factor. Science 1987; 235: 321–324
78 Pittelkow MR, Lindquist PB, Derynck R, Abraham RT, Graves-Deal R,

Coffey RJ. Induction of transforming growth factor α expression in human keratinocytes by phorbol esters. 1988; In press
79 Liebermann TA, Nusbaum HR, Razon N, et al. Amplification, enhanced expression and possible rearrangement of EGF receptor gene in primary human brain tumours of glial origin. Nature 1985; 313: 144–147
80 Malden TM, Novak U, Kaye AH, Burgess AW. Selective amplification of the cytoplasmic domain of the epidermal growth factor receptor in gliobastoma multiforme. Cancer Res 1988; 48: 2711–2714
81 Stromberg K, Hudgins WR, Orth DN. Urinary TGFsα in neoplasia: immunoreactive TGF-α in the urine of patients with disseminated breast carcinoma. Biochem Biophys Res Commun 1987; 144: 1059–1068
82 Barrandon Y, Green H. Cell migration is essential for sustained growth of keratinocyte colonies: the roles of transforming growth factor-alpha and epidermal growth factor. Cell 1987; 50: 1131–1137
83 Elliot JH. Epidermal growth factor: In vivo ocular studies. Trans Am Ophthalmol Soc 1980; 197: 629–656
84 McDonald BJ, Waters MJ, Richards MD, Thorburn GD, Hopkins PD. Effect of epidermal growth factor on wool fibre morphology and skin histology. Res Vet Sci 1983; 35: 91–99
85 Kingsnorth AN, Abu-Khalaf M, Ross JS, Malt RA. Potentiation of 1,2-dimethylhydrazine-induced anal carcinoma by epidermal growth factor. Surgery 1984; 97: 696–699
86 Poulsen SS. On the role of epidermal growth factor in the defence of the gastroduodenal mucosa. Scand J Gastroenterol 1987; 128: 20–23
87 Chaudhary VK, FitzGerald DJ, Adhya S, Pastan I. Activity of a recombinant fusion protein between transforming growth factor type alpha and Pseudomonas toxin. Proc Natl Acad Sci USA 1987; 84: 4538–4542

Transforming growth factors β

J Justin Hsuan
Ludwig Institute for Cancer Research (Middlesex Hospital and University College Branch), London

> Since its discovery as a factor able to induce phenotypic transformation with transforming growth factor α, transforming growth factor β (TGFβ) has been found to have unexpectedly widespread and frequently, seemingly paradoxical effects on a variety of cell types. Thus, a significant property of TGFβ activity is the ability to inhibit cellular growth and transformation. More recently, further important potential roles have also been found for TGFβ including the control of embryonal development, cellular differentiation, hormone secretion and immune function. Multiple forms of both TGFβ and TGFβ receptors are now known to exist, which may generate a complex and diverse range of interacting signals. The multifunctional actions of the TGFβ family are frequently defined in concert with other extracellular factors and much still has to be understood concerning these synergistic processes.

Transforming growth factors were first defined as sarcoma growth factors in the conditioned medium of transformed fibroblasts by their ability to cause reversible phenotypic transformation of cultured fibroblasts. Subsequently two major factors were resolved and termed TGFα and TGFβ. The former is a homologue of epidermal growth factor (EGF) and is quite different to TGFβ. More recently multiple forms of both TGFβ and its receptor have been identified (see below), which complicates the conclusions of many earlier experiments. In this brief review therefore, the general term TGFβ is used where the precise form(s) were not determined, though this will usually mean TGFβ1 as this is the major form to be purified from human platelets.

TGFβ BIOSYNTHESIS AND STRUCTURE

Unlike many other growth factors, TGFβ is synthesised by a wide variety of tissues and cultured cell lines, including both normal and transformed cells.[1,2] Interestingly, elevated levels of TGFβ mRNA can be directly detected at in vivo sites of mitotic activity and cellular differentiation (see below).[1,2]

Major sources for TGFβ purification include the α-granules of platelets, in which the highest levels of TGFβ are to be found, and placentae. The initial purification from human platelets and subsequent cloning of TGFβ showed it to be a disulphide-linked homodimer comprising subunits of 112 amino acid residues, which are derived from the carboxy terminal half of a 391 residue precursor, probably by extracellular proteolysis.[1] Derynck and co-workers have shown that the amino acid residues in the amino terminal half of the human and murine precursors are also conserved,[3] which suggests that this fragment may itself play an as yet undefined biological role. Subsequently it was found that only this latter fragment of simian TGFβ is both glycosylated and phosphorylated when expressed by rodent cells in culture, but the role of these modifications is unknown.

TGFβ is secreted in a latent form and how this is activated remains to be determined, but one pathway is postulated to employ plasmin which causes the release of active TGFβ by proteolysis of the intact complex.[4] Subsequent induction of plasminogen activator inhibitor by TGFβ would then allow control by negative feedback.[5] Similar to EGF and growth hormone for example, mature TGFβ is sequestered as a complex in serum. The TGFβ-binding factor is in fact $α_2$-macroglobulin and complex formation significantly compromises the activity of TGFβ.[6] This association with $α_2$-macroglobulin may thus serve to clear and restrict excess TGFβ activity.

Recently Massague's group has shown by stringent HPLC analysis that porcine platelets actually synthesise three distinct forms of TGFβ from two different subunits.[7,8] Homodimeric TGFβ1 corresponds to the human platelet form used by many workers in the past. The homodimeric TGFβ2 is now known to correspond to several previously identified polypeptide factors, including human glioma-derived T cell suppressor factor, simian BSC-1 cell growth inhibitor, and bovine collagen inducing factor B (polyergin). The novel third form is the heterodimer, termed TGFβ1.2. This system of multiple homologous factors and receptors (see below) can be compared with both the insulin-like growth factors and platelet-derived growth factors (PDGFs) and allows a variable and complex series of distinct signals to be generated, depending on both the type of ligand secreted and the type of receptor expressed.

There are several other factors with sequences that are homologous to TGFβ. These include the inhibins and activins, which antagonistically regulate follicle-stimulating hormone (FSH) secretion by the pituitary gland. This finding has prompted the recognition of a possible use of inhibins in contraception. Inhibins and activins act through distinct receptor mechanisms to TGFβ, although TGFβ itself is able to stimulate FSH secretion and enhance the action of FSH on ovaries. The widespread occurrence of inhibin biosynthesis and the erythropoietic activity of activins suggests that these factors, as well as TGFβ, will prove to have multiple developmental and homeostatic functions. Finally, Mullerian inhibiting substance,[9] the decapentaplegic gene complex of *Drosophila*,[10] and a *Xenopus* mRNA[11] also show sequence homology to TGFβ and in common with TGFβ, are important in the regulation of development and cellular differentiation.[12]

TGFβ RECEPTORS

It is beyond the scope of this review to deal with the functional properties of TGFβ receptors, however a brief summary of receptor structures and expression is included because variations in receptors, as well as ligands, may define the precise action of TGFβ observed in different cell types (Fig. 1).

With the notable exceptions of human retinoblastoma (see below) and rat phaeochromocytoma PC12 cells,[13] cell plasma membrane receptors for TGFβ are ubiquitously expressed by diverse cell types. While early binding studies that used human TGFβ and rodent fibroblasts showed only a single class of receptors, subsequent chemical cross-linking studies revealed the existence of three classes of receptor with quite distinct structures.[14] Type I receptors have M_r approx. 65 000 and type II have M_r approx. 85 000 to 110 000. Both these classes bind TGFβ1 with far higher affinity than TGFβ2. Type III receptors are disulphide-linked proteoglycans of M_r approx. 600 000 that can be reduced to subunits of M_r approx. 280 000 to 330 000. This latter class binds TGFβ1 and β2 with similar affinities and may also interact significantly with the extracellular matrix.

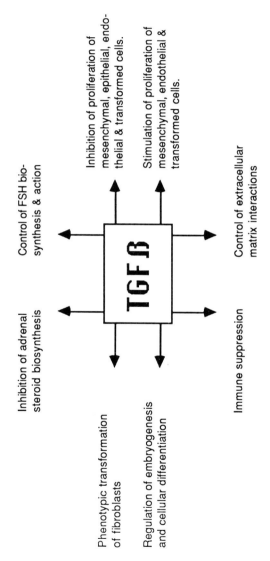

Fig. 1 Summary of the diverse activities of TGFβ.

While all three receptor types are widely expressed, the relative levels of expression by different cell types are variable. Massague's group has proposed that the three classes of receptor have exclusive functions and furthermore, that by comparing the relative activities of TGFβ1 and β2 with receptor expression, functional properties can be assigned to either classes I and II or class III receptors.[7] For example, TGFβ1 and β2 inhibit epithelial cell proliferation equally and the major class of receptors expressed by mammalian epithelial (and fibroblast) cells is class III, which binds TGFβ1 and β2 with equal affinity. Accordingly it is postulated that class III receptors mediate the inhibition of epithelial cell proliferation. In this way type III receptors have also been implicated in modulating the expression of cell adhesion proteins and in adipogenesis,[7] while type I receptors are postulated to mediate the inhibition of colony stimulating factor action on haematopoietic progenitor cells.[15] The differences in receptor affinities also lead to the simple generalization that TGFβ1 has broad actions as it binds to all classes of receptor, while TGFβ2 acts more specifically through type II receptors only.

CELLULAR TRANSFORMATION

Empirical definitions of cellular transformation usually rest upon three types of assay: the ability of cultured cells to grow in soft agar (anchorage-independent growth), the ability to overcome contact inhibition of growth (focus formation), and the generation of solid tumours when cells are injected subcutaneously into nude mice. Clearly, in no case are the assay conditions ideally suited to resemble the variety of in vivo conditions in which tumours can arise. The problem is clearly illustrated by results from studies on the role of TGFβ in cellular transformation, which can be substantially modulated by other factors in the culture medium. Furthermore, many nontransformed cell lines have been generated from primary tissue by continued culture through cell crisis. The basis for spontaneous cell immortalization is still poorly understood but is certainly variable as illustrated particularly well by the variation in responses to TGFβ shown for example by different rodent fibroblast lines. This problem further exacerbates any attempt to define a general role for TGFβ, or even any other growth factor, in cellular transformation. For these reasons the reader is encouraged to consult the original texts in order to appreciate the specific empirical systems and definitions of cellular transformation employed by different workers in this complicated area.

As its name suggests, TGFβ was first described based upon its ability to stimulate anchorage-independent growth of AKR-2B mouse embryo fibroblasts and of normal rat kidney (NRK) fibroblasts, the latter specifically in conjunction with either EGF or TGFα.

Before discussing further examples in which TGFβ contributes to the generation of a transformed phenotype, the bifunctional mitogenic properties of this growth factor must again be emphasised. In many cases TGFβ can inhibit the growth of transformed cells, including melanoma, lung, hepatic, mammary and endometrial carcinoma, fibrosarcoma, osteosarcoma, and possibly mesothelioma cell lines. A particularly interesting example in this area is afforded by the A549 human lung carcinoma line which secretes an inactive form of TGFβ. Activation of this peptide by acid treatment or alternatively by the addition of purified TGFβ results in a potent inhibition of growth, which suggests that perturbation of normal TGFβ biosynthesis can contribute to malignancy.[16] A second example of the loss of TGFβ-mediated inhibition of growth in cellular transformation has been suggested to occur in retinoblastomas. However, in this case resistance to TGFβ is achieved by the complete loss of functional receptor expression.[13] It will be particularly interesting to examine the effect of expressing normal TGFβ receptors in retinoblastoma cells once receptor clones have been obtained.

In contrast to the cases cited above, tumours frequently show elevated synthesis of TGFβ relative to their untransformed counterpart cell types.[17,18] This property is consistent with the original descriptions of TGFβ as a transforming factor for fibroblasts, however more recent work has suggested that in certain cases at least TGFβ may be acting indirectly upon the control of mitosis. In monolayer cultures of AKR-2B cells the mitogenic action of TGFβ has a long prereplicative phase during which the expression of PDGF (a potent fibroblast mitogen) is induced,[19] while in the case of NRK cells, the mitogenic response to TGFβ has been found to depend dramatically upon multiple exogenous and intracellular factors (see below). Indeed it has been suggested that TGFβ can only induce a transformed cellular phenotype in the presence of complete mitogenic stimulation by other growth factors.[20] Reversible phenotypic transformation of NRK cells can be induced by a variety of combinations of growth factors, such as TGFβ with EGF or with PDGF and retinoic acid.[21]

Unlike many immortalised cell lines, normal human fibroblasts do not exhibit anchorage-independent growth in the presence of TGFβ and EGF, but do form foci in culture,[22] thereby again illustrating the empirical problems in defining transformation.

MITOGENIC PROPERTIES OF TGFβ

Work on the mitogenic properties of TGFβ has revealed that TGFβ and other common growth factors found in serum can reciprocally modulate cellular responses. Only recently have defined media become available which allow more precise roles of specific growth factors to be elucidated.

Growth of subconfluent NRK cells is inhibited by human TGFβ by increasing cell cycle time,[23] but growth-arrested NRK, Swiss 3T3 and human lung fibroblasts are stimulated to proliferate in response to rat TGFβ.[24] Thereby TGFβ action defines two distinct responses by the same cell type, dependent upon the mitotic state of the cell. More recently the use of a serum-free medium has led to the conclusion that Swiss 3T3 cells are not stimulated to grow by TGFβ2, unless other growth factors are also present. This activity, as well as the absence of intracellular signal transduction via inositolphospholipid or calcium-dependent pathways, has led to the hypothesis that TGFβ and insulin may activate similar intracellular pathways,[25] which clearly requires further investigation.

The highly diverse actions of TGFβ on fibroblasts suggests that it might not act as a direct cellular mitogen, but may rather modulate other, extracellular factors which in turn influence cellular proliferation. This has been shown in the induction of PDGF expression by AKR-2B cells (see above) and may also involve the observed regulation by TGFβ of the interactions of fibroblasts with extracellular matrix proteins and with EGF. The biosynthesis and secretion of collagen and fibronectin is rapidly enhanced by TGFβ action on many cell types, including fibroblasts, and this pathway has been shown to contribute to the stimulation of anchorage-independent fibroblast growth[26] and would healing.[27] TGFβ is also known to modulate the action of EGF on fibroblasts: treatment of NRK cells with TGFβ causes a rapid and transient loss of high-affinity binding by EGF receptors, followed by a sustained increase in EGF receptor number. This action of TGFβ leads to an initial inhibition followed by an enhancement of EGF-dependent mitogenesis.[28] Control of interactions with extracellular factors also occurs in the EGF-dependent inductions of the metalloproteinases collagenase, stromelysin and transin, which are inhibited by TGFβ,[29,30] while induction of the metalloproteinase inhibitor TIMP by EGF is enhanced.[29] This metalloproteinase/inhibitor system is important in controlling the turnover of connective tissue extracellular matrix and the net effect of TGFβ appears again to be an enhancement of matrix formation. Furthermore, TGFβ induces plasminogen activator inhibitor expression by HT-1080 fibrosarcoma cells,[6] although enhanced plasminogen activator secretion has also been reported for fibroblasts treated with TGFβ.[31]

In addition to fibroblasts, mesenchymal osteoblasts and chondrocytes can be stimulated to proliferate in response to TGFβ, but EGF also is required by chondrocytes.[32] Osteoblasts and articular chondrocytes both synthesize TGFβ1 in vivo,[2] thus Sporn and coworkers have demonstrated that subconfluent bovine osteoblast cultures display autocrine, mitogenic TGFβ action.[33] On the other hand, it has also been shown that confluent rat fetal osteoblasts are stimulated to proliferate by TGFβ, while growth of subconfluent cultures and also of a murine osteoblast cell line are inhibited.[34,35] Interestingly, TGFβ has completely different effects on collagen biosynthesis by rabbit chondrocytes[32] and rat and bovine fetal osteoblasts,[33,34] but at least in the latter case, this probably has no bearing on the mitogenic properties of TGFβ.[34] Nevertheless, by comparison with TGFβ action on AKR-2B cells (see above), the lag phase observed prior to stimulation of osteoblast proliferation by TGFβ[34] suggests that TGFβ may act to induce the expression of a mitogen by osteoblasts.

CELLULAR DIFFERENTIATION AND GROWTH INHIBITION

A particularly useful system for understanding the early control of embryonic differentiation has proven to be the amphibian *Xenopus blastula*. In the course of embryogenesis mesodermal cells appear to be equatorially induced as a result of interactions between the animal and vegetal poles. It seems that certain cells within the animal hemisphere, which would otherwise differentiate to ectodermal tissue, are induced to form the mesoderm by a combination of basic FGF- and TGFβ1-homologous proteins derived from the vegetal hemisphere.[11,36] It was later found that TGFβ2 alone can induce differentiation to mesodermal cells by cultured animal hemisphere progenitors.[37]

The subsequent development of mesenchymal cells in mammals also appears to require TGFβ: by studying immunohistochemical staining densities, areas of mesenchymal differentiation and repair have been shown to correlate with high TGFβ1 expression in bovine and murine tissues.[2,38] In such tissues TGFβ has a multifunctional role: the ability of TGFβ to both stimulate and inhibit proliferation has already been described for several mesenchymal cell types, but the induction of differentiation is commonly associated with inhibition of mesenchymal proliferation. These properties have been demonstrated for TGFβ action in adipogenesis and myogenesis, as well as the responses of epithelial and endothelial cell types. For example TGFβ inhibits differentiation of murine 3T3 preadipocytes[39] and the formation of myotubes from rodent and avian myoblasts[40-42] in culture, while having no effect on their proliferation; conversely, TGFβ stimulates rat muscle mesenchyme chondrogenesis, but no effect on cell proliferation was reported.[43] Direct inhibition of growth by TGFβ occurs with the mitogen induced responses of multipotential haematopoietic progenitor cells[15] and both the EGF-dependent and independent growth of hepatocytes.[44,45]

The correlation between growth inhibition and cellular differentiation is perhaps clearest in the action of TGFβ on epithelial cells, which show high TGFβ1 expression in the kidneys.[2] Rat intestinal, mink lung, and human bronchial epithelial cell growth are all potently inhibited by TGFβ in the presence or absence of mitogens,[46-48] while differentiation and fibronectin synthesis are concomitantly induced.[46,48]

The important role of TGFβ in wound repair has been studied using cultured endothelial cells: TGFβ inhibits endothelial cell growth over a 24 hour period by enhancing fibronectin secretion, decreases cell migration, and abolishes high affinity EGF binding and EGF-dependent competence gene induction.[49-51] These effects would be expected to complement the lack of PDGF receptors on vascular endothelial cells, with the result that stimulation of smooth muscle and connective tissue regeneration would occur more rapidly than reformation of the vascular endothelium in response to platelet degranulation. More recently however, the use of a three-dimensional matrix in which to culture cells has revealed that TGFβ might not inhibit endothelial cell proliferation, but may in fact stimulate angiogenesis.[51]

PROSPECTS

The important understanding that cellular responses must be defined by a complex and interacting set of extracellular factors is largely due to results from work on TGFβ. In order to rationalise the observed range of responses, cloning and characterisation of the three receptor types is particularly important. Once any intrinsic or receptor associated enzymatic activity has been identified, then the intracellular pathways and transmodulation phenomena can be interpreted. The use of defined media and three-dimensional cell cultures will prove particularly useful in this area. Another important application of TGFβ receptor clones will be to transfect or infect receptor-negative cells to elucidate both the roles of different receptor types and the effect of receptor expression in retinoblastoma cells. It will also be interesting to investigate any link between the absence of TGFβ receptor expression and the changes in the retinoblastoma gene product.

Clearly TGFβ plays a critical part in embryogenesis and cellular differentiation. This whole field is particularly complex to model empirically, but the use of blastulae and the cloning of homologous growth factors in Xenopus promises to yield further insights. How far this amphibian system will parallel mammalian embryogenesis remains to be seen.

The potential clinical applications of TGFβ are largely unclear, but tissue repair and control of steroid hormone secretion may prove to be of particular value. Finally, TGFβ may also be of importance in its ability to inhibit B and T-lymphocyte function and proliferation, which may lead to immune suppression by gliomas that secrete TGFβ2,[52] and modulate bone structure.[16] Clearly, not all studies of TGFβ action were able to be discussed here and in general only the most recent results have been cited, but the interested reader is directed several recent reviews.[12,16,53–55]

ACKNOWLEDGEMENT

I am grateful to Anita Roberts for helpful discussions and the generous provision of unpublished material and to Deon Venter for helpful discussions and criticism of this review.

REFERENCES

1 Derynck R, Jarrett JA, Chen EY et al. Human transforming growth factor-β complementary DNA sequence and expression in normal and transformed cells. Nature 1985; 316: 701–705.

2 Ellingsworth LR, Brennan JE, Fok K et al. Antibodies to the N-terminal portion of cartilage-inducing factor A and transforming growth factor β. J Biol Chem 1986; 261: 12362–12367.
3 Derynck R, Jarrett JA, Chen EY, Goeddel DV. The murine transforming growth factor-β precursor. J Biol Chem 1986; 261: 4377–4379.
4 Lyons RM, Keski-Oja J, Moses HL. Proteolytic activation of latent transforming growth factor-β from fibroblast-conditioned medium. J Cell Biol 1988; 106: 1659–1665.
5 Laiho M, Saksela O, Keski-Oja J. Transforming growth factor-β induction of type-I plasminogen activator inhibitor. J Biol Chem 1987; 262: 17467–17474.
6 Huang SS, O'Grady P, Huang JS. Human transforming growth factor β: α_2-macroglobulin complex is a latent form of transforming growth factor β. J Biol Chem 1988; 263: 1535–1541.
7 Cheifetz S, Weatherbee JA, Tsang ML-S et al. The transforming growth factor-β system, a complex pattern of cross-reactive ligands and receptors. Cell 1987; 48: 409–415.
8 Madisen L, Webb NR, Rose TM et al. Transforming growth factor-β2: cDNA cloning and sequence analysis. DNA 1988; 7: 1–8.
9 Fanger BO, Wakefield LM, Sporn MB. Structure and properties of the cellular receptor for transforming growth factor type β. Biochemistry 1986; 25: 3083–3091.
10 Padgett RW, St. Johnston RD, Gelbart WM. A transcript from a Drosophila pattern gene predicts a protein homologous to the transforming growth factor-β family. Nature 1987; 325: 81–84.
11 Weeks DL, Melton DA. A maternal mRNA localized to the vegetal hemisphere in Xenopus eggs codes for a growth factor related to TGFβ. Cell 1987; 51: 861–867.
12 Massague J. The TGF-β family of growth and differentiation factors. Cell 1987; 49: 437–438.
13 Kimchi A, Wang X-F, Weinberg RA, Cheifetz S, Massague J. Absence of TGF-β receptors and growth inhibitory responses in retinoblastoma cells. Science 1988; 240: 196–199.
14 Cheifetz S, Like B, Massague J. Cellular distribution of type I and type II receptors for transforming growth factor-β. J Biol Chem 1986; 261: 9972–9978.
15 Ohta M, Greenberger JS, Anklesaria P, Bassols A, Massague J. Two forms of transforming growth factor-β distinguished by multipotential haematopoietic progenitor cells. Nature 1987; 329: 539–541.
16 Sporn MB, Roberts AB, Wakefield LM, Assoian RK. Transforming growth factor-β: biological function and chemical structure. Science 1986; 233: 532–534.
17 Derynck R, Goeddel DV, Ullrich A et al. Synthesis of messenger RNAs for transforming growth factor a and β and the epidermal growth factor receptor by human tumours. Cancer Res 1987; 47: 707–712.
18 Akhurst RJ, Fee F, Balmain A. Localized production of TGF-β mRNA in tumour promotor-stimulated mouse epidermis. Nature 1988; 331: 363–365.
19 Leof EB, Proper JA, Goustin AS, Shipley GD, DiCorleto PE, Moses HL. Induction of c-sis mRNA and activity similar to platelet-derived growth factor by transforming growth factor β: a proposed model for indirect mitogenesis involving autocrine activity. Proc Natl Acad Sci USA 1986; 83: 2453–2457.
20 Massague J, Kelly B, Mottola C. Stimulation by insulin-like growth factors is required for cellular transformation by type β transforming growth factor. J Biol Chem 1985; 260: 4551–4554.
21 Van Zoelen EJJ, Van Oostwaard TMJ, De Laat SW. The role of polypeptide growth factors in phenotypic transformation of normal rat kidney cells. J Biol Chem 1988; 263: 64–68.
22 Brinckerhoff CE. Morphologic and mitogenic responses of rabbit synovial

fibroblasts to transforming growth factor β require transforming growth factor a or epidermal growth factor. Arthritis Rheum 1983; 26: 1370–1379.
23 Roberts AB, Anzano MA, Wakefield LM, Roche NS, Stern DF, Sporn MB. Type β transforming growth factor: a bifunctional regulator of cellular growth. Proc Natl Acad Sci USA 1985; 82: 119–123.
24 Massague J. Type β transforming growth factor from feline sarcoma virus-transformed rat cells. J Biol Chem 1984; 259: 9756–9761.
25 Brown KD, Holley RW. Insulin-like synergistic stimulation of DNA synthesis in Swiss 3T3 cells by the BSC-1 cell-derived growth inhibitor related to transforming growth factor type β. Proc Natl Acad Sci USA 1987; 84: 3743–3747.
26 Ignotz RA, Massague J. Transforming growth factor-β stimulates the expression of fibronectin and collagen and their incorporation into the extracellular matrix. J Biol Chem 1986; 261: 4337–4345.
27 Mustoe TA, Pierce GF, Thomason A, Gramates P, Sporn MB, Deuel TF. Accelerated healing of incisional wounds in rats induced by transforming growth factor-β. Science 1987; 237: 1333–1336.
28 Assoian RK. Biphasic effects of type β transforming growth factor on epidermal growth factor receptors in NRK fibroblasts. J Biol Chem 1985; 260: 9613–9617.
29 Edwards DR, Murphy G, Reynolds JJ et al. Transforming growth factor beta modulates the expression of collagenase and metalloproteinase inhibitor. EMBO J 1987; 6: 1899–1904.
30 Machida CM, Muldoon LL, Rodland KD, Magun B. transcriptional modulation of transin gene expression by epidermal growth factor and transforming growth factor beta. Mol Cell Biol 1988; 8: 2479–2483.
31 Laiho M, Saksela O, Kesi-Oja J. Transforming growth factor β alters plasminogen activator activity in human skin fibroblasts. Exp Cell Res 1986; 164: 399–407.
32 Skantze KA, Brinckerhoff CE, Collier JP. Use of agarose culture to measure the effect of transforming growth factor β and epidermal growth factor on rabbit articular chondrocytes. Cancer Res 1985; 45: 4416–4421.
33 Robey PG, Young MF, Flanders KC et al. Osteoblasts synthesize and respond to transforming growth factor-type β (TGF-β) in vitro. J Cell Biol 1987; 105: 457–463.
34 Centrella M, McCarthy TL, Canalis E. Transforming growth factor β is a bifunctional regulator of replication and collagen synthesis in osteoblast-enriched cell cultures from fetal rat bone. J Biol Chem 1987; 262: 2869–2874.
35 Noda M, Rodan GA. Type-β transforming growth factor inhibits proliferation and expression of alkaline phosphatase in murine osteoblast-like cells. Biochem Biophys Res Commun 1986; 140: 56–65.
36 Kimelman D, Kirschner M. Synergistic induction of mesoderm by FGF and TGF-β and the identification of an mRNA coding for FDG in the early Xenopus embryo. Cell 1987; 51: 869–877.
37 Rosa F, Roberts AB, Danielpour D, Dart LL, Sporn MB, Dawid IB. Mesoderm inductionin amphibians: the role of TGF-β2-like factors. Science 1988; 139: 783–785.
38 Heine UI, Munoz EF, Flanders KC et al. Role of transforming growth factor-β in the development of the mouse embryo. J Cell Biol 1987; 105: 2861–2876.
39 Ignotz RA, Massague J. Type β transforming growth factor controls the adipogenic differentiation of 3T3 fibroblasts. Proc Natl Acad Sci USA 1985; 82: 8530–8534.
40 Florini JR, Roberts AB, Ewton DZ, Falen SL, Flanders KC, Sporn MB. Transforming growth factor-β. J Biol Chem 1986; 261: 16509–16513.
41 Massague J, Cheifetz S, Endo T, Nadal-Ginard B. Type β transforming growth factor is an inhibitor of myogenic differentiation. Proc Natl Acad Sci USA 1986; 83: 8206–8210.

42 Olsen EN, Sternberg E, Hu JS, Spizz G, Wilcox C. Regulation of myogenic differentiation by type β transforming growth factor. J Cell Biol 1986; 103: 1799–1805.
43 Sneydin SM, Thompson AY, Bentz H et al. Cartilage-inducing factor-A. J Biol Chem 1986; 261: 5693–5695.
44 Shiota K, Nakamura T, Ichihara A. Distinct effects of transforming growth factor-β on EGF receptors and EGF-induced DNA synthesis in primary cultured rat hepatocytes. Biochem Int 1986; 13: 893–901.
45 Wollenberg GK, Semple E, Quinn BA, Hayes MA. Inhibition of proliferation of normal, preneoplastic, and neoplastic rat hepatocytes by transforming growth factor-β. Cancer Res 1987; 47: 6595–6599.
46 Kurokawa M, Lynch K, Podolsky DK. Effects of growth factors on an intestinal epithelial cell line: transforming growth factor β inhibits proliferation and stimulates differentiation. Biochem Biophys Res Commun 1987; 142: 775–782.
47 Like B, Massague J. The antiproliferative effect of type β transforming growth factor occurs at a level distal from receptors for growth-activating factors. J Biol Chem 1986; 261: 13426–13429.
48 Massui T, Wakefield LM, Lechner JF, LaVeck MA, Sporn MB, Harris CC. Type β transforming growth factor is the primary differentiation-inducing serum factor for normal human bronchial epithelial cells. Proc Natl Acad Sci USA 1986; 83: 2438–2442.
49 Heimark RL, Twardzik DR, Schwartz SM. Inhibition of endothelial cell regeneration by type-beta transforming growth factor from platelets. Science 1986; 233: 1078–1080.
50 Takehara K, LeRoy EC, Grotendorst GR. TGF-β inhibition of endothelial cell proliferation: alteration of EGF binding and EGF-induced growth-regulatory (competence) gene expression. Cell 1987; 49: 415–422.
51 Madri JA, Pratt BM, Tucker AM. Phenotypic modulation of endothelial cells by transforming growth factor-β depends upon the composition and organization of the extracellular matrix. J Cell Biol 1988; 106: 1375–1384.
52 de Martin R, Haendler B, Hofer-Warbinek R et al. Complementary DNA for human glioblastoma-derived T cell suppressor factor, a novel member of the transforming growth factor-β gene family. EMBO J 1987; 6: 3673–3677.
53 Moses HL, Coffey RJ, Leof EB, Lyons RM, Keski-Oja J. Transforming growth factor-β regulation of cell proliferation. J Cell Physiol 1987; S5: 1–7.
54 Massague J, Cheifetz S, Ignotz RA, Boyd FT. Multiple type-β transforming growth factors and their receptors. J Cell Physiol 1987; S5: 43–47.
55 Sporn MB, Roberts AB, Wakefield LM, de Crombrugghe B. Some recent advances in the chemistry and biology of transforming growth factor-beta. J Cell Biol 1987; 105: 1039–1045.

Fibroblast growth factors

Andrew Baird[1]
Patricia A Walicke[2]

[1]*Laboratories for Neuroendocrinology, Salk Institute* and [2]*Department of Neuroscience, University of California at San Diego, La Jolla, California, USA*

> The existence of fibroblast growth factors (FGFs) was proposed over 40 years ago to account for the ability of tissue extracts to stimulate fibroblast proliferation. In the 1970s it became clear that preparations containing FGF activity were in fact pleiotropic, affecting the growth and function of a wide variety of mesenchymal, endocrine and neural cells. Their angiogenic effects have promoted research in cardiology and neurology because of their proposed role in stimulating collateral vascularisation and recovery from ischemia. Their identity with a component of tumour angiogenesis factor activity has stimulated research in oncology and their capacity to enhance wound healing, nerve regeneration and cartilage repair has affected research in neurology, orthopaedic medicine and pathology. The potential therapeutic value of FGFs is just beginning to be realized and will be dependent on a concerted effort to establish their function in the regulation of normal cell homeostasis and the pathophysiology of disease.

DISCOVERY OF FIBROBLAST GROWTH FACTORS

A combination of astute observations in clinical and basic research led to the proposal that specific molecules were responsible for regulating fibroblast proliferation, wound healing and blood vessel growth.[1] The purification and identification of some of the factors involved in these processes has required almost half a century and has identified several families of structurally distinct growth factors including acidic and basic FGFs and the fibroblast growth factor family. Their physiological functions remain only partly understood. The purpose of this review is not to survey the wealth of information in the current literature, but to give an overview of the most active areas in FGF research. As such, readers are referred to formal reviews[1-3] for a comprehensive bibliography.

Both acidic and basic FGFs have the same range of biological activities although the basic form is usually 10 to 100-fold more potent than the acidic form in in vitro assays.[4] Heparin, a glycosaminoglycan (GAG) with which both mitogens interact, increases the activity of acidic FGF, making it nearly equipotent with basic FGF. This interaction with heparin has become a hallmark characteristic of the FGF family of growth factors. Another feature of FGFs is the remarkable number of cell types whose growth and/or function they affect. These include mesenchymal cells such as vascular and capillary endothelial cells, smooth muscle cells, chondrocytes and fibroblasts; endocrine cells such as Leydig, granulosa, and adrenocortical cells and the lactotrophs and thyrotrophs of the pituitary; and neural cells such as astrocytes, oligodendrocytes and neurons in the central nervous system, retina and peripheral ganglia (Table 1).

The initial discovery of FGFs suggested that the pituitary and brain were rich sources of the growth factors. With the chemical, biochemical and immunological tools made available from their isolation and structural characterization, it has become apparent that they are both widely distributed. In fact, in almost every tissue that has been reported to contain an 'FGF-like' activity, it has been possible to identify acidic FGF and/or basic FGF in the extract. In view of the pleiotropic activity of FGFs described above, the observation that FGFs were widely distributed meant that many researchers in different fields had unknowingly been studying the biological and biochemical characteristics of these same molecules. Within a short period of time following their structural characterization, the work of several research groups soon suggested that a variety of partially purified trophic factors were all in fact acidic FGF or basic FGF.

THE FIBROBLAST GROWTH FACTOR FAMILY

Even as biological activities were being assigned an identity with acidic FGF or basic FGF, gene transfection experiments were identifying new FGFs and establishing the notion that acidic FGF and basic FGF were only two members of a large family of structurally related trophic factors. The members of this family include an oncogene called 'hst' characterized from a stomach carcinoma, and which encodes a protein that shares about 50% structural identity with basic FGF.[5] An identical oncogene has been described in fibroblasts derived from Kaposi's sarcoma[6] and a distinct gene (int-2) has been identified that encodes yet another potential oncogene.[7] Even more recently, Goldfarb and colleagues[8] have described a gene that encodes FGF-5, which, based on its homology to basic FGF, is a fifth member of

Table 1 Pleiotropic activities of FGFs on normal cells

Tissue target	In Vitro		In Vivo[1]	
	Mitogenic Activity	Non-Mitogenic Activity	Mitogenic Activity	Non-Mitogenic Activity
fibroblasts	+	+	+	
endothelial	+	+	+	
smooth muscle	+	+	+	
pericytes	+			
myocytes				
chondrocytes	+	+	+	+
keratinocytes	+	+		
myoblasts	+			
osteoblasts	+			
neuroblasts	+			
blastema	+			
adrenocortical	+	+		
granulosa	+	+		
thyroid	+			
lactotrophs				
thyrotrophs				
melanocytes	+			
neurons	−	+		+
astrocytes	+	+		
oligodendrocytes	+	+		
Schwann	+	+	+	+
adrenomedullar				
hepatocytes	+			
epithelial lens	+	+		
epithelial cornea	+	+	+	
epithelial prostatic	+			
hair bulb papillary	+			
tumour cells[2]	±	±		

[1]The effects of FGFs on cell types in vivo are not necessarily direct and may involve secondary or tertiary reponses mediated by other growth factors (i.e. TGFβ, epidermal growth factor. . .) over the time course of the experiments (3–20 days).
[2]FGFs have mitogenic and non-mitogenic effects on a wide range of tumour cell types and have been purified from several tumours. In some instances, the mitogens are anti-mitogenic, emphasizing their pleiotropic activity. Target tumour cells include PC-12 (pheochromocytoma), glioma, cervical carcinoma, mammary tumours, prolactinoma, and transformed fibroblasts. Not all tumour cells produce, have receptors for, or respond to FGFs.

the FGF family of mitogens. Finally, the FGFs show approximately 25% homology with interleukin-1 (IL-1), a lymphokine classically considered hematopoietic, but that also stimulates some FGF target cells.[9]

Because the identification of the FGF-related proteins is relatively new, this review describes the activities and potential applications of basic FGF. This molecule was sequenced in 1985[4] and has been produced as a recombinant protein in yeast and *Escherichia coli* in sufficient quantities to permit an extensive examination of its biological activities in vitro and in vivo.[10]

BIOLOGICAL FUNCTIONS OF FIBROBLAST GROWTH FACTORS

Tissue repair in the reticulo-endothelium

Both acidic FGF and basic FGF are potent stimuli for cell components of the vascular wall.[4] The FGFs are chemotactic and mitogenic for endothelial cells and enhance expression of differentiated function (i.e. plasminogen activator). Because basic FGF is also a mitogen for vascular smooth muscle cells and is found in macrophages,[11] it has also been implicated in the development of atherosclerosis.

Basic FGF can stimulate neovascularization in all models tested to date, including the rabbit cornea, hamster cheek pouch and chick chorioallantoic membrane. It is also active in more physiological models of angiogenesis. The infusion of basic FGF onto the external wall of the carotid artery increases growth of the vasa vasorum (Cuevas et al., unpublished observations) suggesting that it may play a role in the establishment and regulation of collateral circulation (Fig. 1a, b). It is interesting to speculate that basic FGF might have important therapeutic applications in clinical paradigms where an enhancement of vascularization is beneficial. In this context, one of the most striking applications of basic FGF would be in wound healing. This includes the recovery from ischemic lesions[12] as well as from traumatic wounds.[13] As is often true in the development of therapeutics, the design of the appropriate systems to deliver growth factor to the locus of the lesion will be the next technological challenge. In the ischemic lesion, this will mean delivery to the heart and brain.

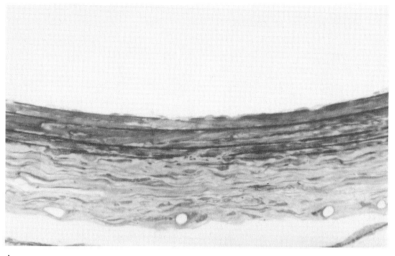

A

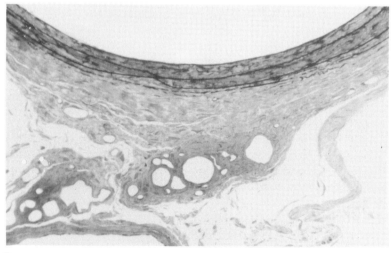

B

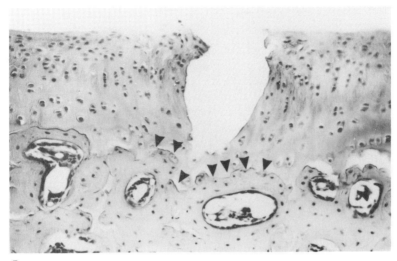

C

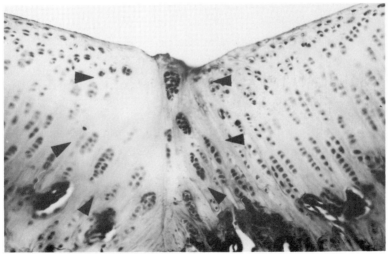

D

Fig. 1 Effect of basic FGF on tissue repair.
Saline (A,C) or basic FGF (B,D) were infused onto the outside of a rat carotid artery (A,B) or onto the lesioned articular cartilage of a rabbit knee (C,D) for 7 and 14 days. Tissues were collected and assessed by standard histological tests.

Repair of connective tissue

As mentioned earlier, FGFs are mitogens for many types of mesenchymal cells, including fibroblasts, smooth muscle cells, skeletal myoblasts, and chondrocytes. As in most cell types affected by FGFs, these cells are not only stimulated to proliferate, but also show enhanced differentiated function in cell culture. The presence in and effects of basic FGF on melanocytes, keratinocytes and in chondrocytes suggests a physiological function for basic FGF in the repair of connective tissue. To date, much of the inferred in vivo activities of basic FGF and its potential therapeutic benefits are extensions of its in vitro activities. Some preliminary work with basic FGF has confirmed its potential use.[14] As an example, local administration of basic FGF into a lesioned rabbit knee can stimulate cartilage repair (Fig. 1c, d). By virtue of its capacity to stimulate the differentiated functions of cells in connective tissue, the possibility that FGFs can increase the compressive and tensile strength of cartilage and ligaments is currently under examination. In such an instance, the availability of large quantities of basic FGF for experimentation will have a large impact on dermatology, and in particular surgery, orthopaedics and even veterinary medicine.

FGF and the modulation of the endocrine response

Basic FGF is a trophic factor for a variety of endocrine cells including adrenocortical cells, ovarian granulosa cells, testicular Leydig cells and pituitary lactotrophs and thyrotrophs. In most instances, however, the effects of basic FGF are on the differentiated function of these cells rather than on cell proliferation. Thus, at this point in time, it seems reasonable to propose that pituitary, ovarian and testicular FGFs are not exclusively involved in the local tissue repair response, but are available to modulate local endocrine function. As such, the primary function of FGFs would be to modulate the response of cells to primary endocrine signals.

The physiological function of pituitary and adrenal derived basic FGF is unclear. In vitro, the growth factor enhances synthesis and release of prolactin (PRL) from lactotropes and thyrotropin (TSH) from thyrotropes.[15] It has no known effects on other endocrine types of the pituitary. In as much as both the thyrotroph and lactotroph are closely associated with whole animal reproductive and developmental biology, it is of more than passing interest that these two hormones are affected by pituitary-derived basic FGF.

In vitro studies have established the capacity of basic FGF to stimulate adrenocortical cell proliferation and to delay their senescence. It is not clear how these in vitro activities translate into a physiological function, but it is interesting to speculate that local factors like basic FGF and transforming growth factor beta (TGFβ) modulate the adrenocortical response to ACTH in vivo. This hypothesis would account for the endocrine changes linked to adrenocortical rhythmicity, development of the adrenal fetal zone and the onset of adrenarche. It would also support the notion that one of the functions of basic FGF is to act as a local modulator of the endocrine response. By virtue of its effect as a mitogen for endothelial cells, it is also important to consider the possibility that basic FGF plays a function in maintaining the vascular integrity of highly vascular endocrine tissues.

Reproductive biology

In vitro, basic FGF is a potent inhibitor of aromatase activity in cultured granulosa cells as well as peripheral fibroblasts (*see* Ref. 16 for review). Basic FGF is also a potent inhibitor of testosterone synthesis in vitro, an observation that, to date is of unknown physiological significance. Because basic FGF is angiogenic and is present in the corpus luteum, there is considerable interest in the possibility that it is associated with the neovascular response that underlies normal menses, implantation and fetal development. Although there are no direct physiological experiments to support this hypothesis, basic FGF has all of the necessary prerequisites to fit the description of an ovarian angiogenic factor. For these same reasons, it also fulfills the criteria necessary to be implicated in the etiology of some types of ovarian dysfunction (i.e. endometriosis). Many of these disorders can be traced to problems in vascularization.

FGF and neurology

In tissue culture, basic FGF has trophic effects on neurons from the cortex, hippocampus, stratum, cerebellum, spinal cord and parasympathetic ganglia.[17] It is a mitogen for neuroblasts from young embryos and enhances survival of post-mitotic differentiated neurons. As in most tissues, basic FGF is generally more potent than acidic FGF, but there is evidence to suggest that some neurons, such as retinal ganglion cells, might specifically require acidic FGF. Both FGFs also enhance the growth of neuritic processes. Since trophic factors for many of these neurons had not previously been identified, these observations have potentially significant implications for growth regulation in the brain.

Neurons are not the only FGF-responsive cells in the brain. Astrocytes proliferate, adopt a fibrillar morphology and increase their content of some differentiated products in the presence of basic FGF. Similarly, oligodendrocytes proliferate and increase their content of myelin-related proteins and lipids. There is considerable interest in the potential use of basic FGF to try and improve neuronal recovery after brain lesions. Recent studies have suggested that basic FGF can be administered to the central and peripheral nervous system with beneficial results. As an example, infusion of basic FGF into the ventricle has been reported to prevent the death of cholinergic septal neurons after lesions to the hippocampus.[18] The infusion of basic FGF to the severed sciatic nerve has been observed to enhance the rate of nerve regeneration[19] and basic FGF administered to the stump of the severed optic nerve can increase survival of retinal ganglion cells.[20,21] Thus, it seems reasonable to suggest that the FGFs may provide a useful therapeutic tool to approach the problems associated with injury to the nervous system.

FGFs in embryonic development

The studies described here have all emphasized the wide range effects of basic FGF on both cell proliferation and in maintaining cell differentiated function. It has now been established that FGFs are also an important developmental morphogen.[22] They stimulate the differentiation of mesenchyme and antibodies to the growth factor prevent this process. It will be important to determine exactly how this activity can be applied clinically. It is perhaps worthy to note that the possibility of stimulating the differentiation of tissues in vivo offers a new approach to tissue transplantation.[23]

PATHOPHYSIOLOGY OF FGFs

As in the case for all biologically active materials, for every in vivo activity that has therapeutic value, there is the potential that this same activity is responsible for the etiology of disease. FGFs are no exception and have been implicated in the pathophysiology of diseases of neovascularization. These include tumour angiogenesis, reproductive dysfunction and the complications of diabetes.

FGFs as oncogene proteins

The observation from several groups that over expression of FGF by cells can lead to transformation is a strong suggestion that FGFs can act as proto-oncogenes.[24,25] The characterization of the FGF-related oncogenes hst, int-2, and FGF-5 also support this notion since each is associated with cell transformation. Many tumour cells have been shown to synthesize FGFs and in many instances, the FGFs are mitogens for the untransformed cell. On this basis, it will be important to define the steps that lead to over expression of FGFs and FGF-dependent tumour growth.

Tumour angiogenesis

A second mechanism through which FGFs might participate in tumour growth is in their capacity to stimulate new vessel growth.[1] Under these circumstances, FGF need not be trophic for the tumour cell itself, but need only vascularize the invading tissue. Over the last twenty years, Folkman and colleagues (*see* Ref. 1 for review) have established the importance of angiogenesis in the development of solid tumours. FGFs may well present a component of the activity attributed to tumour angiogenesis factor. This is supported by the observation that many, but not all, tumour cells produce FGFs. In this instance where the tumour itself is not making the angiogenic factor, local 'host' FGFs could be mobilized by the invading tumour cells in order to vascularize the tumour. In this paradigm, which is a variant of the tumour angiogenic factor hypothesis, it becomes of paramount importance to understand the regulation of endogenous FGF (see below). Any factor capable of mobilizing endogenous FGFs would effectively recruit their angiogenic potential.

FGFs and the complications of diabetes

Many of the complications of diabetes are associated with a distinct microvascular pathology. Although it is not known whether FGFs are responsible for the progression of this disease, these molecules possess the features that make them attractive candidates. They are angiogenic, located in the tissues affected (eye, kidney, peripheral nerve, etc.) and they interact with carbohydrates, the major disorder underlying diabetes. In view of the fact that carbohydrates, GAGs and the extracellular matrix (ECM) are all thought to regulate the bioavailability of endogenous FGFs (see below), and that each of these elements is modified in diabetes, there is compelling indirect evidence that some of the complications of diabetes are in fact mediated by FGFs.

ACTIVITIES AND REGULATION OF ENDOGENOUS FGFs

All of the studies summarized above suggest potential therapeutic applications of FGFs. With the exception of current ideas regarding their contribution in the etiology of disease, relatively little is known about the actions and regulation of endogenous FGFs. As a family of pluripotent, widely distributed factors, major questions must be addressed regarding their regulation and physiological function.

Activities of endogenous FGFs

There is excellent biochemical and immunohistochemical data to support the presence of basic FGF essentially in all tissues of the body. And yet there is little if any work aimed at establishing a function for the endogenous FGFs. Experiments using passive immunization and transgenic animals may eventually establish this role. Until such a time, it might be necessary to leave its endogenous role to conjecture. It seems likely, however, that FGFs are participating in vascular homeostasis; this includes the heart's role to conjecture. It seems likely, however, that FGFs are participating in vascular homeostasis; this includes the heart's ability to elicit collateral vessels, the capacity of tissues to repair and the ability of the female reproductive system to undergo normal menses.

Regulation of FGF production

Although acidic and basic FGFs are widely distributed, it has been very difficult to detect the presence of the mRNA required for its synthesis in most tissues (with the possible exception of brain).

This has led to the hypothesis that FGFs may be normally present in a storage form and saved for emergencies such as wound repair.[26–28] In this paradigm, the bioavailability of the FGFs would be locally regulated at the target cell. Since FGFs are pleiotropic, the restrictions on their availability would ensure that their effects are not systemic.

Some unusual biochemical properties of basic FGF have suggested a model to account for the regulation of their bioavailability (Fig. 2). The affinities of acidic and basic FGFs for GAGs (particularly heparin) have suggested that these cell-associated complex carbohydrates and the ECM can function as a storage depot and serve as a local source of growth factor (Fig. 2A). Basic FGF, which has been located in the ECM produced by endothelial cells, could be made bioavailable to the target cell by one of several mechanisms. Increased expression of high affinity receptors on the target cell would effectively remove the FGF bound to lower affinity sites by kinetic equilibrium (Fig. 2B). A second mechanism that might mobilize basic FGF from the ECM could be mediated by any post-translational modification that would alter its affinity for the ECM (Fig. 2C). Finally, a third mechanism

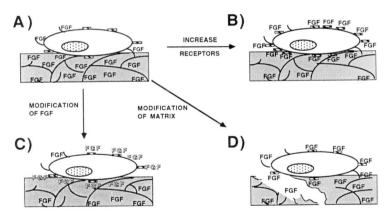

Fig. 2 Regulation of FGF bioavailability.
(A) Normal cell: FGF available if needed.
(B) Receptor number increased. FGF binding equilibrium is shifted from low affinity (GAG) sites to high affinity receptor sites.
(C) FGF is modified. The post translational change results in a decreased affinity for GAGs and increased availability for high affinity receptors.
(D) The ECM/GAGs are modified. Degradation of the ECM and/or modification of the GAGs and ECM proteins results in release of FGFs and availability for their high affinity receptors

leading to the bioavailability of FGFs involves damage to the matrix, whether physical (as during injury) or biochemical (as during tissue remodelling), and would be mediated via degradation of the ECM by proteases and/or heparinases secreted by target cells, invading tumour cells or macrophages (Fig. 2D). The attractive aspects of this model are that it accounts for many of the proposed physiological and pathological functions of FGFs. On one hand, cells could respond to an external stimulus by increasing their numbers of high affinity FGF receptors and obtaining trophic relief. Enzymes, known to be secreted by macrophages and tumour cells could activate the host mitogen and exploit its angiogenic potential to invade tissues. Finally, diseases associated with changes in the ECM (e.g. diabetes) could disturb the basement membrane's ability to regulate FGF activity and lead to characteristic complications of cell proliferation. In this paradigm, the long-term changes in the ECM (i.e. glycation, etc.) would also coincide with the long-term nature of the progression of the complications of diabetes (retinopathies, nephropathies and neuropathies).

CONCLUSIONS

It should be recognized that neither the FGFs, or in fact any other trophic factor, exerts its influence in isolation from other hormones and cytokines. Instead, the in vivo response is the result of the combined effects of all of the components in a complex homeostatic system. The target cell is akin to a microprocessor acting in response to the integrated signals from many trophic inputs. The time and concentration dependent changes in all of the trophic stimuli acting on the cell ultimately define its cellular response. It will be necessary to understand the nature and regulation of these interactions before a more unified and realistic appreciation of the role of trophic factors in growth control can be realized. Until that time, as experimental data suggest,[1,11-23] FGFs will remain potentially important therapeutic tools in the management of disease.

REFERENCES

1 Folkman J, Klagsbrun M. Angiogenic Factors. Science 1987; 235: 442–446
2 Gospodarowicz D, Ferrara N, Schweigerer L, Neufeld G. Structural characterization and biological functions of fibroblast growth factor. Endocr Rev 1987; 8: 95–114

3 Baird A, Esch F, Mormède P, et al. Molecular characterization of fibroblast growth factor: Distribution and biological activities in various tissues. Recent Prog Horm Res 1986; 42: 143–205
4 Esch F, Baird A, Ling N, et al. Primary structure of bovine pituitary basic fibroblast growth factor (FGF) and comparison with the amino-terminal sequence of bovine brain acidic FGF. Proc Natl Acad Sci USA 1985; 82: 6507–6511
5 Taira M, Yoshida T, Miyagawa K, Sakamoto H, Terada M, Sugimura T. cDNA sequence of human transforming gene hst and identification of the coding sequence required for transforming activity. Proc Natl Acad Sci USA 1987; 84: 2980–2984
6 Delli-Bovi P, Curatola AM, Kern FG, Greco A, Ihman M, Basilico C. An oncogene isolated by transfection of Kaposi's sarcoma DNA encodes a growth factor that is a member of the FGF family. Cell 1987; 50: 729–737
7 Dickson C, Peters G. Potential oncogene product related to growth factors. Nature 1987; 326: 833
8 Zhan X, Bates B, Hu X, Goldfarb M. The human FGF-5 encogene encodes a novel protein related to fibroblast growth factors. Mol Cell Biol 1988; 8: 3487–3497
9 Thomas KA. Fibroblast growth factors. FASEB J 1987; 1: 434–440
10 Barr PJ, Cousens LS, Lee-Ng CT, et al. Expression and processing of biologically active fibroblast growth factors in the yeast *Saccharomyces cerevisiae*. J Biol Chem 1988; (In press)
11 Baird A, Mormède P, Böhlen P. Immunoreactive fibroblast growth factor in cells of peritoneal exudate suggests its identity with macrophage-derived growth factor. Biochem Biophys Res Commun 1985; 126: 358–364
12 Cuevas P, Baird A, Guillemin R. Angiogenic response to fibroblast growth factor in the rat brain in vivo. In: Gagliardi R, Benvenuti L, eds. Controversies in EIAB for Cerebral Ischemia. Florence Monduzzi Editore, 1988, pp.731–737
13 Cuevas P, Carceller, Esteban A, Baird A, Guillemin R. Basic fibroblast growth factor (bFGF) enhances epithelial wound healing in alkali-burned corneas. VIIIth Congress of the European Society of Opthalmology, Intl Fair, Lisbon, Portugal, May 16–20, 1988
14 Cuevas P, Burgos J, Cuevas B, Baird A, Guillemin R. Basic fibroblast growth factor (bFGF) stimulates cartilage regeneration. XXVI World Congr Int Coll Surg, Milan, Italy, 1988
15 Baird A, Mormède P, Ying S-Y, et al. A nonmitogenic function of fibroblast growth factor: Regulation of thyrotropin and prolactin secretion. Proc Natl Acad Sci USA 1985; 82: 5545–5559
16 Baird A, Emoto N, Shimasaki S, Gonzales AM, Fauser B, Hsueh AJW. Fibroblast growth factors as local mediators of gonadal function. VII Ovarian Workshop, Paracrine Communication in the Ovary: Ontogenesis and Growth Factors: Tacoma, WA
17 Walicke P. Novel neurotrophic factors, receptors and oncogenes. Annu Rev Neurosci 1988; 12: (In press)
18 Anderson KJ, Dam D, Lee S, Cotman CW. Basic fibroblast growth factor prevents death of lesioned cholinergic neurons in vivo. Nature 1988; 332: 360–361
19 Cuevas P, Carceller F, Baird A, Guillemin R. Basic fibroblast growth factor (bFGF) increases peripheral nerve regeneration rate. 7th Gen Meeting Europ Soc Neurochem, Goteborg, 1988
20 Cuevas P, Carceller F, Esteban A, Baird A, Guillemin R. Basic fibroblast growth factor (bFGF) enhances retinal ganglion cells survival and promotes axonal growth of rat transected optic nerve. Third Joint Meeting on Neurochemical Approaches to the Understanding of Cerebral Disorders, European Society for Neurochemistry, June 9–12, Copenhagen, 1988

21 Sievers J, Hausmann B, Unsicker K, Berry M. Fibroblast growth factors promote the survival of adult rat retinal ganglion cells after transection of the optic nerve. Neurosci Lett 1987; 76: 157
22 Slack JMW, Darlington BG, Heath JK, Godsave SF. Mesoderm induction in early Xenopus embryos by heparin binding growth factors. Nature 1987; 326: 197–200
23 Hayek A, Culler FL, Beattie GM, Lopez AD, Cuevas P, Baird A. An in vivo model for study of the angiogenic effects of basic fibroblast growth factor. Biochem Biophys Res Commun 1987; 147: 876–880
24 Rogelj S, Weinberg RA, Fanning P, Klagsburn M. Basic fibroblast growth factor fused to a signal peptide transforms cells. Nature 1988; 331: 173–175
25 Jaye M, Lyall RM, Mudd R, Schlessinger J, Sarver N. Expression of acidic fibroblast growth factor cDNA confers growth advantage and tumorigenesis to Swiss 3T3 cells. EMBO J 1988; 7: 963–969
26 Baird A, Ling N. Fibroblast growth factors are present in the extracellular matrix produced by endothelial cells in vitro: Implications for a role of heparinase-like enzymes in the neovascular response. Biochem Biophys Res Commun 1987; 142: 428–435
27 Vlodavsky I, Folkman J, Sullivan R, et al. Endothelial cell-derived basic fibroblast growth factor: Synthesis and deposition into subendothelial extracellular matrix. Proc Natl Acad Sci USA 1987; 84: 2292–2296
28 Folkman J, Klagsbrun M, Sasse I, Wadzinski M, Ingber D, Vlodavsky I. A heparin-binding angiogenic protein—basic fibroblast growth factor—is stored within basement membrane. Am J Pathol 1988; 130: 393–400

Platelet-derived growth factors: A family of isoforms that bind to two distinct receptors

Carl-Henrik Heldin
Ludwig Institute for Cancer Research, Biomedical Center, Uppsala, Sweden

Bengt Westermark
Department of Pathology, University Hospital, Uppsala, Sweden

> Platelet-derived growth factor (PDGF) is a mitogen for connective tissue cells and occurs as disulphide-bonded homodimers or heterodimers of related polypeptide chains. Recent data indicate that the isoforms have different functional activities due to the fact that they bind with different affinities to two distinct receptor types. The frequent expression of PDGF and PDGF receptors in normal as well as transformed cells, suggests roles for PDGF in autocrine and paracrine stimulation of cell growth in vivo.

Platelet-derived growth factor (PDGF) is a polypeptide mitogen that originally was purified from human platelets, but which subsequently has been found to be produced also by a number of other cell types (reviewed in Refs 1 & 2). PDGF acts primarily on connective tissue cells and glial cells, and is the major mitogen in serum for these cell types.

In 1983 the amino acid sequence of PDGF was found to be homologous to that of $p28^{sis}$, the transforming protein of simian sarcoma virus (SSV).[3,4] Subsequently, it was demonstrated that SSV-transformation is exerted by a PDGF-like growth factor via autocrine stimulation of growth (reviewed in Ref. 5). This finding exemplified how oncogenes may act, e.g. by directing the synthesis of proteins that subvert the mitogenic pathway of growth factors (reviewed in Ref. 6). In addition, it stimulated work to elucidate whether PDGF, or other growth factors, are involved in autocrine stimulation also in human tumours.

In this communication we will briefly review the structure and mechanism of action of PDGF, and discuss the possible involvement of PDGF in autocrine and paracrine stimulation of growth of normal and malignant cells.

DIFFERENT ISOFORMS OF PDGF

PDGF is a dimeric molecule which is composed of disulphide-bonded A chains and B chains. The cDNA sequences of the two PDGF chains predict hydrophobic signal sequences, which indicates that the protein products are secreted. The two chains are synthesized as precursors which are proteolytically processed to mature polypeptide chains of slightly more than 100 amino acids each.[7-9] In the mature polypeptide, the A and B chains are 60% similar in their amino acid sequences with a perfect conservation of the eight cysteine residues in each chain.

The A chain gene is located on chromosome 7[8] and the B chain gene on chromosome 22.[10,11] In support of the notion the genes have a common evolutionary origin, their exon/intron organizations have been found to be similar.[12,13] The A chain occurs in two variants that are formed as a result of differential splicing;[12,13] the three most C-terminal amino acids in the shorter variant are replaced in the longer variant by 18 different amino acids derived from an extra exon. Whether functional differences occur between the two variants of the A chain remains to be elucidated. The human B chain mRNA has been identified as a single 3.5 kb species,[14,15] whereas the A chain mRNA occurs as three species, ranging from 1.9 to 2.8 kb.[8] This is most likely due to an alternative use of polyadenylation signals, several of which are found in the 3' end of the A chain gene.[12,13]

The PDGF chains are assembled as homodimers or heterodimers; PDGF-AA, PDGF-AB, as well as PDGF-BB, have been identified and purified from natural sources.[16-18] Interestingly, the various isoforms of PDGF were found to have different functional effects. Thus, in contrast to PDGF-AB, PDGF-AA had only a low mitogenic activity, and no effect on chemotaxis and actin reorganization of human fibroblasts.[19]

TWO DISTINCT PDGF RECEPTOR TYPES

A possible basis for the differences in functional effects of the isoforms of PDGF, was revealed by their binding to cultured fibroblasts; two distinct PDGF receptor types were identified and denoted type A and type B.[20,21] Cross-competition experiments revealed that the A type receptor binds all isoforms of PDGF whereas the B type receptor binds only PDGF-BB with high affinity; PDGF-AB is bound with a ten-fold lower affinity and PDGF-AA with more than a hundred-fold lower affinity[20–22] (Fig. 1).

The B type PDGF receptor is a transmembrane glycoprotein of about 180 kD, which has a ligand-activated protein tyrosine kinase activity (reviewed in Ref. 23). The cDNA sequence of the receptor predicts that the protein backbone is about 120 kD.[24–26] The cytoplasmic part of the receptor contains a stretch of amino acids with homology to other tyrosine kinases. The PDGF B type

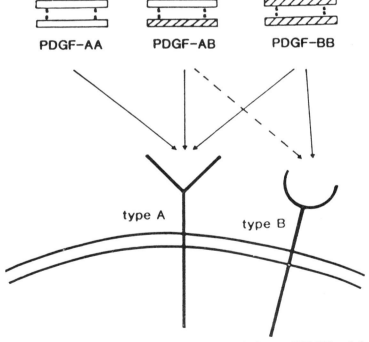

Fig. 1 Schematic illustration of the different dimeric forms of PDGF and their binding affinities to two distinct receptor types. Solid arrows indicate affinities of K_d:s of 0.2–0.5 nM, broken arrow indicates an affinity of a K_d of about 5 nM.

receptor is closely related to the receptor for colony stimulating factor-1 and the c-*kit* product, a receptor-like structure with unknown ligand. In particular, two structural features are shared. Firstly, the kinase domains contain insert sequences without homologies to other kinases. Secondly, the deduced sequences for the extracellular parts of the receptors predict that each of them is composed of five immunoglobulin-like domains.

The biosynthesis of the B type PDGF receptor has been studied through the use of specific antisera. The human receptor is synthesized as a 160 kD precursor containing up to 11 N-linked carbohydrate groups; after maturation of the carbohydrate complexes and possibly other post-translational modifications, the receptor reaches its final size of 180 kD.[27-29] The A type receptor is slightly smaller than the B type receptor; it is synthesized as a precursor of 140 kD which is converted to a mature size of 170 kD.[30] The A type receptor has not been further characterized.

Transfection of Chinese hamster ovary cells with a B type PDGF receptor cDNA construct, induced the synthesis of functionally active receptors.[31] Interestingly, deletion of the insert sequence in the receptor kinase domain led to the synthesis of a receptor which retained kinase activity and ability to stimulate phosphatidylinositol turnover, but which could not transduce a mitogenic signal.[32]

ACTIVATION OF THE B TYPE PDGF RECEPTOR

PDGF-BB has recently been found to induce dimerization purified B type receptors in a concentration-dependent manner, as analyzed by SDS-gel electrophoresis after covalent cross-linking with disuccinimidyl suberate.[33] The fact that dimerization decreased at high ligand concentrations indicates that each dimeric complex contains one PDGF-BB molecule and two receptors; most likely each subunit in the PDGF molecule binds one receptor molecule. The dimerization correlated perfectly with activation of the receptor kinase suggesting that the dimerization induced the activation. It is possible that ligand-induced dimerization causes an interaction between the internal domains of the receptors, leading to their activation. A similar mechanism has previously been proposed for the activation of the EGF receptor.[34]

SSV-TRANSFORMATION IS EXERTED BY EXTERNALIZED PDGF-BB

Amino acid sequencing of PDGF revealed that the B chain of PDGF is virtually identical to p28^{sis}, the transforming protein of SSV, an acutely transforming retrovirus that gives rise to glioblastomas and fibrosarcomas of infected monkeys.[3,4] This finding suggested that SSV-transformation is exerted by a PDGF-like factor, a notion that has received support from several subsequent observations. Firstly, SSV-transformed cells in culture produce a factor similar to PDGF-BB that binds to and activates PDGF receptors. Secondly, only cell types that respond to PDGF, i.e. that have PDGF receptors, are transformed by SSV. Finally, SSV-transformation can be reverted by agents that prevent the binding of PDGF to the receptor (for references see Ref. 5).

Structural analysis of c-*sis* in comparison to the SSV proviral genome shows that SSV has acquired all of the protein coding sequences except for the first exon that encodes the signal sequence.[15] This deletion is compensated for by a hydrophobic helper-virus-derived upstream *env*-sequence. Deletion mutants that lack the hydrophobic sequence have lost their transforming activity, indicating that the transforming protein has to reach the endoplasmic lumen in order to be active.[35,36] Evidence has been presented that the PDGF-like factor of SSV-transformed cells need not be secreted to the extracellular space in order to be active, but can activate its receptor already inside the cell.[37,38] On the other hand, PDGF antibodies[39] and suramin[40,41] inhibit SSV-transformation, suggesting that a ligand-receptor interaction at the cell surface is necessary. Further studies are needed to determine whether the mitogenic signal can be initiated in an intracellular compartment, or the ligand has to reach the cell surface to be functionally active.

The morphological and functional characteristics of acutely SSV-transformed human fibroblasts indicate that the infected cells receive a powerful autocrine growth signal, but other features that have been associated with transformation, e.g. immortalization, do not occur.[42] Therefore, in order to explain the development of malignant glioblastomas and fibrosarcomas in marmoset monkeys infected by SSV, one has to propose that the autocrine growth stimulation be complemented by additional genetic alterations that are responsible for the development of the fully malignant phenotype.

POSSIBLE AUTOCRINE AND PARACRINE EFFECTS OF PDGF IN HUMAN TUMORS

The finding that a factor similar to PDGF-BB functions in an autocrine manner in SSV-transformation has prompted experiments to determine the transforming effect also of the A chain of PDGF. Transfection into Rat-1 cells of PDGF A chain cDNA under the control of a viral LTR induced growth to higher cell densities, but in contrast to similar experiments with B chain constructs, no foci were found.[43] Using human fibroblasts as target cells, it was found that neither expression of PDGF A chain nor B chain had any immortalizing effect, but the transfected cell cultures changed morphology, an effect which was more pronounced in cells expressing the B chain.[43] Constructs of PDGF chains under the control of the inducable metallothionein promoter transfected into NIH3T3 cells, gave similar results; the transforming efficiency of the B chain was 20–40 fold higher than that of the A chain, when estimated as the ability to change cell morphology.[44] Those findings are consistent with the lower mitogenic activity of PDGF-AA on these cell types. In addition, the fact that the PDGF-BB remained cell associated to a large extent, while PDGF-AA was secreted, may contribute to the higher focus forming activity of the B chain.[43,44] Similarly, the transforming protein of SSV-transformed cells has been found to remain cell associated, rather than being secreted into the cell culture medium.[45]

Investigations aimed at elucidating whether PDGF is involved also in stimulation of growth of human tumors have been initiated. Expression of PDGF A and B chain mRNA, or production of PDGF receptor competing activity, have been found in a variety of human tumour cell lines (reviewed in refs. 1,2,6).

There are several examples of PDGF producing cell lines that are derived from connective tissue tumors and gliomas.[1,2,6] Since the normal counterparts of these cells respond to PDGF, it is possible that the endogenous growth factor production has an autocrine effect and drives tumor growth. As an example, out of 23 investigated human glioma cell lines, most of which express PDGF B type receptor mRNA, 17 were found to express B chain mRNA while all expressed A chain mRNA.[46] PDGF and PDGF receptor mRNA was also found, by *in situ* hybridization, in biopsies of human glioblastomas. In addition to the expression detected in tumor cells, PDGF B chain and B type receptor mRNA was found in proliferating endothelial cells.[47] These results suggest that PDGF may have a role in autocrine stimulation of malignant as well as normal cell types of human gliomas.

PDGF production is common also in cell lines derived from PDGF receptor negative cell types, e.g. carcinomas and leukemias.[1,2,6] In one study, expression of PDGF A and B chain mRNA was found in 8 and 9, respectively, of 10 investigated human mammary carcinoma cell lines.[48] Since these cell lines lack PDGF receptors, it is highly unlikely that the endogenously produced PDGF has any autocrine effect. However, if PDGF production also occurs in vivo, it is possible that it stimulates stroma cell proliferation, which is a common finding in many carcinomas.

PDGF IN AUTOCRINE AND PARACRINE STIMULATION OF NORMAL CELLS

Smooth muscle cells[49,50] and placental cytotrophoblasts[51] have been found to produce PDGF under certain conditions. Since these cell types also respond to PDGF, it is possible that the PDGF produced serves an autocrine function in pathophysiological reactions in the vessel wall and in placental growth, respectively. Such autocrine systems in normal cells appear to be subject to regulation; PDGF expression occurs only in response to external stimuli or in a defined phase of the development. Mitogen stimulated fibroblasts also express PDGF A chain mRNA and protein.[52] Although the interpretation of this finding remains unclear, it suggests the presence of a positive feed-back mechanism which may amplify the mitogenic signal.

Endothelial cells[53] and activated macrophages[54,55] are examples of normal cells that produce PDGF but do not have PDGF receptors. It is possible that PDGF released from these cell types stimulates neighbouring cells in a paracrine fashion. Thus, PDGF secreted by regenerating endothelial cells in the vessel wall could stimulate the proliferation of underlying smooth muscle cells, and PDGF secreted by activated macrophages could be involved in the stimulation of connective tissue cells that is often seen in chronic inflammatory processes.

PDGF IN VIVO

Although its in vivo function remains to be elucidated, the fact that PDGF is a release product of blood platelets and is secreted also by certain other cell types (see above), suggests beneficial effects of PDGF in wound healing and in placenta development, as well as adverse reactions in fibrotic lesions, atherosclerosis and tumor growth. A role for PDGF in tissue repair processes is also supported by the observations that PDGF stimulates not only growth of connective cells, but also production of matrix proteins, and chemotaxis of fibroblasts as well as monocytes and neutrophils (reviewed in Ref. 1). Initial in vivo studies showed that when PDGF was placed in porous chambers inserted subcutanously, it led to an increase in the number of cells and in the amount of granulation tissue formed in the chambers.[56]

A role for PDGF in gliogenesis has recently been implicated, since PDGF has been found to be produced by a certain type of rat astrocytes (type-1 astrocytes) and to act on 0-2A progenitor cells that differentiate into oligodendrocytes and type-2 astrocytes.[57,58] PDGF was also found to induce the normal timing of differentiation of the progenitor cells.[59] It is thus possible that PDGF is involved in regulation of growth and differentiation of cells in the central nervous system during development via paracrine, and possibly also autocrine, mechanisms.

The recent observation that the B type PDGF receptor is not expressed, or only expressed at low levels, on cells in normal connective tissue, is of significance for the understanding of the in vivo effects of PDGF. The receptor was found to be induced, e.g. in inflammatory lesions,[60,61] or when cells were explanted into tissue culture.[62] Thus, the response to PDGF-BB in vivo is dependent not only on the availability of the ligand, but also on the induction of the receptor. Whether the expression of the A type PDGF receptor is regulated in a similar manner is not known.

Since large quantities of pure and functionally active recombinant PDGF isoforms recently have become available[63] (also Östman et al., submitted), it will now be possible to address several important questions regarding the in vivo function of the various isoforms of PDGF, and to determine the effect of PDGF administered in vivo.

ACKNOWLEDGEMENTS

We thank L Baltell for valuable help in the preparation of this manuscript.

REFERENCES

1. Heldin C-H, Wasteson, Westermark B. Platelet-derived growth factor. Mol Cell Biol 1985: 3: 169–187
2. Ross R, Raines EW, Bowen-Pope DF. The biology of platelet-derived growth factor. Cell 1986; 46: 155–169
3. Waterfield MD, Scrace GT, Whittle N et al. Platelet-derived growth factor is structurally related to the putative transforming protein p28^{sis} of simian sarcoma virus. Nature 1983; 304: 35–39
4. Doolittle RF, Hunkapiller MW, Hood LE et al. Simian sarcoma virus oncogene, v-sis, is derived from the gene (or genes) encoding a platelet-derived growth factor. Science 1983; 221: 275–277
5. Westermark B, Betsholtz C, Johnsson A, Heldin C-H. Acute transformation by simian sarcoma virus is mediated by an externalized PDGF-like growth factor. In: Kjeldgard NO, Forchhammer J, eds. Viral Carcinogenesis. Copenhagen: Munksgaard. 1987: pp. 445–457
6. Heldin C-H, Betsholtz C, Claesson-Welsh L, Westermark B. Subversion of growth regulatory pathways in malignant transformation. Biochim Biophys Acta 1987; 907: 219–244
7. Josephs SF, Guo C, Ratner L, Wong-Staal F. Human protooncogene nucleotide sequences corresponding to the transforming region of simian sarcoma virus. Science 1984; 223: 487–490
8. Betsholtz C, Johnsson A, Heldin C-H et al. cDNA sequence and chromosomal localization of human platelet-derived growth factor A-chain and its expression in tumor cell lines. Nature 1986; 320: 695–699
9. Johnsson A, Heldin C-H, Wasteson et al. The c-sis gene encodes a precursor of the B chain of platelet-derived growth factor. EMBO J 1984; 3: 921–928
10. Dalla Favera R, Gallo RC, Giallongo A, Croce CM. Chromosomal localization of the human homolog (c-sis) of the simian sarcoma virus onc gene. Science 1982; 218: 686–688
11. Swan DC, McBride OW, Robbins KC, Keithley DA, Reddy EP, Aaronson SA. Chromosmal mapping of the simian sarcoma onc gene analogue in human cells. Proc Natl Acad Sci USA 1982; 79: 4691–4695
12. Rorsman F, Bywater M, Knott TJ, Scott J, Betsholtz C. Structural characterization of the human platelet-derived growth factor A-chain cDNA and gene: alternative exon usage predicts two different precursor proteins. Mol Cell Biol 1988; 8: 571–577
13. Bonthron DT, Morton CC, Orkin SH, Collins T. Platelet-derived growth factor A chain: Gene structure, chromosomal location, and basis for alternative mRNA splicing. Proc Natl Acad Sci USA 1988; 85: 1492–1496
14. Collins T, Ginsburg D, Boss JM, Orkin SH, Pober JS. Cultured human endothelial cells express platelet-derived growth factor B chain; cDNA cloning and structural analysis. Nature 1985; 316: 748–750
15. Rao CH, Igarashi H, Chiu IM, Robbins KC, Aaronson SA. Structure and sequence of the human c-sis/platelet-derived growth factor 2 (SIS/PDGF 2) transcriptional unit. Proc Natl Acad Sci USA 1986; 83: 2392–2396
16. Heldin C-H, Johnsson A, Wennergren S, Wernstedt C, Betsholtz C, Westermark B. A human osteosarcoma cell line secretes a growth factor structurally related to a homodimer of PDGF A chains. Nature 1986; 319: 511–514
17. Hammacher A, Hellman U, Johnsson A et al. A major part of PDGF purified from human platelets is a heterodimer of one A chain and one B chain. J Biol Chem 1988; 263: 16493–16498

18 Stroobant P, Waterfield MD. Purification and properties of porcine platelet-derived growth factor. EMBO J 1984; 3: 2963–2967
19 Nistér M, Hammacher A, Mellström K et al. A glioma-derived PDGF A chain homodimer has different functional activities than a PDGF AB heterodimer purified from human platelets. Cell 1988; 52: 791–799
20 Heldin C-H, Bäckström G, Östman A et al. Binding of different dimeric forms of PDGF to human fibroblasts: Evidence for two separate receptor types. EMBO J 1988; 7: 1387–1394
21 Hart CE, Forstrom JD, Kelly RA et al. Two classes of PDGF receptors recognize different isoforms of PDGF. Science 1988; 240: 1529–1531
22 Escobedo JA, Navankasatussas S, Cousens LS, Coughlin SR, Bell GI, Williams LT. A common PDGF receptor is activated by homodimeric A and B forms of PDGF. Science 1988; 240: 1532–1534
23 Heldin C-H, Rönnstrand L. The platelet-derived growth factor receptor. In: Moudgil VK, ed. Receptor Phosphorylation. CRC press, 1989 (in press)
24 Yarden Y, Escobedo JA, Kuang W-J et al. Structure of the receptor for platelet-derived growth factor helps define a family of closely related growth factor receptors. Nature 1986; 323: 226–232
25 Claesson-Welsh L, Eriksson A, Morén A et al. cDNA cloning and expression of a human PDGF receptor specific for B chain containing PDGF molecules. Mol Cell Biol 1988; 8: 3476–3486
26 Gronwald RGK, Grant FJ, Haldeman BA et al. Cloning and expression of a cDNA coding for the human platelet-derived growth factor receptor: Evidence for more than one receptor class. Proc Natl Acad Sci USA 1988; 85: 3435–3439
27 Hart CE, Seifert RA, Ross R, Bowen-Pope DF. Synthesis, phosphorylation and degradation of multiple forms of the platelet-derived growth factor receptor studied using a monoclonal antibody. J Biol Chem 1987; 262: 10780–10785
28 Keating MT, Williams LT. Processing of the platelet-derived growth factor receptor. Biosynthetic and degradation studies using anti-receptor antibodies. J Biol Chem 1987; 262: 7932–7937
29 Claesson-Welsh L, Rönnstrand L, Heldin C-H. Biosynthesis and intracellular transport of the receptor for platelet-derived growth factor. Proc Natl Acad Sci USA 1987; 84: 8796–8800
30 Claesson-Welsh L, Hammacher A, Westermark B, Heldin C-H, Nistér M. Identification and structural analysis of the A type receptor for PDGF. Similarities with the B type receptor. J Biol Chem 1989 (in press)
31 Escobedo JA, Keating MT, Ives HE, Williams LT. Platelet-derived growth factor receptors expressed by cDNA transfection couple to a diverse group of cellular responses associated with cell proliferation. J Biol Chem 1988; 263: 1482–1487
32 Escobedo JA, Williams LT. A PDGF receptor domain essential for mitogenesis but not for many other responses to PDGF. Nature 1988; 335: 85–87
33 Heldin C-H, Ernlund A, Rorsman C, Rönnstrand L. Dimerization of B type PDGF receptors occur after ligand binding and is closely associated with receptor kinase activation. J Biol Chem 1989 (in press)
34 Schlessinger J. Allosteric regulation of the epidermal growth factor receptor kinase. J Cell Biol 1986; 103: 2067–2072
35 Hannink M, Donoghue DJ. Requirement for a signal sequence in biological expression of the v-sis oncogene. Science 1984; 230: 1197–1199
36 King CR, Giese NA, Robbins KC, Aaronson SA. In vitro mutagenesis of the v-sis transforming gene defines functional domains of its growth factor-related product. Proc Natl Acad Sci USA 1985; 82: 5295–5299
37 Keating MT, Williams LT. Autocrine stimulation of intracellular PDGF receptors in sis-transformed cells. Science 1988; 239: 914–916
38 Huang SS, Huang JS. Rapid turnover of the platelet-derived growth factor receptor in sis-transformed cells and reversal by suramin. Implications for the mechanism of autocrine transformation. J Biol Chem 1988; 263: 12608–12618

39 Johnsson A, Betsholtz C, Heldin C-H, Westermark B. Antibodies against platelet-derived growth factor inhibit acute transformation by simian sarcoma virus. Nature 1985; 317: 438–440
40 Betsholtz C, Johnsson A, Heldin C-H, Westermark B. Efficient reversion of simian sarcoma virus transformation and inhibition of growth factor-induced mitogenesis by suramin. Proc Natl Acad Sci USA 1986; 83: 6440–6444
41 Hannink M, Donoghue DJ. Autocrine stimulation by the v-sis gene product requires a ligand-receptor interaction at the cell surface. J Cell Biol 1988; 107: 287–298
42 Johnsson A, Betsholtz C, Heldin C-H, Westermark B. The phenotypic characteristics of simian sarcoma virus-transformed human fibroblasts suggest that the v-sis gene product acts solely as a PDGF receptor agonist in cell transformation. EMBO J 1986; 5: 1535–1542
43 Bywater M, Rorsman F, Bongcam-Rudloff E et al. Expression of recombinant platelet-derived growth factor A- and B-chain homodimers in Rat-1 cells and human fibroblasts reveals differences in protein processing and autocrine effects. Mol Cell Biol 1988; 8: 2753–2762
44 Beckmann MP, Betsholtz C, Heldin C-H et al. Comparison of biological properties and transforming potential of human PDGF-A and PDGF B-chains. Science 1988; 241: 1346–1349
45 Robbins KC, Leal F, Pierce JH, Aaronson SA. The v-sis/PDGF-2 transforming gene product localizes to cell membranes but is not a secretory product. EMBO J 1985; 4: 1783–1792
46 Nistér M, Libermann T, Betsholtz C et al. Expression of messenger RNAs for platelet-derived growth factor and transforming growth factor-α and their receptors in human malignant glioma cell lines. Cancer Res 1988; 48: 3910–3918
47 Hermansson M, Nistér M, Betsholtz C, Heldin C-H, Westermark B, Funa K. Endothelial cell hyperplasia in human glioblastoma; Co-expression of mRNA for PDGF B chain and PDGF receptor suggests autocrine growth simulation. Proc Natl Acad Sci USA 1988; 85: 7748–7752
48 Perez R, Betsholtz C, Westermark B, Heldin C-H. Frequent expression of growth factors for mesenchymal cells in human mammary carcinoma. Cancer Res 1987; 47: 3425–3429
49 Seifert RA, Schwartz SM, Bowen-Pope DF. Developmentally regulated production of platelet-derived growth factor-like molecules. Nature 1984; 311: 669–671
50 Nilsson J, Sjölund M, Palmberg L, Thyberg J, Heldin C-H. Arterial smooth muscle cells in primary culture produce a platelet-derived growth factor-like protein. Proc Natl Acad Sci USA 1985; 82: 4418–4422
51 Goustin AS, Betsholtz C, Pfeifer-Ohlsson S et al. Co-expression of the sis and myc proto-oncogenes in human placenta suggest autocrine control of trophoblast growth. Cell 1988; 41: 301–312
52 Paulsson Y, Hammacher A, Heldin C-H, Westermark B. Possible autocrine feed-back in the prereplicative phase of human fibroblasts. Nature 1987; 328: 715–717
53 DiCorleto PE, Bowen-Pope DF. Cultured endothelial cells produce a platelet-derived growth factor-like protein. Proc Natl Acad Sci USA 1983; 80: 1919–1923
54 Shimokado K, Raines EW, Madtes DK, Barrett TB, Benditt EP, Ross RA. A significant part of macrophage-derived growth factor consists of at least two forms of PDGF. Cell 1985; 43: 277–286
55 Martinet Y, Bitterman PB, Mornex J-F, Grotendorst G, Martin GR, Crystal RG. Activated human monocytes express the c-sis proto-oncogene and release a mediator showing PDGF-like activity. Nature 1986; 319: 158–160

56 Sprugel KH, McPherson JM, Clowes AW, Ross R. Effects of growth factors in vivo. I. Cell ingrowth into porous subcutaneous chambers. Am J Pathol 1987; 129: 601–613
57 Richardson WD, Pringle N, Mosley MJ, Westermark B, Dubois-Dalcq M. A role for platelet-derived growth factor in normal gliogenesis in the central nervous system. Cell 1988; 53: 309–319
58 Noble M, Murray K, Stroobant P, Waterfield M, Riddle P. Platelet-derived growth factor promotes division and mobility and inhibits premature differentiation of the oligodendrocyte/type-1 astrocyte progenitor cell. Nature 1988; 333: 560–562
59 Raff MC, Lillien LE, Richardson WD, Burne JF, Noble MD. Platelet-derived growth factor from astrocytes drives the clock that times oligodendrocyte development in culture. Nature 1988; 333: 562–565
60 Rubin K, Terracio L, Rönnstrand L, Heldin C-H, Klareskog L. Expression of platelet-derived growth factor receptor is induced on connective tissue cells during chronic synovial inflammation. Scand J Immunol 1988; 27: 285–294
61 Rubin K, Tingström A, Hansson K. et al. Induction of PDGF B-type receptors in vascular inflammation: possible implications for the development of vascular proliferative lesions. Lancet 1988; 1: 1353–1356
62 Terracio L, Rönnstrand L, Tingström A. et al. Induction of PDGF receptor expression in smooth muscle cells and fibroblasts upon tissue culturing. J Cell Biol 1987; 107: 1947–1957
63 Östman A, Rall L, Hammacher A et al. Synthesis and assembly of a functionally active recombinant PDGF-AB heterodimer. J. Biol Chem 1988; 263: 16202–16208

Structural and functional analysis of insulin-like growth factors

D R Clemmons
Department of Medicine, University of North Carolina School of Medicine, Chapel Hill, North Carolina, USA

The insulin and insulin-like growth factor family of peptides are proteins with similar structural characteristics whose functions have diverged during evolution. Recent studies have provided a great deal of information regarding structural characteristics of these peptides, the structures of the genes that control their biosynthesis, and determination of their receptor structures. Initially these factors were believed to function as classical hormones and the endocrine regulation of their blood concentrations was studied intensively. More recently several cell types have been shown to secrete these peptides and the autocrine and paracrine regulation of insulin-like growth factor secretion by cells and tissues has received extensive characterization. Following secretion into interstitial fluids the IGF's associate with high affinity, soluble binding proteins. These proteins are capable of modulating receptor binding and growth factor biological activity. The structure of these proteins and the variables that control their secretion are currently being determined. In spite of this information significant gaps in our knowledge exist regarding the mechanisms by which these peptides stimulate replication.

The term insulin-like growth factor (IGF) was proposed to denote a class of compounds whose structure was highly similar to proinsulin (e.g. 50% amino acid sequence homology) but whose functional characteristics differed. The significant differences between these two families of molecules are:

(1) insulin levels fluctuate widely in response to variations in carbohydrate intake;

(2) the IGF's circulate bound to carrier proteins and their blood concentrations are more stable;

(3) insulin and the IGF's have strucurally distinct receptors;

(4) following receptor association insulin stimulates glucose transport and metabolic processes, such as glycogen and lipid synthesis, whereas, the IGF's stimulate cellular replication.

These functional and structural distinctions appear to be very important for both the maintenance of normal carbohydrate homeostasis and long-term growth.

STRUCTURAL CHARACTERIZATION

Insulin-like growth factor I is a peptide that contains 70 amino acids[1] which shares 48% amino acid sequence homology with human pro-insulin (see Fig. 1). The A and B domains have 60–70% homology with each other while there is no homology in the connecting peptide region. IGF-I also contains an 8 amino acid extension at the carboxy terminus termed the D domain. IGF-I is a basic protein with an isoelectric point of 8.6 and has three disulfide bridges. The first 16 residues of the B domain in IGF-I and II contain the region that is critical for binding to carrier proteins.[2] Mutants that have had this portion of the sequence deleted have no binding protein activity. Likewise, insulin which does not bind to binding proteins, has significant differences in the structure of this region. IGF-II in contrast to IGF-I contains only 67 amino acids. There is approximately 50% structural identity of IGF-II with IGF-I and insulin.[3] The connecting peptide domain shows significant sequence divergence although the disulfide structure is identical. Like IGF-I the critical B chain residues that are necessary for the capacity to bind the binding proteins are preserved.

The genes that encode these molecules have recently been structurally characterized.[4,5] Both the IGF-I and II genes have three introns and four exons. The protein coding sequence of each is contained in two exons. Pro-insulin has two introns and like the IGF gene the protein coding sequence is contained in two exons. The IGF-I gene has been shown to transcribe at least five distinct forms of messenger RNA that contain exons 1–3. The high

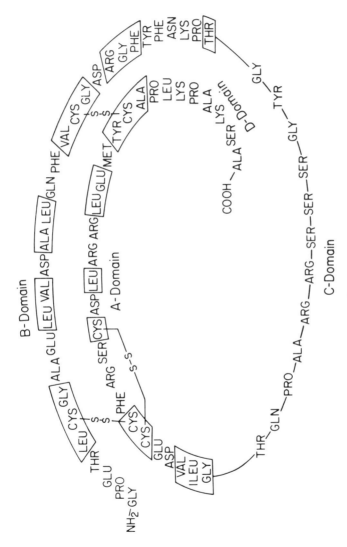

Fig. 1 The structure of insulin-like growth factor I.

molecular weight forms of messenger RNA for both IGF-I and II are not translated, the significance of this is uncertain. There is alternative splicing that occurs at the end of the third exon of IGF-I and a fourth and fifth exon have been shown to be present in human liver genomic library.[6] These forms are termed IGF-I A and B. These alternatively processed mRNA's have been shown to be translatable in in vitro test systems. IGF-II transcripts also show evidence of alternative splicing and multiple sizes of messenger RNA.[7] Furthermore, the IGF-II gene has at least 3 distinct promoters, at least one of which encodes a fetal specific 5.6 kb transcript. In the rat this promoter is activated during development.[8] Activation of this promoter apparently terminates at the end of gestation and the translation product that is obtained in the post-fetal animal is different than that observed in the fetal blood. This change occurs concommitantly with a 20-fold reduction in plasma IGF-II concentrations.

CONTROL OF SYNTHESIS AND SECRETION

The initial classical studies of IGF regulation focused on the endocrine mechanisms that controlled the blood concentration of IGF-I and II. Growth hormone was shown to be the most important factor controlling IGF-I secretion although other hormones were also shown to be important (Table 1). The control of

Table 1 Factors that control blood IGF-I concentrations

	Factor	Comment
1	Age	Peak at adolescence
2	Sex	Females $20\% >$ males
3	Pregnancy	Levels highest 3rd trimester
4	Nutritional status	Fasting causes 70% decline in 10 days. Refeeding response requires $\approx 15-18$ kcal/kg energy and 1.0 gm/kg protein
5	Growth hormone	Decreased by hypophysectomy. Increased by GH producing tumors
6	Thryoxine	Decrease in hypothyroidism in proportion to the decrease in GH secretion
7	Prolactin	In the absence of GH prolactin is a weak stimulus
8	Oestrogen	Physiologic oestrogen replacement causes an increase
9	Negative feedback	IGF-I suppresses GH secretion by the pituitary and therefore, indirectly controls IGF-I secretion

blood IGF concentrations has been extensively reviewed[9] and will not be detailed herein.

In vitro translation studies of IGF-II mRNA have shown that a 22 000 M_r prepro translation product is generated in rat liver cells.[10] Following transport across the endoplasmic reticulum a 26 amino acid leader sequence is clipped resulting in pro-IGF-II (20 000 M_r) that is further processed to 16 and 18 kD forms following secretion. Likewise, both alternatively processed forms of IGF-I mRNA can be translated in vitro.[11] Fibroblasts have been shown to secrete a 20 kD pro-IGF-I form that has been purified from conditioned medium.[12] This form has an amino acid composition similar to that predicted for the IGF-I-B sequence and is biologically active. Higher molecular weight forms of IGF-II have been shown to be present in plasma and one 16 700 M_r form has been purified and shown to have biologic activity.[13]

The role of various tissues in contributing to the blood pool of the IGFs has been a point of intensive investigation. Specifically the autocrine/paracrine hypothesis has been applied to the analysis of IGF synthesis and secretion. The initial studies demonstrated that rat lung and liver IGF-I concentrations increased after GH administration prior to an increase in blood concentrations, indicating that this increase was due to tissue synthesis of IGF rather than to transport from blood. Recently the induction of IGF-I mRNA in non-hepatic tissues after GH has been shown by Northern blotting. IGF-like peptides have been shown to be secreted by multiple types of cells in culture (Table 2). More importantly the factors that stimulate secretion of the IGF's by cells such as platelet derived growth factor, have been shown to be distinct from those that increase plasma concentrations of IGF-I, such as GH. Subsequently many cell types have been shown to

Table 2 Partial list of the cell types that have been shown to secrete IGF-I

1	Human skin fibroblasts	10	Rat pancreatic beta cells
2	Rat hepatocytes	11	Human connective tissue explants (e.g. aponeurosis)
3	Human fetal myoblast	12	Rat thyroid follicular cells (FRTL5)
4	Human glial cells	13	Corneal lens epithelial cells
5	Rat and pig granulosa cells	14	Mammary epithelial cells
6	Rat leydig cells	15	Lung epithelial cells
7	Rat mesangial cells	16	Rat skeletal muscle cells
8	Corneal epithelial cells	17	Rat chondrocytes
9	Rat GH_3 pituitary cells	18	Porcine smooth muscle cells

respond to specific trophic stimuli for that organ with an increase in the secretion of IGF-like peptides. Two of the best studied systems are the granulosa cells and thyroid follicular cell, FRTL-5. The granulosa cell responds to LH with increased IGF secretion[14] while FRTL-5 responds to TSH.[15] Fetal rat fibroblasts have been shown to secrete increased amounts of IGF-II in response to human placental lactogen, whereas, post-natal fibroblasts do not, indicating that IGF-II secretion is developmentally regulated.[16] Based on these results a hypothesis of dual control mechanisms of IGF secretion has been proposed.[17] This hypothesis states that cell type specific trophic stimuli are dominant in controlling IGF secretion in the local microenvironment and that paracrine regulatory mechanisms might be important in processes such as wound healing, whereas, in balanced systemic growth sustained increases in blood IGF concentrations would be the most important variable.

The autocrine/paracrine hypothesis has been further strengthened by immunoinhibition and *in situ* hybridization studies. In in vitro test systems the addition of anti-IGF antibodies or antireceptor antibodies can block DNA synthesis in cell types that secrete these peptides.[18] It is presumed that these antibodies interfere with the ability of the IGF to interact directly with its receptor. Regional infusion of IGF-I antibodies into a perfused limb has been shown to block both IGF-I and GH stimulated growth, suggesting that the paracrine increase in IGF-I secretion in response to GH infusion, may also be a growth regulatory signal.[19] *In situ* hybridization studies have shown that IGF-I and II mRNA's can be detected in fibroblast-like cells of multiple tissues.[20] In contrast, if immunocytochemical localization studies are performed, IGF-I is detected at the surface of many cell types that do not express its mRNA. This is believed to be due to transport of locally synthesized IGF-I by carrier proteins and co-localization or association of the IGF-I with the carrier protein on the cell surface. These results suggest that IGF-I and II may function as paracrine regulators of growth in cell types that do not actually synthesize these growth factors.

Recent studies have demonstrated that the paracrine hypothesis of IGF action may provide insight into understanding the mechanisms that regulate tissue repair after injury. Following balloon denudation of the rat aorta, IGF-I mRNA is increased in aortic smooth muscle cells and this increase is accompanied by an increase in IGF-I peptide. This response is not reduced by hypophysectomy. Likewise, following toxic injury to skeletal muscle there is muscle cell regeneration accompanied by expression of high levels of IGF mRNA by satellite cells.[21] These cells subsequently differentiate into myotubes under the direct influence of IGF-I. The studies in these injury models suggest that these regulatory mechanisms are independent of GH secretion and changes in blood IGF concentrations.

IGF RECEPTORS

Three distinct types of receptors have been characterized that bind the peptides in this family. The insulin and Type I IGF receptors have a high degree of structural homology.[22] The primary amino acid sequences show approximately 50% homology. Both receptors are heterotetramers containing two alpha subunits and two beta subunits. The alpha subunits contain the peptide binding site and each binds all three peptides. There is a high degree of specificity with the type I receptor binding IGF-I > IGF-II > insulin whereas, the insulin receptor binds insulin > IGF-I > IGF-II.[23] The affinity of the type I IGF receptor is reduced four fold for IGF-II and 800-fold for insulin. The insulin receptor shows a 100-fold reduction in affinity for IGF-I and 200-fold for IGF-II. Receptor specificity studies have been further strengthened by showing that anti-insulin receptor antibodies will block IGF-I binding to the insulin receptor only at supraphysiologic concentrations and likewise a monoclonal antibody directed against the Type I IGF receptor will block insulin binding only at supraphysiologic concentrations. This specificity of binding is critical to maintenance of the specificity of metabolic actions of each peptide.

Following binding there are multiple transmembrane signalling events that are believed to be mediated through the beta subunit. The beta subunits of both receptors contain tyrosine protein kinase activity and autophosphorylate tyrosine residues in response to IGF or insulin binding. The most important phosphorylations occur on the tyrosines at positions 1146, 1150 and 1151 of the insulin receptor.[24] Following autophosphorylation the kinase is activated and phosphorylates other cellular proteins. The best described example is pp185 that is phosphorylated within fifteen minutes after IGF-I or insulin binding to their respective receptors. Blocking this reaction has been shown to inhibit insulin action.[25]

Regulation of the cell surface abundance of both receptors has been demonstrated. Following insulin or IGF binding there is down regulation of each receptor and this may function as a mechanism for protecting cells from over stimulation. Likewise, there appears to be heterologous receptor regulation, since platelet derived growth factor exposure to cells can stimulate an increase in the quantity of Type I IGF receptor detected and exposure to dexamethasone also increases Type I receptor number.[26]

Although IGF-II can bind to the Type I IGF and the insulin receptor, another type of receptor, the Type II IGF receptor has also been identified. In contrast to the other two receptors it is a single chain 260 000 kD monomeric unit. It binds IGF-II with approximately three times greater affinity than IGF-I and does not bind insulin. Recently the structure of this protein has been analyzed and it has been shown to be identical with the cation independent Type II mannose-6-phosphate receptor.[27] The protein is a multifunctional protein which binds not only the insulin-like growth factors but also mannose-6-phosphate and following mannose-6-phosphate binding there is an increase in affinity for IGF-II. The exact function of this protein is unknown, however it is believed to be intimately involved in binding specific proteins that have been transported to lysosomes for degradation. Several agents have been shown to stimulate the translocation of this protein from lysosomes to the cell surface. The most interesting is insulin which induces translocation of approximately 50% of the Type II receptors to the cell surface within 10 minutes. The Type II receptor can be cleaved from the cell surface resulting in 200 kD form that is water soluble and circulates in blood.[28] This cleavage occurs at the transmembrane domain junction and the cleaved fragment has been shown to function as an IGF-II binding protein in rat plasma. The role of the Type II receptor in regulating IGF induced growth has not been established. Antibody blocking studies have shown that both IGF-I and II mediate their growth promoting effects through the Type I receptor and not through binding to the Type II receptor.[29] Therefore the exact functional role of the receptor, its relationship to lysosomal degradation of proteins, and whether or not this effect is related to IGF cellular growth stimulation has not been defined.

IGF BINDING PROTEINS

In addition to their respective receptors IGF-I and II bind to several carrier proteins that are present in blood and extracellular fluids. Due to structural differences outlined previously, insulin does not associate with these carrier proteins. The role of these carrier proteins in modulating IGF action is the subject of intense interest. At present two distinct IGF binding protein species have been identified by cDNA sequence analysis. One protein (53 000 M_r) is the predominant species found in plasma and its serum concentrations are growth hormone dependent.[30] This protein binds both IGF-I and II with high affinity and its concentrations increase approximately 6-fold after growth hormone administration. It is present in extracellular fluids and is secreted by several types of cells in culture. Structural analysis shows that the protein contains 291 amino acids and has three carbohydrate chains.[31] Impure preparations of this protein have been shown to inhibit insulin-like actions of IGF-I on fat cells. In plasma the protein is saturated with IGF-I and II and coincubation of radiolabelled IGF-I with normal human plasma followed by chromatography shows that most of the unsaturated binding sites are due to binding to other forms of IGF-BP's. Since this form is the most abundant IGF binding protein in plasma, it acts as the principle carrier of endogenously secreted IGF-I and II. This protein has been shown to be secreted by the liver and hepatic secretion is under growth hormone control. Following secretion into blood the BP-53 subunit associates with a heat labile subunit (M_r 100 000) to form a large complex and formation of this complex is also GH dependent.

Plasma and extracellular fluids also contains a 25 kD IGF binding protein whose plasma concentrations appear to be inversely related to growth hormone. This protein binds IGF-II and IGF-I with equal affinity and is the most abundant IGF binding protein in amniotic fluid. The decidual cells of the human placenta have been shown to be a major source of this binding protein.[32] This protein is also synthesized in the liver and cultured hepatoblastoma cells. The protein has been purified to homogeneity and recently its complete amino acid sequence has been reported.[33,34] The protein contains 18 cysteines that align with the cysteines in the growth hormone dependent IGF–BP, suggesting that the preservation of the cysteine placement is necessary for secondary structure and IGF binding. Plasma concentrations of this protein are regulated not only by growth hormone, but also by nutritional intake. After an overnight fast the plasma concentration rises approximately 8 fold and it is reduced following ingestion of a mixed meal or glucose infusion.[35] Levels are elevated in Type II diabetes and are reduced with improved control. The protein is translated from a single 1.5 kb mRNA species that is present in liver and decidua. An interesting structural feature of this protein is the presence of Arg-Gly-Asp sequence near the carboxy terminus.[33] This RGD sequence has been shown to be important for cellular attachment of matrix proteins and coincubation of cells with synthetic RGD peptides will inhibit binding of this form of binding protein to cell surfaces. The protein can also be detected in association with extracellular matrix. These findings suggest that like other matrix proteins the RGD sequence is important for IGF-BP-cell association.

One of the striking findings of this particular binding protein is that it potentiates the effect of IGF-I on DNA synthesis.[36] Cultured human, chick and mouse embryo fibroblasts as well as porcine aortic smooth muscle cells are normally responsive to IGF-I but their responses can be potentiated 4 to 5-fold by the addition of low concentrations (1–20 ng/ml) of this binding protein. The exact molecular mechanism by which DNA synthesis is stimulated has not been determined, however potentiation of the IGF-I response does require that the IGF-BP associate with the cell surface or matrix and failure of the binding protein to associate with one of these components results in failure to potentiate the DNA synthesis response.[37] Therefore variables that control the concentration of this protein or its capacity to adhere to cell surfaces may be important growth potentiating factors.

The 25 kD protein is present in amniotic fluid, lymph and acites fluid. It has been shown to be secreted by many types of cells in culture. The factors that stimulate its secretion have not been determined, however, IGF-I itself is a stimulant of synthesis of this protein by muscle cells and fibroblasts. In L6 myoblasts, secretion of the protein can be stimulated by insulin or IGF-I, and the capacity of these factors to stimulate its synthesis is associated with rapid cellular proliferation.[38] In contrast, when L6 cells fuse into myotubes and no longer can enter the cell cycle they lose their sensitivity to insulin or IGF-I stimulation. These findings suggest that this protein may be involved not only in cell growth control but also in maintaining the differentiated state.

Another form of IGF binding protein has been identified by its binding specificity pattern. A 34 kD protein that is present in plasma is the major species in cerebrospinal fluid. More importantly, this protein prefers IGF-II with a 6-fold greater affinity than IGF-I.[39] This protein has not been structurally characterized at the present time, and the variables controlling its secretion have not been identified. Electrophoretic separation of plasma and extracellular fluids also shows a 25 000 M_r form of IGF binding protein. This protein appears to be preferentially secreted by tumor cells and not stimulated by IGF-I secretion. Therefore based on size and functional criteria it may be a distinct form of IGF binding protein. The determination of the functional roles of the IGF binding proteins and their ability to modulate IGF contact with the type I receptor are important areas of future investigation.

TARGET CELL ACTIONS

The insulin-like growth factors were originally isolated on the basis of their ability to stimulate sulfate incorporation into cartilidge (termed sulfation factor activity). Although insulin also mimicked this effect it was noted in earlier studies that this required suraphysiologic concentrations of this hormone. Another assay that was used to monitor purification measured the transport of glucose into fat cells in the presence of anti-insulin antiserum, termed non-suppressible insulin-like activity. With structural identification of these proteins it was determined that these two activities were due to the same proteins and that sufficient structural homology existed for the IGF's to interact directly with insulin receptor and vice versa. Functional specificity has been preserved however, since supraphysiologic concentrations of insulin are required to activate DNA synthesis to the same extent as IGF-I or II in most cell types. Specifically, cultured fibroblasts, muscle cells, hepatocytes, ovarian cells, gastrointestinal epithelial cells, lung and renal epithelial cells all require concentrations of insulin greater than 500 ng/ml in order to stimulate DNA synthesis. At these concentrations, insulin is known to bind to the Type I IGF receptor and its effects can be blocked with anti-Type I receptor antibodies. IGF-I stimulation of glycogen synthesis in the liver or glucose oxidation and lipid synthesis in fat cells requires IGF-I concentrations in excess of 100 ng/ml, concentrations that bind to the insulin receptor.[40] Certain cell lines, such as the Ruber H35 rat hepatoma cell, contain no Type I IGF receptors and respond to 1.5 ng/ml concentrations of insulin. The exact mutation that is allowing this cell line to grow in the absence of Type I IGF receptors and respond to low concentrations of insulin is unknown. Recently a glial cell line that contains only Type II IGF receptors and responds to low concentrations of IGF-II has been identified.[41] However, most cell types that grow in response to IGF-II appear to be responding through its binding to the Type I receptor.

The effects of IGFs and insulin appear to be cell cycle specific. Neither IGF-I nor II can act as competence factors, that is they are not able to recruit quiescent cells into the cell cycle, and thereby facilitate DNA synthesis. Instead, they require prior exposure to growth factors such as, platelet derived growth factor or fibroblast growth factor.[42] Following removal of these mitogens however, the IGFs can act as potent mitogens and function synergistically with competence factors to stimulate a rapid increase in cellular proliferation. The range of target cells in which IGFs are active is extensive and has been published in other recent review articles.[43] The IGFs appear to be important mitogens for a wide variety of cells including those derived from all three types of embryonic germ cell lines. In general, the IGFs function in a synergistic manner with other growth factors, such as those previously mentioned, although there are instances where they can function in isolation to achieve the same degree of stimulation of replication.

The IGFs are unique in that they stimulate not only growth, but can stimulate differentiation. In the L6 myoblast the IGFs are a potent stimuli of cell fusion and the expression of muscle specific proteins, such as CPK. The IGFs appear to be important potentiators of other differentiated functions such as FSH and LH stimulated steroidogenesis by ovarian granuloses cells.[44] These results suggest that IGFs may be necessary for maintenance of the synthesis of differentiation-associated proteins. This concept is consistent with the concept that growth hormone stabilizes the concentration of specific proteins by preferentially stimulating the synthesis of specific protease inhibitors. Likewise IGF-I itself has been shown to stabilize specific messenger RNA's in Balb/C 3T3 cells, suggesting that an important mechanism of action of these compounds may be to increase the abundance of labile mRNA's and proteins by preventing their degradation.[45] Since the rapid degradation of specific messages such as *c-fos* has been shown to be an important growth regulatory event this could be an important function of the IGF's in modulating growth regulation.

IN VIVO ACTIONS

Infusion of IGF-I into hypophysectomized rats for 6 days results in weight gain and long bone growth.[46] Likewise, infusion of IGF-I into normal control rats has been shown to cause small increases in body weight, tail length and tibial thickening—but the percentage increase is not as great as in the hypophysectomized animal. In both cases infusions of growth hormone are more potent by a factor of 10–15-fold and it is difficult for IGF-I to completely mimic the actions of growth hormone in stimulating all growth parameters. The exact explanation for this failure is not entirely known, however it suggests one of three hypotheses:

(1) IGF-I itself cannot mimic all the growth promoting actions of growth hormone;

(2) some other growth hormone dependent protein is required for IGF-I actions to be manifested;

(3) the IGF's work primarily by autocrine/paracrine mechanisms and in vivo infusions do not mimic these actions.

Possible candidates for proteins that function to potentiate IGF actions are the IGF binding proteins themselves. Indirect evidence favoring this theory is provided by the observation that in normal rat plasma the growth hormone dependent forms of IGF binding proteins are completely saturated. In contrast, in diabetic or malnourished rats these proteins are unsaturated and these animals respond with a greater percentage increase in growth in response to IGF-I than normal rats.[47] This suggests a correlation between the ability of IGF to optimally stimulate growth and the level of unsaturated binding protein. Alternatively, Issakson has proposed that growth hormone stimulates precommitted cells into a differentiation pathway that enables them to respond to locally produced IGF-I.[48] Since GH exposure is required for these cells to become sensitized to the effects of IGF-I, administration of IGF-I alone is insufficient for a maximal effect. Since GH receptors are not ubiquitous, however, other mechanisms of growth regulation that require IGF-I but also require other growth factors unrelated to growth hormone may be important particularly with respect to paracrine growth regulation. Recent studies have shown that exposure of rat skin wounds to the combination of PDGF plus IGF-I results in maximal rates of connective tissue division within the wound and re-epithelialization after injury.[49] Thus the synergism that was first demonstrated in an in vitro test system has been demonstrated in an in vivo wound healing model. Extension of these experiments to the analysis of the mechanism of IGF action in other in vivo test systems is an important area of future investigation.

ACKNOWLEDGMENTS

The author gratefully acknowledges the secretarial assistance of Anne Myers who aided in the preparation of this manuscript. This work was supported by grants from the National Institute of Health (AG-02331, HL-36313).

REFERENCES

1. Rinderknecht E, Humbel RE. The amino acid sequence of human insulin-like growth factor I and its structural homology with proinsulin. J Biol Chem 1978; 253: 2769–2776
2. Bayne MJ, Applebaum J, Chicchi GG, Hayes NS, Green BG, Cascieri MP. Structural analogues of human insulin like growth factor one with reduced affinity for serum binding protein and the type II insulin-like growth factor receptor. J Biol Chem 1988; 263: 6233–6239
3. Rinderknecht E, Humbel RE. Primary structure of human insulin-like growth factor II. FEBS Letters 1978; 89: 283–286
4. Rotwein P, Pollack KM, Didier DK, Krivi GC. Organization and sequence of the human insulin-like growth factor I gene. J Biol Chem 1986; 261: 4828
5. Pagter-Holthuizen P de, van Schaik FMA, Verduijn GH, van Ommen GJB, Bouma BN, Jansen M, Sussenback JS. Organization of the human genes for insulin-like growth factors I and II. FEBS Letters 1986; 195: 179–184
6. Rotwein P. Two insulin-like growth factor I messenger RNAs are expressed in human liver. Proc Nat Acad Sci USA 1986; 83: 77–81
7. Chairotti L, Brown AL, Frunzio R, Clemmons DR, Rechler MM, Bruni CB. Structure of the rat insulin-like growth factor II transcriptional unit. Mol Endocrinol; 2: 1115–1122.
8. Pagter-Holthuizen P de, Jansen M, van Schaik FMA, Van der Kammen R, Oosterwijk C, Van der Brande JL, Sussenback JS. The human insulin like growth factor II gene contains two development-specific promoters. FEBS Lett 1987; 214: 259–264
9. Clemmons DR, Van Wyk JJ. Factors controlling blood concentrations of somatomedin-c. Clin Endocrinol Metab 1984; 13: 113–143
10. Yang YH-H, Rechler MM, Nissley SP, Coligan JE. Biosynthesis of rat insulin-like growth factor II. J Biol Chem 1985; 260: 2578–2582
11. Rotwein P, Folz RH, Gordon JI. Biosynthesis of human insulin-like growth factor I (IGF-I). J Biol Chem 1987; 262: 11807–11812
12. Clemmons DR, Shaw DS. Purification and biologic properties of fibroblast somatomedin. J Biol Chem 1986; 263: 2841–2849
13. Gowan LK, Hampton B, Hill DJ, Schleutter RJ, Perdue JF. Purification and characterization of a unique high molecular weight form of insulin-like growth factor II. Endocrinology 1987; 121: 449–458
14. Adashi EY, Resnick CE, D'Ercole AJ, Svoboda ME, Van Wyk JJ. Insulin-like growth factors as intra-ovarian regulators of granulosa cell growth and function. Endocrinol Rev 1985; 6: 400–420.

15 Tramontano D, Moses AC, Venezani BM, Ingbar SH. Adenosine 3'5' monophosphate mediates both the mitogenic effect of TSH and its ability to amplify the responses to insulin-like growth factor I in FRTL-5 cells. Endocrinology 1988; 122: 127–132
16 Adams SO, Nissley SP, Handwerger S, Rechler MM. Developmental patterns of insulin-like growth factor I and II synthesis and regulation in rat fibroblasts. Nature 1983; 302: 150–153
17 Clemmons DR. Multiple hormones stimulate the production of somatomedin by cultured human fibroblasts. J Clin Endocrinol Metab 1984; 58: 850–856
18 Clemmons DR, Van Wyk JJ. Evidence for a functional role of endogenously produced somatomedin-like peptides in the regulation of DNA synthesis in cultured human fibroblasts and porcine smooth muscle cells. J Clin Invest 1985; 75: 1914–1918.
19 Schlecter NL, Russell SM, Spencer EM, Nicoll CS. Evidence suggesting that the direct growth promoting effect of growth hormone on cartilage in vivo is mediated by local production of somatomedin. Proc Natl Acad Sci USA 1986; 83: 7932–7938
20 Han VKM, D'Ercole AJ, Lund PK. Cellular location of somatomedin (insulin-like growth factor) messenger RNA in the human fetus. Science 1987; 236: 193–197
21 Jennische E, Hannson HA. Regenerating skeletal muscle cells express insulin-like growth factor I. Acta Physiol Scand 1987; 130: 327–332
22 Ullrich A, Gray A, Tam AW et al. Insulin-like growth factor I receptor primary structure: comparison with insulin receptor suggests structural determinants that define functional specificity. EMBO J 1986; 5: 2503–2512
23 Nissley SP, Rechler MM. Somatomedin/insulin-like growth factor tissue receptors. Clin Endocrinol Metab 1984; 13: 13–68
24 Ellis LE, Claussen DO, Morgan M, Edey M, Bota AA, Rutter WJ. Replacement of insulin receptor tyrosine residues 1162 and 1163 compromises insulin stimulated kinase activity and uptake of 2 deoxyglucose. Cell 1986; 45: 721–732
25 Kadowaki T, Koyasu S, Nishida E et al. Tyrosine phosphorylation of common specific sets of cellular proteins rapidly induced by insulin, insulin-like growth factor I and epidermal growth factor in an intact cell. J Biol Chem 1987; 262: 7342–7350
26 Kaplowitz P. Glucocorticoids enhance somatomedin-C binding and stimulation of amino acid uptake in human fibroblasts. J Clin Endocrinol Metab 1987; 64: 563–571
27 Tong PK, Tollefsen S, Kornfeld S. The cation independent mannose 6 phosphate receptor binds insulin-like growth factor II. J Biol Chem 1987; 263: 2585–2588
28 Kiess W, Greistein LA, Lee L, White RM, Rechler MM, Nissley SP. The type II insulin like growth factor (IGF) receptor protein in rat serum. Proc Natl Acad Sci USA 1987; 84: 7720–7721
29 Kiess W, Haskell JF, Lee L et al. An antibody that blocks insulin-like growth factor (IGF) binding to the type II IGF receptor is neither against nor an inhibitor of IGF stimulated biologic responses in L-6 myoblasts. J Biol Chem 1987; 262: 12745–12751
30 Baxter RC, Martin JL. Radioimmunoassay of growth hormone dependent insulin-like growth factor binding protein in human plasma. J Clin Invest 1986; 78: 1504–1512
31 Wood WI, Cathianos G, Hummel WJ et al. Cloning and expression of the GH dependent insulin-like growth factor binding protein. Mol Endocrinol; In press
32 Rutanen EM, Koistinon R, Wahlstrom T, Bohn H, Ranta T, Seppala M. Synthesis of placental protein 12 by human decidua. Endocrinology 1985; 116: 1304–1309

33 Brewer MT, Stetler GL, Squires CH, Thompson RC, Busby WT, Clemmons DR. Cloning characterization and expression of a human insulin-like growth factor binding protein. Biochem Biophys Res Commun 1988; 152: 1289–1297
34 Lee YL, Hintz RL, James DM, Lee PDK, Shively JE, Powell DR. Insulin-like growth factor IGF binding protein complementary deoxyribonucleic acid from human Hep G_2 hepatoma cells: predicted protein sequence suggests an IGF binding domain different from those of IGF-I and IGF-II receptors. Mol Endo 1988; 3: 404–411
35 Baxter RC, Colwell CT. Diurnal rhythm of growth hormone dependent binding protein for insulin-like growth factors in human plasma. J Clin Endocrinol, Metab 1987; 65: 432–440
36 Elgin RG, Busby WH, Clemmons DR. An insulin-like growth factor binding protein enhances the biogic response to IGF-I. Proc Natl Acad Sci 1987; 84: 3313–3318
37 Busby WH, Klapper DG, Clemmons DR. Purification of a 31000 dalton insulin like growth factor binding protein from human amniotic fluid. J Biol Chem 1988; 263: 14203–14210
38 McCusker RH, Camacho-Huber C, Clemmons DR. Identification of insulin-like growth factor binding proteins that are secreted by muscle cells in vitro. J Cell Physiol; 137: 505–512
39 Binoux M, Hardouin S, Lassare C, Hossenlopp P. Evidence for production by the liver of two IGF binding proteins with similar molecular weights but different affinities for IGF-I and IGF-II. Their relationship with serum and cerebrospinal fluid binding proteins. J Clin Endocrinol Metab 1982; 55: 600–602
40 King GL, Kahn CR. Non parallel evolution of metabolic and growth promoting factors of insulin. Nature 1981; 292: 644–646
41 Tally M, Li CH, Hall K. IGF-2 stimulated growth mediated by the somatomedin type 2 receptor. Biochem Biophys Res Commun 1987; 148: 811–814
42 Stiles CD, Capone GT, Scher CD et al. Dual control of cell growth by somatomedin and platelet derived growth factor. Proc Natl Acad Sci USA 1979; 76: 1279–1283
43 Van Wyk JJ. The somatomedins: biological actions and physiologic control mechanisms. In: Li CH ed. Hormonal Proteins and Peptides. Orlando: Academic Press, 1985; pp.81–125
44 Veldheiss JD, Rogers RJ. Mechanisms subserving the steroidogenic synergism between follicle stimulating hormone and insulin-like growth factor I. J Biol Chem 1987; 262: 7658–7664
45 Zumstein P, Stiles CD. Molecular cloning of gene sequences that are regulated by insulin like growth factor I. J Biol Chem 1987; 262: 11252–11260
46 Schoenle E, Zapf J, Hauri G, Steiner T, Froesch ER. Comparison of in vivo effects of insulin-like growth factors I and II and of growth hormone in hypophysectomized rats. Acta Endocrinol 1985; 108: 167–174
47 Schweller E, Guler HP, Merryweather J et al. Growth restoration of insulin deficit diabetic rats by recombinant human insulin-like growth factor I. Nature 1986; 323: 169–171
48 Nilsson A, Isgaard J, Lindahl A, Dahlstrom A, Skottner A, Isaksson OG. Regulation by growth hormone of number of chondrocytes containing IGF-I in rat growth plate. Science 1986; 233: 571–574
49 Calvin RB, Antoniades HN. Role of platelet-derived growth factor in wound healing: Synergistic effects with other growth factors. Proc Natl Acad Sci USA 1987; 84: 7696–7700

Scatter factor and other regulators of cell mobility

Michael Stoker
Ermanno Gherardi
Department of Pathology, University of Cambridge, UK, and Imperial Cancer Research Fund, London, UK

> The scatter factor is a basic protein with an apparent molecular weight of about 62K, which is released from certain strains and lines of cultured fibroblasts. It affects the mobility, morphology, and cell to cell attachment of epithelial cells in culture and there is some evidence of an effect on early embryo development. Fibroblasts are unaffected by the factor and there is a negligible effect on cell growth. The scatter factor differs from a similar agent, the autocrine motility factor, in its paracrine role, its lack of association with tumour cells, and in some biochemical features, but both may be representatives of a group of cytokines which regulate cell motility.

This article has a very doubtful claim to inclusion in an issue of the British Medical Bulletin devoted to growth factors, because it is mostly about agents which have little or no effect on growth. Our particular concern is with the agent termed scatter factor which affects cell movement and topography, especially in cultures of epithelial cells, and which, since it is derived from cultured fibroblastic cells, appears to be involved in the phenomenon of mesenchymal epithelial interaction. Nevertheless, we cannot rule out the possibility that cell movement may play a part in growth regulation. Thus one of the first growth factors to be discovered, nerve growth factor (NGF), affects movement and outgrowth of neurites, while epidermal growth factor (EGF) apparently stimulates epithelial cell movement besides growth,[1,2] and platelet-derived growth factor (PDGF) is strongly chemotactic.[3]

Although we shall concentrate on the scatter factor, we will also discuss other motility factors, and in particular the autocrine motility factor (AMF) isolated from certain tumour cells by Liotta and his colleagues.[4] We will not however consider the extensive studies on motility of circulating cells such as granulocytes and macrophages.

SCATTER FACTOR

Our studies stemmed from the observation that conditioned medium from human embryo fibroblasts promoted clonal growth of human mammary epithelium as colonies of scattered cells, quite unlike the colonies of tightly adjoining cells which grew in conditioned medium from other cell types. Existing sheets of joined cells were also scattered when exposed to embryo fibroblast medium.[5] The effect of this medium was not limited to human mammary epithelium, however, and other epithelial cells from different species were found to be sensitive to the scattering activity.[6] In particular the MDCK line of dog kidney cells, was particularly responsive and was used for a simple multiwell plate assay giving arbitrary activity units (Fig. 1). With this assay it was found that in addition to embryo fibroblasts (human and mouse) some variants of the mouse 3T3 cell lines released the activity. Several of these cell lines produced about 500 units of scattering activity per million cells over 48 hours, but for regular production of conditioned medium for purification, a fast growing ras oncogene transformed NIH 3T3 cell line has been used as a regular source.

PURIFICATION AND CHARACTERISTICS OF SCATTER FACTOR

The scatter factor activity is due to a protein with a M_r of about 50K as determined by gel filtration chromatography in the presence of guanidinium chloride. The activity requires intact disulphide bonds, and is lost at 60°C for 30 minutes.

Purification of scatter factor from the medium conditioned by ras transformed NIH 3T3 cells has recently been achieved by a combination of ion exchange and reverse phase chromatography. The final preparation has a specific activity in the order of 1 unit per ng in the MDCK assay, and shows one major band in non-reducing SDS gels with a M_r of about 62K, from which the scatter activity can be recovered by elution.

SCATTER FACTOR AND REGULATORS OF MOTILITY 483

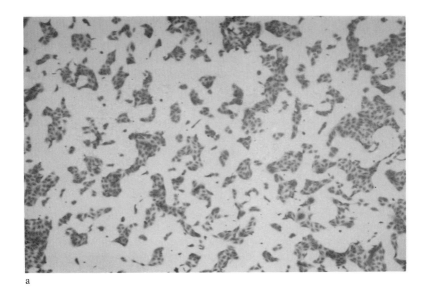

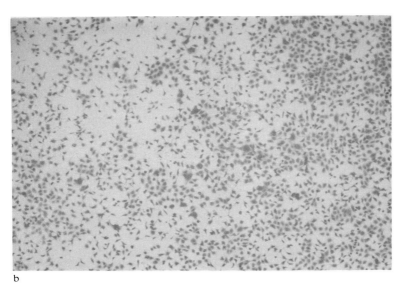

Fig. 1 Assay of scatter factor using MDCK in 96 well plate: (a) well without addition; and (b) well with partially purified scatter factor, 1000 units (approx. 1 µg). Giemsa stain × 130.

ACTION OF SCATTER FACTOR ON EPITHELIAL CELLS

The effects of scatter factor, either in native conditioned medium or after purification, may be observed on isolated epithelial cells or on sheets with intact junctions. Thus after exposure of MDCK cells to the factor, isolated cells and those in small islands rapidly change from the normal 'poached egg' or rounded morphology into a multipolar form with extensive ruffling and pseudopodia, which extend and retract very rapidly (Fig. 2). Though this form of local movement is greatly increased, distant translocation is still restricted, apparently by anchorage to the substrate. Enhanced motility can also be measured by penetration of filters in Boyden chambers. This enhanced penetration is markedly dose dependent, with a maximal effect at 30 to 100 units per ml but diminishing at higher concentrations. Movement is enhanced more by exposure of the cells to a gradient than to a uniform concentration of scatter factor, indicating some chemotactic as well as a chemokinetic effect.

When intact, confluent, sheets of cells are exposed to the factor, there may be no obvious change in cell morphology. If there is free space around the cells, however, as at the edge of an isolated colony, the area of the colony and of its constituent cells begin to increase a few minutes after exposure. There is at first no change in cell shape, or loss of junctional contact, but about 6 hours after exposure, cell separation occurs, with the subsequent morphological changes described above for individual cells. The expansion of the cell sheet and rapid invasion of adjoining free space, may also be seen when the scatter factor is added to freshly wounded confluent cells, resulting in increased emigration from the wound edge. Finally, in confluent sheets of secretory epithelium, which form domes either spontaneously or after induction, the factor inhibits or delays the formation of these structures.

The changes observed with MDCK cells are also found in various degrees with most other normal epithelial cells which have been tested. But the effects vary with different cell types, some mainly showing centrifugal colony expansion, others a more obvious change in cell morphology. The few cell types tested so far in Boyden chambers all show increased motility when exposed to the factor.

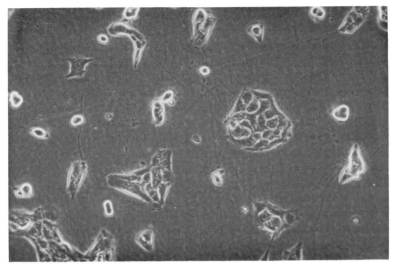

a

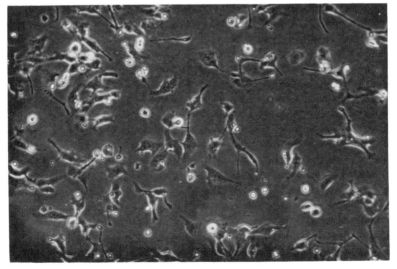

b

Fig. 2 Morphology of MDCK cells: (a) without addition; and (b) 24 hours after addition of partially purified scatter factor, 1000 units (approximately 1 µg). Phase contrast × 640.

SCATTER FACTOR AND FIBROBLASTS

When scatter factor is added to cultured fibroblasts no obvious change in behaviour is seen either in morphology or in movement of isolated cells, or those at the edges of colonies or wounded cell sheets. Fibroblasts unlike epithelial cells have a high spontaneous rate of penetration through Boyden chamber filters, and the presence of the scatter factor has hardly any additional effect. However, the apparent lack of action of the factor on fibroblasts and some other cell types is difficult to assess. This is because such cells are often bipolar or multipolar, with high motility rates compared to epithelial cells, and they do not form the tightly adherent sheets of cells in which scattering can be observed.

Fibroblasts indeed behave in many ways like epithelial cells exposed to scatter factor, and one may ask if their behaviour is due in part to an endogenous or autocrine effect of scatter factor or a related molecule. Some fibroblasts release the factor but others do not, and there is no correlation with their morphology or motility. This does not exclude the possibility of an intracellular autocrine loop, or perhaps more likely, constitutive expression in fibroblasts but not epithelial cells, of pathways affecting shape and motility through which the scatter factor may act.

SCATTER FACTOR AND GROWTH

As already mentioned PDGF is chemotactic as well as mitogenic, and EGF can also affect movement as well as growth. So is the scatter factor simply another growth factor which happens to stimulate movement as well? The characteristics of the molecule already suggest that it is not one of the known growth factors. Conditioned medium containing scatter activity did originally increase the cloning efficiency of mammary epithelial cells, but scattering of MDCK cells was accompanied by only slight inhibition of growth, and this was lost on purification, and was presumably due to another substance. Although thymidine incorporation is slightly increased by purified factor in certain experimental conditions, we have been unable to detect any regular enhancement of a number of MDCK cells exposed to the scatter factor in association with the increased motility, nor is there stimulation of growth of 3T3 cells.

SPECIFICITY OF ACTION

Some 60 cell strains and lines from different sources have been examined for release of scatter factor and sensitivity to its action.[7] In general normal epithelial cells, whether freshly isolated or as continuous lines, respond to the factor by one or more of the changes described above. None of these responsive epithelial cells release detectable scatter factor.

Established lines from epithelial tumours, mostly mammary, have been unresponsive, and are also non yielders. They include (otherwise responsive) mammary epithelium transformed by SV40 virus. Nevertheless some recent observations have shown that cells from chemically induced rat mammary and liver tumours do retain some sensitivity to the factor as do SV40 transformed mouse keratinocytes, and chemically transformed bladder epithelial cells.

Fibroblastic cells, both freshly isolated and as cell lines, are, as noted above, unresponsive to added factor. On the other hand, some fibroblasts release substantial quantities of the factor (500 units per million cells). These include cell strains from embryos, human and mouse, and some variants of Swiss mouse cell lines, such as the NIH 3T3 line. Other fibroblastic cell lines from mice and hamsters, and freshly isolated fibroblasts derived postnatally from humans of varying ages, including some with epithelial cancers, release no detectable factor (less than 5 units per million cells). We do not yet know whether any of these cells synthesise the factor without releasing it.

One may well ask whether the scatter factor is simply a product of laboratory culture without relevance to the living animal. Recently however we have found that fetal calf serum contains the factor. Its action is apparently blocked in the native serum, since it would otherwise interfere with various assay systems in which the serum is present. But ion exchange chromatography allows isolation of the active factor or a related molecule. Interestingly, similarly treated postnatal calf serum contains little or no activity, possibly connected with the absence of factor production by cultured postnatal cells.

EFFECT ON EMBRYONIC DEVELOPMENT

The source of scatter factor in fetal cells and fetal serum, has suggested a possible importance in embryonic development, and has led to collaborative research on the developing chick embryo with Dr C Stern and Dr G Ireland in Oxford.[8] So far it has been found that when fibroblasts which release the factor are implantated near the early primitive streak a second primitive streak and/or neural plate develops, while implantation of non-releasing cells has no effect. Currently partially purified scatter factor, bound to beads, is being implanted into the early embryos, and preliminary results show the same effect (C. D. Stern and G. W. Grenham, unpublished observations). The role of scatter factor in normal embryogenesis must now be further investigated—for example by attempts to influence development with antibody to the factor.

REGULATION OF MOTILITY

It is hardly necessary to emphasize the importance of regulation of cell movement, and consequently cell position, starting with the very earliest stages of fetal development, and continuing in processes of reconstruction and repair, inflammation, and tumour invasion in adult life. Cell movement is imperfectly understood but is thought to occur by forward protrusion of lamellae displaying adhesion plaques. These plaques are linked to the main skeletal proteins of the cell, which are presumably involved in the transfer of the cell mass.

Studies at various research centres have shown that cell movement can be regulated at different levels. For example there is ample evidence of the important roles of the substrates such as laminin, fibronectin, vitronectin and collagen, and their cellular receptors, the integrins, in direction movement.[9] There is also evidence of the importance of cell adhesion molecules (CAMs)[10] which provide for specificity of interaction of different cell types and which must surely affect movement as well as topography. Movement of epithelial cells is particularly limited by their specialized junctional systems, which are known to be affected, for example, by calcium ions.

MOTILITY FACTORS

In addition there is now evidence that cell mobility, like growth and differentiation, may be affected by cytokines, or hormone like factors, freely circulating in the external environment of the cells. The first evidence of such factors came from Yoshida and colleagues in 1970[11] who showed that certain metastatic tumour cells released an activity which increased their mobility. Subsequently, as already mentioned, Liotta and his colleagues have isolated a protein released by melanoma and certain other metastatic tumour cells, which is capable of increasing the ability of the same cells to penetrate Boyden chamber filters.[4] This factor, appropriately named the autocrine motility factor (AMF) is similar to a factor obtained by Nicholson and his colleagues from breast tumour cells.[12] The AMF may turn out to be of great importance if its expression and release by tumour cells is at least in part responsible for their ability to migrate and penetrate the normal surrounding tissue. Whether the factor has a role in normal regulation of movement is not yet reported.

The scatter factor is another hormone-like agent which affects cell movement, and Table 1 shows a comparison of its main characteristics with AMF and with two growth factors, EGF and PDGF, which also affect cell movement. Table 1 shows that the scatter factor differs from these other motility factors, and in particular from AMF both in molecular weight and biological activity.

Whether or not scatter factor and AMF are members of a related group, there is an intriguing difference in the cell specificity of these two agents. The AMF is autocrine because the factor acts on the cells that produce it. The scatter factor on the other hand is paracrine in that the producer cells and the target cells are distinct. Moreover its derivation from fibroblasts, and its action on epithelial cells, suggest that it is a mediator of mesenchymal-epithelial interaction. In contrast to AMF there is as yet no evidence to suggest a role in neoplasia, but this cannot be ruled out at present, nor can a possible role in tissue repair processes—for example following epithelial wounds.

The mechanism by which these factors affect motility is as yet

Table 1 Characteristics of some cytokines affecting cell motility

	Scattering of MDCK cells	M_r
Scatter factor	+	62K
AMF	−	55K (Ref 4)
EGF	−	6K (Ref. 14)
PDGF	−	30K (Ref. 15)

The M_r indicated for scatter factor, AMF and PDGF is from non-reducing SDS gels. The AMF used in the MDCK assay was a sample of serum-free conditioned medium of human A2058 melanoma cells kindly supplied by Dr L Liotta. Purified EGF and PDGF were kindly supplied by Drs S Cohen and R Ross, respectively.

unclear. It seems unlikely that the scatter factor, for example, constitutes a substrate for cell adhesion, since it is active at picomolar concentrations, where it would not provide a sufficient density of binding sites. It does not simply remove epithelial junction proteins of the zonula occludens or desmosomes because it can act on single cells. The factor also acts independently of calcium concentration, and there is no evidence that it is a protease. It is perhaps most likely that the motility factors act directly on the cells, probably via specific receptors, and that they alter the ability of the cells to respond to substrate binding via the adhesion plaques and the associated cytoskeletal assemblies. Indeed it has already been reported that AMF may affect the distribution of fibronectin binding sites on the pseudopodia of affected cells.[13]

In this article we have described an endogenous factor which affects mobility and topography of epithelial cells in culture, and have discussed its relationship to other motility factors. They may represent a new group of cytokines, which could play an important role in normal development and in pathological conditions. Indeed, we respectfully suggest that they may one day be almost as important as the growth factors which are the subject of this issue of the Bulletin.

REFERENCES

1 Blay J, Brown KD. Epidermal growth factor promotes the chemotactic migration of cultured rat intestinal epithelial cells. J Cell Physiol 1985; 124: 107–112.
2 Barrandon Y, Green, H. Cell migration is essential for sustained growth of keratinocyte colonies: the role of transforming growth factors- and epidermal growth factor. Cell 1987; 50: 1131–1137.
3 Grotendorst GR, Seppa HEJ, Kleinman HK, Martin GR. Attachment of smooth muscle cells to collagen and their migration toward platelet-derived growth factor. Proc Natl Acad Sci USA 1981; 78: 3669–3672.
4 Liotta LA, Mandler R, Murano G, Katz DA, Gordon RK, Chiang PK, Schiffmann E. Tumour cell autocrine motility factor. Proc Natl Acad Sci USA 1986; 83: 3302–3306.
4 Stoker M, Junctional competence in clones of mammary epithelial cells and modulation by conditioned medium. J Cell Physiol 1984; 121: 174–183.
5 Stoker M, Perryman M. An epithelial scatter factor released by embryo fibroblasts. J Cell Sci 1985; 77: 209–223.
6 Stoker M, Gherardi E. Factors affecting epithelial interactions. In: Junctional complexes of epithelial cells (Ciba Foundation Symposium 125). Chichester: Wiley, 1987; p. 219.
7 Stoker M, Gherardi E, Perryman M, Gray J. Scatter factor is a fibroblast-derived modulator of epithelial cell mobility. Nature 1987; 327: 239–242.
8 Ireland GW, Stern CD, Stoker M. Human MRC5 cells induce a secondary primitive streak when grafted into chick embryos. J Anat 1987; 152: 223–224.
9 Ruoslahti E, Pierschbacher MD. New perspectives in cell adhesion: RGD and integrins. Science 1987; 238: 491–497.

10 Edelman GM. Cell adhesion molecules in the regulation of animal form and tissue pattern. Ann Rev Cell Biol 1986; 2: 81–116.
11 Yoshida K, Ozaki T, Ushijima K, Hayashi H. Studies on the mechanisms of invasion in cancer. I. isolation and purification of a factor chemotactic for cancer cells. Int J Cancer 1970; 6: 123–132.
12 Atnip KD, Carter LM, Nicolson GL, Dabbous MK. Chemotactic response of rat mammary adenocarcinoma cell clones to tumour-derived cytokines. Biochem Biophys Res Commun 1987; 146: 996–1002.
13 Guirguis R, Margulies I, Taraboletti G, Schiffmann E, Liotta L. Cytokine-induced pseudopodial protrusion is coupled to tumour cell migration. Nature 1987; 329: 261–263.
14 Taylor JM, Mitchell WM, Cohen S. Epidermal growth factor: physical and chemical properties. J Biol Chem 1972; 247: 5928–5934.
15 Heldin K-H, Westermark B, Wasteson A. Platelet-derived growth factor, purification and partial characterization. Proc Natl Acad Sci USA 1979; 76: 3722–3726.

Neuropeptides as growth regulators

Penella J Woll
Enrique Rozengurt
Growth Regulation Laboratory, Imperial Cancer Research Fund, Lincoln's Inn Fields, London, UK

> The classical role of neuropeptides as fast-acting neurohumoral signallers has recently been challenged by the discovery that many neuropeptides are also growth factors stimulating slow-acting mitogenesis. Their mechanisms of action have been studied in cell culture, and their cell-surface receptors have been characterized pharmacologically using agonists and antagonists. We describe the mitogenic effects of bombesin, vasopressin, bradykinin and vasoactive intestinal peptide in murine fibroblasts. We suggest that the receptors for bombesin, vasopressin and bradykinin have more than one binding site, permitting modulation of transmitted signals. As these neuropeptide receptors share the ability to mobilize intracellular Ca^{2+}, their common domain may be essential to G-protein coupling.

Cells in a living organism exist in a dynamic equilibrium. In most tissues cell turnover is slow, with the majority of cells viable and metabolically active but in a non-proliferating state. Many cells, however, retain the capacity to respond, by division, to extracellular signals such as hormones, antigens and growth factors. Thus the growth of individual cells is regulated according to the functional requirements of the organism. These conditions can be simulated in vitro using cell culture techniques, and we have found mouse fibroblasts (Swiss 3T3 cells) a particularly useful model. Confluent cultures of these cells cease to proliferate when they deplete the medium of its growth-promoting activity and can be stimulated to resume DNA synthesis and cell division by the addition of serum or defined growth factors. In addition to the polypeptide growth factors (including platelet-derived growth factor, PDGF; epidermal growth factor, EGF) and pharmacological agents (such as phorbol esters, diacylglycerol), increasing numbers of neuropeptides have been shown to act as growth factors (see Ref. 1 for review).

Neuropeptides are small regulatory peptides localized in neurones of the central and peripheral nervous system. They are classically released by electrical stimulation and may act on postganglionic receptors (neurotransmitters), nearby cells (paracrine hormones) or distant target organs (endocrine hormones). These types of signal elicit a rapid response, such as the secretion of pancreatic amylase stimulated by bombesin. This contrasts with the long-term response of mitogenesis. The variety among neuropeptides and the diversity of their effects suggests a rich network of control, permitting fine homeostatic adjustments. We have tested a wide variety of neuropeptides for growth promoting activity in Swiss 3T3 cells (Table 1), and here we describe those found to be mitogenic and characterize their receptors using antagonists. We suggest that the receptors for the Ca^{2+}-mobilizing mitogenic neuropeptides have more than one binding site, allowing modulation of the transmitted signal.

Table 1 Neuropeptides tested for growth-promoting activity in Swiss 3T3 cells[*]

Mitogenic	Non-mitogenic
Bombesin-like peptides	[Ser^1,Thr^8]angiotensin II
bombesin	atrial natriuretic peptide
GRP	atriopeptin I
litorin	atriopeptin II
neuromedin B	atriopeptin III
neuromedin C	cholecystokinin
	dynorphin A
Vasopressin	α-endorphin
	[Leu^5]-enkephalin
Bradykinin	galanin
	gastric inhibitory polypeptide
VIP	gastrin
	neurotensin
PHI	physalaemin
	serotonin
	substance P

[*]Peptides were tested in assays of DNA synthesis[4] alone and with insulin, at concentrations ranging from 0.1 ng/ml to 10 μg/ml[27]

BOMBESIN

Bombesin is a 14-amino acid peptide first isolated from the skin of the European frog *Bombina bombina* (Table 2). Structurally-related peptides are found in other amphibians (ranatensin, alytesin, litorin) and mammals (gastrin-releasing peptide, GRP; neuromedin B; neuromedin C). The functions of these peptides in amphibians remain obscure, but they have been extensively studied in mammals. Bombesin-like peptides are found in the central and peripheral nervous systems, principally in the intrinsic neurones of the gut.[2] Here they have secretory effects, stimulating the release of gastrin and cholecystokinin from the gut and pancreas.[3]

Bombesin is a potent mitogen for Swiss 3T3 cells.[4] In serum-free medium it stimulates DNA synthesis and cell division in the absence of other growth-promoting agents. The ability of bombesin, like PDGF, to act as a sole mitogen for these cells contrasts with other growth factors which are active only in synergistic combinations.[5] The mitogenic effects of bombesin are markedly potentiated by insulin, which both increases the maximal response and reduces the bombesin concentration required for half-maximal effect from 1nM to 0.3nM. The other bombesin-like peptides, including GRP, have similar mitogenic effects (Table 1).

Bombesin-like peptides are abundant in human fetal lung and the mRNA for GRP is maximally expressed at 16–30 weeks gestation.[6] Thereafter levels decline rapidly, and in adulthood these peptides are found sparsely in bronchial neuroendocrine cells. Speculation that bombesins may be growth factors for fetal lung has been supported by their paucity of expression in the

Table 2 Structural formulae of the neuropeptides bombesin, vasopressin, bradykinin and VIP

Bombesin:
pGlu-Gln-Arg-Leu-Gly-Asn-Gln-Trp-Ala-Val-Gly-His-Leu-Met-NH$_2$

Vasopressin:

┌─────────────────────────┐
Cys-Tyr-Phe-Gln-Asn-Cys-Pro-Arg-Gly-NH$_2$

Bradykinin:
Arg-Pro-Pro-Gly-Phe-Ser-Pro-Phe-Arg

VIP:
His-Ser-Asp-Ala-Val-Phe-Thr-Asp-Asn-Tyr-Thr-Arg-Leu-Arg-Lys-Gln-Met-Ala-Val-Lys-Lys-Tyr-Leu-Asn-Ser-Ile-Leu-Asn-NH$_2$

immature lungs of infants with respiratory distress syndrome.[7] Human small cell lung cancers (SCLC) are rich in bombesin-like peptides, which may act as autocrine growth factors for these tumours.[8]

Bombesin receptors

To determine how bombesin/GRP stimulates mitogenesis, we sought specific receptors on Swiss 3T3 cells, using radiolabelled [^{125}I]GRP. This binds to the quiescent cells in a specific, saturable and reversible manner.[9] Scatchard analysis indicates the presence of a single class of high-affinity sites of K_d about 1nM and about 1.25×10^5 binding sites per cell. [^{125}I]GRP binding is not inhibited by other mitogens for Swiss 3T3 cells including PDGF, fibroblast-derived growth factor, EGF, insulin or the neuropeptides vasopressin, bradykinin, vasoactive intestinal peptide (VIP) and substance P. Various bombesin-like peptides inhibit [^{125}I]GRP binding in proportion to their ability to stimulate DNA synthesis, suggesting that the receptors are specific and distinct from those for other mitogens. The possibility that different subtypes of bombesin receptor exist in different tissues, perhaps mediating different functions, is attracting interest,[10] but is at present unresolved.

We have investigated the physical properties of the bombesin/GRP receptor in Swiss 3T3 cells using an affinity-labelling method. Quiescent cells were incubated with [^{125}I]GRP then treated with disuccinimidyl cross-linking agents. The cells were then solubilized and the extracts electrophoresed on a polyacrylamide gel. A major band was seen migrating with apparent M_r 75 000–85 000.[11] This M_r 75 000–85 000 protein was not found in cell lines lacking bombesin receptor. Its expression was inhibited by the addition of unlabelled GRP in a dose-dependent manner, but not by other hormones or mitogens, supporting the conclusion that the M_r 75 000–85 000 protein is a component of the bombesin receptor. A solubilized preparation of the radiolabelled protein binds to wheatgerm lectin/sepharose columns and can be eluted with N-acetyl-D-glucosamine, suggesting that it is a glycoprotein. In addition, treatment with endo-β-N-acetyl glycosaminidase F reduced the M_r of the affinity-labelled band from 75 000–85 000 to 42 000, indicating the presence of N-linked oligosaccharide groups.[12] Thus the bombesin/GRP receptor appears to be a glycoprotein of M_r 75 000–85 000 with N-linked carbohydrate side-chains and a protein core of M_r 42 000. This would be consistent with a receptor of the type recently described for substance K[13] and serotonin (5-hydroxytryptamine).[14]

The binding of polypeptide growth factors such as EGF and PDGF to their receptors is followed by rapid internalization and intracellular degradation of receptor and ligand. This causes a marked reduction in the number of cell-surface binding sites (down-regulation). We have shown that, unlike these, bombesin does not cause down-regulation of its receptor. Exposure of cells to mitogenic concentrations of bombesin for up to 24 hours does not alter the number of binding sites or the affinity cross-linking of the M_r 75 000–85 000 component of the receptor.[15] Thus receptor down-regulation is not necessary for mitogenic signalling.

The binding of bombesin to its receptor elicits an array of signals in the membrane, cytosol and nucleus, leading to cell proliferation.[5] These are described elsewhere in this volume (*see* Rozengurt, this Issue).

VASOPRESSIN

Vasopressin exemplifies neurohumoral control mechanisms. The cyclic nonapeptide (Table 2) is secreted in the hypothalamus and then passes down neural axons to the posterior pituitary before being released into the circulation. As an endocrine hormone it has antidiuretic effects on the kidney, pressor effects mediated through arteriolar smooth muscle, and stimulates hepatic glycogenolysis. Vasopressin is a mitogen in vitro for Swiss 3T3 cells[16] at nanomolar concentrations, acting synergistically with insulin. In vivo it facilitates the proliferative responses to haemorrhage[17] and partial hepatectomy.[18] It has also been implicated in the control of brain development in fetal rats.[19]

The mechanism of the growth promoting effects of vasopressin in Swiss 3T3 cells has been studied in detail in our laboratory. Vasopressin binds to specific, high-affinity receptors[20] and elicits an array of biological responses including Ca^{2+} mobilization, inositol phosphate production, activation of protein kinase C, accumulation of cAMP and c-*fos* oncogene induction (*see* Rozengurt, this Issue).

Two types of vasopressin receptor have been distinguished functionally and pharmacologically. The V_1 receptor mediates the vascular and hepatic effects of vasopressin by activating Ca^{2+}-dependent inositol phosphate turnover. In contrast, V_2

receptors are coupled to adenylate cyclase and mediate the antidiuretic response of the kidney. Recently, subtypes of these receptors have been identified in other tissues including adenohypophysis[21] and mammary tumour cell lines.[22] The receptors present in Swiss 3T3 cells, which mediate a mitogenic response, are of the V_1 type[23] which is blocked by the antagonist [1-(β-mercapto-β, β-cyclopentamethylene propionic acid), 2-(0-methyl)tyrosine]Arg^8-vasopressin (denoted by [Pmp^1, OMeTyr^2,Arg^8]vasopressin).[24] As yet the molecular structure of these receptors is unknown.

BRADYKININ

The nonapeptide bradykinin (Table 2) is generated in the circulation, particularly at sites of tissue damage. It is one of the most potent pain-producing substances known and bradykinin receptors are localized to the nocioceptive sensory pathways.[25] In addition, bradykinin mediates smooth muscle contraction, vasodilation and vascular permeability. It has been shown to be a weak mitogen for human fibroblasts[26] and we have recently demonstrated that it is also a potent mitogen for Swiss 3T3 cells.[27] Acting synergistically with insulin, bradykinin achieves a response at 10nM with insulin equivalent to that obtained with serum. Like bombesin and vasopressin, its effects in Swiss 3T3 cells are mediated in part by rapid Ca^{2+} mobilization.

Many synthetic bradykinin analogues have been used as agonists and antagonists to classify bradykinin receptors in various tissues and species.[28] B_1 and B_2 receptor types have been distinguished pharmacologically, although there is no clear functional separation. It now appears that the B_2 receptors can be further divided into subtypes.[29,30] The receptor mediating mitogenesis in Swiss 3T3 cells is a B_2 subtype as shown by the effectiveness of the antagonist [DArg^0,Hyp^3,Thi^{5,8}, DPhe^7]bradykinin but the absence of the effect of [desArg^9,Leu^8]bradykinin and [Thi^{5,8},DPhe^7]bradykinin.[27]

VASOACTIVE INTESTINAL PEPTIDE (VIP)

This 28-amino acid polypeptide (Table 2) is closely related to secretin, glucagon, PHI (porcine histidine, isoleucine amide-containing peptide) and PHM (peptide histidine methionine). It is found in large amounts in the mammalian brain and in the mucosa and muscle of the gastrointestinal tract, where it is localized to postganglionic nerves. In addition it is found in the salivary glands, pancreas, respiratory and urogenital tracts.[31] Neural stimulation causes release of VIP, which binds to specific receptors that can also bind the related hormones with lower affinity. In Swiss 3T3 cells, VIP stimulates mitogenesis in the presence of insulin and cAMP phosphodiesterase inhibitors. In contrast to bombesin, vasopressin and bradykinin, VIP is a weak mitogen, and its effects are mediated by the elevation of cAMP without Ca^{2+} mobilization or protein kinase C activation.[32] We have found that the related polypeptide PHI can also act as a mitogen for these cells.

NEUROPEPTIDE RECEPTOR ANTAGONISTS

The three mitogenic neuropeptides bombesin, vasopressin and bradykinin share the ability to mobilize Ca^{2+} in Swiss 3T3 cells. It is therefore important to determine whether they bind to a common or different receptors. Binding studies using radiolabelled ligands have shown that GRP does not interfere with [^{3}H]vasopressin binding, nor does vasopressin interfere with [^{125}I]GRP binding to Swiss 3T3 cells.[24] We have also shown that bradykinin has no effect on either [^{3}H]vasopressin binding or [^{125}I]GRP binding[27] suggesting that the three mitogens have distinct receptors in these cells. Further evidence in support of this contention has been provided using ligand analogues that can act as specific antagonists for each of these three mitogens.

[Leu^{13}-ψ(CH$_2$NH)Leu^{14}]bombesin belongs to a new class of peptide analogues in which a peptide bond in the backbone has been reduced to produce a closely-related 'pseudopeptide'.[33] This analogue has no agonist activity, but is a potent bombesin antagonist both in short-term assays of pancreatic cell secretion[33] and in long-term assays of mitogenesis.[34] It is effective against other bombesin-like peptides including GRP and litorin but is ineffective against other growth factors, including vasopressin and bradykinin (Fig. 1).

The vasopressin analogue [Pmp^1,OMeTyr^2,Arg^8]vasopressin is a potent V_1-receptor antagonist active against both the vasopressor and mitogenic effects[24] of vasopressin mediated through the V_1 receptor. It is a specific vasopressin antagonist showing no inhibition of GRP or bradykinin-induced mitogenesis (Fig. 1).

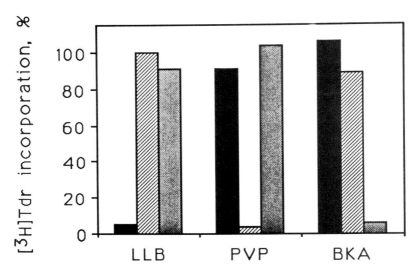

Fig. 1 Effects of ligand-specific antagonists on DNA synthesis stimulated by GRP, vasopressin and bradykinin. Quiescent cultures of Swiss 3T3 cells were incubated in Dulbecco's modified Eagle's/Waymouth medium containing [^{3}H]thymidine ([^{3}H]Tdr) 1μCi/ml and insulin 1μg/ml with GRP 3.6 nM (■), vasopressin 14 nM (▨) or bradykinin 9.4 nM (▩) and the antagonists indicated. LLB = [Leu^{13}-ψ(CH$_2$NH)Leu^{14}]bombesin   1μM;   PVP = [Pmp^1,OMeTyr^2, Arg^8]vasopressin 20 nM; BKA = [DArg^0, Hyp^3,Thi^{5,8}, DPhe^7]bradykinin 210 nM. DNA synthesis was estimated by incorporation of [^{3}H]Tdr into acid precipitable material.[4] Values represent the mean of at least 2 determinations (100% = 4.4 × 10^5 cpm).

The bradykinin analogue [DArg^0,Hyp^3,Thi^{5,8},DPhe^7]bradykinin is a B$_2$-receptor antagonist active in assays both of vascular permeability and mitogenesis.[27] It shows no cross-reactivity against mitogenesis stimulated by GRP or vasopressin (Fig. 1). The demonstration of ligand-specific antagonists for each of these mitogens strongly supports the view that they have distinct receptors in Swiss 3T3 cells.

Common antagonists

The tachykinin substance P has minimal amino acid homology with bombesin and neither inhibits the binding of [^{125}I]GRP nor stimulates DNA synthesis in Swiss 3T3 cells. Unexpectedly, the substance P antagonist [DArg^1,DPro^2,DTrp^{7,9},Leu^{11}]substance P was found to block the secretory effects of bombesin in pancreatic acinar cells, and subsequently, to reversibly block the mitogenic effects of both bombesin and vasopressin in Swiss 3T3 cells (Fig. 2).[9,24,35] The binding of both [^{125}I]GRP and [^{3}H]vasopressin are inhibited in a dose-dependent and competitive manner, and all the early events leading to mitogenesis with each ligand are blocked. [DArg^1,DPhe^5,DTrp^{7,9},Leu^{11}]substance P has now been shown to be consistently 5–10 fold more potent than [DArg^1,DPro^2,DTrp^{7,9},Leu^{11}]substance P, with similar activity against the mitogenic effects of bombesin and vasopressin (Fig. 2).[35] On discovering that bradykinin is also mitogenic for Swiss 3T3 cells, we tested [DArg^1,DPhe^5,DTrp^{7,9},Leu^{11}]substance P for inhibitory effects against this mitogen[27] (Fig. 2). Bradykinin induced mitogenesis is inhibited by both substance P antagonists in a competitive and reversible manner. Moreover, [DArg^1,DPhe^5,DTrp^{7,9},Leu^{11}]substance P is 5–10 fold more potent than [DArg^1,DPro^2,DTrp^{7,9},Leu^{11}]substance P in inhibiting bradykinin-induced mitogenesis.

These findings imply that the substance P antagonists can block the mitogenic effects of three neuropeptides at their distinct receptors, although they have no effect on mitogenesis induced by a wide range of other mitogens including polypeptide growth factors and pharmacological agents.[27] The observation that the two substance P antagonists have a consistent difference in potency against each mitogen suggests that they recognize a common domain in the three receptors. This putative shared domain must be separate from the ligand binding site because the ligands are structurally unrelated (Table 2) and the ligand-specific antagonists show no cross-reactivity.

The substance P antagonists show no inhibitory activity against VIP-induced mitogenesis. VIP differs from bombesin, vasopressin and bradykinin in its signalling pathway — it does not mobilize Ca^{2+} or activate protein kinase C, but acts by stimulating cAMP accumulation.[32] In view of this, it is tempting to speculate that the substance P antagonists recognize a domain common to the bombesin, vasopressin and bradykinin receptors that is essential to the coupling of G-proteins required for Ca^{2+} mobilization.

SMALL CELL LUNG CANCER (SCLC)

Lung cancer is the commonest fatal malignancy in the developed world. SCLC constitutes 25% of lung cancers; it follows an aggressive course and, despite being initially chemosensitive, only

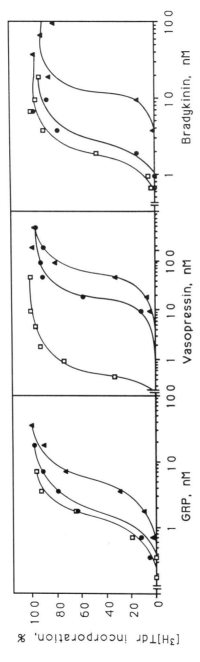

Fig. 2 Effects of substance P antagonists on DNA synthesis stimulated by GRP, vasopressin and bradykinin. DNA synthesis was estimated (as in Fig. 1) in the presence of [^{3}H]Tdr 1μCi/ml; insulin 1μg/ml and the mitogens indicated, in the absence (□) or presence of [DArg^1,DPro^2,DTrp^{7,9},Leu^{11}]substance P 20μM (●) or [DArg^1,DPhe^5,DTr^{7,9},Leu^{11}]substance P 20μM (▲). Values represent the mean of 2 determinations. (100% = 8.24 × 10^5 cpm).

5% of patients survive 2 years after diagnosis. These tumours are associated with ectopic production of many hormones including vasopressin, adrenocorticotrophin (ACTH) and bombesin, causing characteristic clinical syndromes. Bombesin-like peptides are found in specimens of SCLC and secreted by SCLC cell lines in vitro.[37] In view of the potent growth-promoting effects of bombesin in Swiss 3T3 cells, we suggested that it might be an autocrine growth factor for SCLC.[4] This was substantiated by Cuttitta et al.,[8] who demonstrated that a monoclonal antibody to bombesin could inhibit the growth of SCLC cell lines in vitro and in nude mice. We have now shown that [DArg^1,DPro^2,DTrp^{7,9}, Leu^{11}]substance P and [DArg^1,DPhe^5,DTrp^{7,9},Leu^{11}]substance P can reversibly inhibit the growth of SCLC cell lines in vitro[36] with relatively little effect on non-SCLC lung tumour cell lines.[38] It is not yet known whether this results from blockade of bombesin receptors or those of another secreted neuropeptide.

DISCUSSION

There is accumulating evidence that many neuropeptides can act as growth factors including not only those detailed here, but also substance P, substance K, β-endorphin and gastrin (see Ref. 1 for review). This appears to be a general phenomenon and suggests that these peptides have multiple signalling actions, fast and slow, throughout the body. In this way proliferative responses might be subjected to fine co-ordination. For example, release of bradykinin at sites of tissue damage might mediate a proliferative wound healing response in addition to transmitting pain sensation. In this context, the model of a neuropeptide receptor with two binding sites, described here, offers interesting possibilities for the modulation of transmitted signals. A similar model has been developed for the N-methyl-D-aspartate receptors.[39]

As the molecular structures of the receptors for bombesin, vasopressin and bradykinin are as yet unknown, it is not possible to predict the nature of the proposed common binding sites. We have been able to define the receptors pharmacologically and to establish the apparent M_r and physical composition of the bombesin receptor. The available evidence is consistent with receptors of a type increasingly described for neuropeptides. cDNA cloning of the adrenergic, muscarinic, rhodopsin, substance K and serotonin receptors shows a remarkable degree of amino acid homology between them. They are glycoproteins of core M_r 40 000–50 000 which are thought to traverse the cytoplasmic membrane seven times. The transmembrane loops are clustered to form a ligand-binding pocket. Most interestingly, each appears to be coupled to Ca^{2+}-mobilizing G-proteins.[40,41] The availability of specific and common antagonists such as those we have described will be invaluable in defining the structure-function relationships of neuropeptides and their receptors. It is also possible to envisage therapeutic applications for such antagonists in the treatment of SCLC.

ACKNOWLEDGEMENT

We thank Theresa Higgins for expert assistance.

REFERENCES

1 Zachary I, Woll PJ, Rozengurt E. A role for neuropeptides in the control of cell proliferation. Dev Biol 1987; 124: 295–308
2 Panula P. Histochemistry and function of bombesin-like peptides. Med Biol 1986; 64: 177–192
3 Knigge U, Holst JJ, Knuhtsen S et al. Gastrin-releasing peptide: pharmacokinetics and effects on gastro-entero-pancreatic hormones and gastric secretion in normal men. J Clin Endocrinol Metab 1984; 59: 310–315
4 Rozengurt E, Sinnett-Smith J. Bombesin stimulation of DNA synthesis and cell division in cultures of Swiss 3T3 cells. Proc Natl Acad Sci USA 1983; 80: 2936–2940
5 Rozengurt E. Early signals in the mitogenic response. Science 1986; 234: 161–166
6 Spindel ER, Sunday ME, Hofler H, Wolfe HJ, Habener JF, Chin WW. Transient elevation of messenger RNA encoding gastrin-releasing peptide, a putative pulmonary growth factor in human fetal lung. J Clin Invest 1987; 80: 1172–1179
7 Ghatei MA, Sheppard MN, Henzen-Logman S, Blank MA, Polak JM, Bloom SR. Bombesin and vasoactive intestinal polypeptide in the developing lung: marked changes in acute respiratory distress syndrome. J Clin Endocrinol Metab 1983; 57: 1226–1232
8 Cuttitta F, Carney DN, Mulshine J et al. Bombesin-like peptides can function as autocrine growth factors in human small-cell lung cancer. Nature 1985; 316: 823–826
9 Zachary I, Rozengurt E. High-affinity receptors for peptides of the bombesin family in Swiss 3T3 cells. Proc Natl Acad Sci USA 1985; 82: 7616–7620
10 Erspamer GF, Severini C, Erspamer V, Melchiorri P, Fave GD, Nakajima T. Parallel bioassay of 27 bombesin-like peptides on 9 smooth muscle preparations. Structure-activity relationships and bombesin receptor subtypes. Regul Pept 1988; 21: 1–11
11 Zachary I, Rozengurt E. Identification of a receptor for peptides of the bombesin family in Swiss 3T3 cells by affinity cross-linking. J Biol Chem 1987; 262: 3947–3950
12 Sinnett-Smith J, Zachary I, Rozengurt E. Identification of a bombesin receptor on Swiss mouse 3T3 cells by affinity cross-linking: Further studies and characterization as a glycoprotein. J Cell Biochem 1988; In press
13 Masu Y, Nakayama K, Tamaki H, Harada Y, Kuno M, Nakanishi S. cDNA

cloning of bovine substance K receptor through oocyte expression system. Nature 1987; 329: 836–838
14 Julius D, Macdermott AB, Axel R, Jessell TM. Molecular characterization of a functional cDNA encoding the serotonin 1c receptor. Science 1988; 241: 558–564
15 Zachary I, Rozengurt E. Internalization and degradation of peptides of the bombesin family in Swiss 3T3 cells occurs without ligand-induced receptor down-regulation. EMBO J 1987; 6: 2233–2239
16 Rozengurt E, Legg A, Pettican P. Vasopressin stimulation of mouse 3T3 cell growth. Proc Natl Acad Sci USA 1979; 76: 1284–1287
17 Hunt NH, Perris AD, Sandford PA. Role of vasopressin in the mitotic response of rat bone marrow cells to haemorrhage. J Endocrinol 1977; 72: 5–16
18 Russell WE, Bucher NLR. Vasopressin modulates live regeneration in the Brattleboro rat. Am J Physiol 1983; 245: G321–G324
19 Boer GJ. Vasopressin and brain development: studies using the Brattleboro rat. Peptides 1985; 6(Suppl 1): 49–62
20 Collins MKL, Rozengurt E. Vasopressin induces selective desensitization of its mitogenic response in Swiss 3T3 cells. Proc Natl Acad Sci USA 1983; 80: 1924–1928
21 Jard S, Gaillard RC, Guillon G et al. Vasopressin antagonists allow demonstration of a novel type of vasopressin receptor in the rat adenohypophysis. Mol Pharmacol 1986; 30: 171–177
22 Woods DJ, Monaco ME. Characterization of the vasopressin receptor on WRK-1 cells. Mol Endocrinol 1988; 2: 350–354
23 Rozengurt E, Brown KD, Pettican P. Vasopressin inhibition of epidermal growth factor binding to cultured mouse cells. J Biol Chem 1981; 256: 716–722
24 Zachary I, Rozengurt E. A substance P antagonist also inhibits specific binding and mitogenic effects of vasopressin and bombesin-related peptides in Swiss 3T3 cells. Biochem Biophys Res Commun 1986; 137: 135–141
25 Steranka LR, Manning DC, DeHaas CJ et al. Bradykinin as a pain mediator: receptors are localized to sensory neurons, and antagonists have analgesic actions. Proc Natl Acad Sci USA 1988; 85: 3245–3249
26 Owen NE, Villereal ML. Lys-Bradykinin stimulates Na^+ influx and DNA synthesis in cultured human fibroblasts. Cell 1983; 32: 979–985
27 Woll PJ, Rozengurt E. Two classes of antagonist interact with receptors for the mitogenic neuropeptides bombesin, bradykinin and vasopressin. Growth Factors; In press.
28 Vavrek RJ, Stewart JM. Competitive antagonists of bradykinin. Peptides 1985; 6: 161–164
29 Whalley ET, Nwator IA, Stewart JM, Vavrek RJ. Analysis of the receptors mediating vascular actions of bradykinin. N S Arch Pharmac 1987; 336: 430–433
30 Braas KM, Manning DC, Perry DC, Snyder SH. Bradykinin analogues: differential agonist and antagonist activities suggesting multiple receptors. Br J Pharmacol 1988; 94: 3–5
31 Fahrenkrug J, Emson PC. Vasoactive intestinal peptide: functional aspects. Br Med Bull 1982; 38: 265–270
32 Zurier RB, Kozma M, Sinnett-Smith J, Rozengurt E. Vasoactive intestinal peptide synergistically stimulates DNA synthesis in mouse 3T3 cells: role of cAMP, Ca^{2+} and protein kinase C. Exp Cell Res 1988; 176: 155–161
33 Coy DH, Heinz-Erian P, Jiang N-Y, et al. Probing peptide backbone function in bombesin: a reduced peptide bond analogue with potent and specific receptor antagonist activity. J Biol Chem 1988; 263: 5056–5060
34 Woll PJ, Coy DH, Rozengurt E. [Leu^{13}-$\psi(CH_2NH)Leu^{14}$]bombesin is a specific bombesin receptor antagonist in Swiss 3T3 cells. Biochem Biophys Res Comm 1988; 155: 359–365

35 Corps AN, Rees LH, Brown KD. A peptide that inhibits the mitogenic stimulation of Swiss 3T3 cells by bombesin or vasopressin. Biochem J 1985; 231: 781–784
36 Woll PJ, Rozengurt E. [D-Arg^1,D-Phe^5,D-Trp^{7,9},Leu^{11}]substance P, a potent bombesin antagonist in murine Swiss 3T3 cells, inhibits the growth of human small cell lung cancer cells in vitro. Proc Natl Acad Sci USA 1988; 85: 1859–1863
37 Moody TW, Pert CB, Gazdar AF, Carney DN, Minna JD. High levels of intracellular bombesin characterize human small cell lung carcinoma. Science 1981; 214: 1246–1248
38 Woll PJ, Rozengurt E. Bombesin and bombesin antagonists: studies in Swiss 3T3 cells and human small cell lung cancer. Br J Cancer 1988; 57: 579–586
39 Foster AC, Fagg GE. Taking apart NMDA receptors. Nature 1987; 329: 395–396
40 Dohlman HG, Caron MG, Lefkowitz RJ. A family of receptors coupled to guanine nucleotide regulatory proteins. Biochem 1987; 26: 2657–2664
41 Lefkowitz RJ, Caron MG. Adrenergic receptors: models for the study of receptors coupled to guanine nucleotide regulatory proteins. J Biol Chem 1988; 263: 4993–4996

Erythropoietin

G R Johnson
The Walter and Eliza Hall Institute of Medical Research, Royal Melbourne Hospital, Melbourne, Australia

> Erythropoietin mRNA is detected primarily in kidney peritubular cells in response to hypoxia, and this tissue is the major adult source of the hormone. Erythropoietin can be assayed by in vivo or in vitro biological methods, or by radioimmunoassay, but only the in vivo assay can distinguish the most biologically active forms. The mature hormone consists of 166 amino acids and approximately 50% of the mature molecule (M_r 39 000) consists of carbohydrate. The gene is highly conserved among species studied, and is located on human chromosome 7, region q11–q22. Recombinant erythropoietin has been administered to haemodialysis patients and shown to increase haemoglobin levels, reticulocyte numbers and haematocrit. In transfusion-dependent patients, the need for regular transfusions was abrogated. Problems with hypertension have been noted in previously hypertensive patients, but the results of clinical trials with erythropoietin suggest that it will provide a valuable alternative therapy, for correcting some disorders of erythropoiesis.

This brief review will outline recent observations on the molecular cloning, structure and biological properties of erythropoietin- (Epo). These studies have identified that Epo alone, acting as a hormone, is able to produce the effects on erythropoiesis initially postulated by Carnot and Deflandre (1901). The recent availability of large quantities of pure Epo have enabled its use in clinical trials, suggesting an important role for this glycoprotein in alleviating anaemia.

PHYSIOLOGY OF ERYTHROPOIETIN AND RED CELL PRODUCTION

Because the principal function of erythrocytes is to transport oxygen, changes in oxygen levels, erythrocyte mass and Epo levels are intimately linked.[2-4] Thus, decreased oxygen stimulates, whereas excess oxygen availability suppresses Epo production. That hypoxia produces a blood-born erythropoietic stimulus was first demonstrated by Reissmann (1950)[5] and subsequently it was shown that a similar stimulus was present in the plasma of anaemic animals.[6] In adult life, Epo is produced primarily by the kidneys as was first clearly demonstrated in 1951.[7]

It has been suggested that the kidneys' unique ability to adjust oxygen demand to oxygen supply is the reason for this organ being the primary erythropoietin-producing tissue.[5] Decreased kidney blood flow decreases glomerular filtration and consequently kidney oxygen demand, such a mechanism preventing the hyperviscosity and subsequent decreased blood flow associated with erythrocytosis from increasing Epo production and subsequently enhancing the erythrocytosis.[9]

Confirmation that the kidney produces Epo has come from studies where Epo mRNA was detected in the kidney shortly after anaemia induction[10,11] increasing up to 200-fold.[11] Kinetic studies have shown that circulating Epo levels, with appropriate lag times, parallel the changes in renal Epo and mRNA content,[12] suggesting that renal Epo production in response to hypoxia is by *de novo* synthesis and not release of stored hormone. By use of *in situ* hybridization on kidney tissue from anaemic animals, Epo mRNA has been localized to peritubular cells occurring primarily in the cortex.[13,14] The location of the positive cells outside the tubule basement membrane suggesting a subset of interstitial or endothelial cells[13,14] as the major site of Epo production in the hypoxic kidney.

EXTRARENAL ERYTHROPOIETIN PRODUCTION

Erythropoietin although present at reduced levels, can still be detected in anephric animals. Embryonic and early fetal erythroid cells respond to Epo suggesting that this hormone may be present during fetal life at a time prior to kidney development. These observations suggest that tissues other than the kidney can produce Epo. Fetal liver cells in vitro can be shown to produce Epo,[15] although recent studies in normoxic and hypoxic fetal rats suggest that before day 17 of gestation, the rat fetus has hypoxia-independent, extrahepatic Epo which is followed by hepatic and renal Epo production.[16] Whether this Epo is maternally derived has yet to be determined.

In neonatal rats, more Epo originates from the liver than the kidneys until day 10, although the switch from hepatic to renal Epo production occurred earlier under hypoxic conditions.[16] Recent studies have also suggested that the switch of Epo production, from the hepatic to renal site, was not due to suppression of hepatic Epo production by renal Epo production.[17] Transplantation into adult sheep, of fetal lamb livers obtained prior to onset of renal Epo production, was associated with increases in serum Epo levels and a reticulocytosis, irrespective of the presence or absence of kidneys in the adult recipients.[17] These data suggest that the liver to kidney switch of Epo production, during ontogeny, may represent a genetically determined event.

ERYTHROPOIETIN PRODUCTION BY TRANSFORMED CELLS

As both the kidney and liver are known sites of Epo production, it is not surprising that neoplastic transformation of certain cells from these tissues is associated with an erythrocytosis.

Elevated erythropoietin is of value as a biologic marker in some renal cell cancers,[18] and cell lines developed from these renal carcinomas provide model systems for the study of erythropoietin synthesis and secretion.[19,20] Erythrocytosis is also a well described paraneoplastic phenomenon in patients with hepatocellular carcinoma,[21,22] and cell lines derived from these neoplastic cells display both constitutive and regulated production of Epo.[23]

Capillary haemangioblastoma is also a tumour known to be associated with secondary polycythaemia,[24] and these tumours have been shown to contain scattered cells binding anti-erythropoietin antibodies.[24]

ASSAYS FOR ERYTHROPOIETIN

Erythropoietin can be assayed by its ability to stimulate erythropoiesis in vivo or in vitro or by radioimmunoassay. Each assay however, has its limitations, and until antibodies known to react only with biologically-active Epo are developed, a combination of various assays is required to determine biologically-active and inactive Epo.

The in vivo assay relies upon artificially suppressing Epo levels, e.g. by hypertransfusion[25] or reduced air pressure.[26] The substance to be tested is then injected into animals, and at varying periods later the incorporation of Fe^{59} into stimulated erythroid cells is measured. Although this assay primarily measures Epo, it is not absolutely specific as a number of other haemopoietic growth factors (e.g. GM-CSF, IL-3) can perturb erythropoiesis in vivo[27,28] and would result in Fe^{59} incorporation into erythroblasts.

In vitro proliferation assays, involving incorporation of a radioisotope preferentially into dividing erythroblasts, have also been developed.[29,30] An alternative in vitro assay, relying upon the ability of murine erythroid progenitor cells, immobilized in semi-solid medium, to differentiate into clones of haemoglobinized erythroid cells in response to Epo, also provides a sensitive (able to detect approx. 1 milliunit) assay for Epo.[31,32] This latter assay directly scores haemoglobinization, thus determining specificity of cell types responding, but as with all in vitro assays, is limited if nonspecific inhibitory materials are present in the material being assayed.

Radioimmunoassays for Epo have been developed,[33–35] but these detect multiple forms of Epo which may or may not have biological activity.[36] Loss of biological activity in vivo is associated with loss of the carbohydrate moiety of the Epo molecule, which although not having a role in the interaction between Epo and its target cells,[37] markedly reduces biological half-life.[38,39]

In vitro assays are also unable to distinguish between normal and asialo Epo, thus only the in vivo assay is able to distinguish the most biologically-active forms of Epo. These problems need to be recognized if only in vitro or presently available immunoreactive assays for Epo are used.

STRUCTURE OF ERYTHROPOIETIN AND GENE CLONING

Erythropoietin purified from human urine has a molecular weight of 39 000.[40] The mature hormone is 166 amino acids in length (calculated M_r of 18 399.[41,42] Thus approximately 50% of the native molecule is due to carbohydrate of which 40% is sialic acid[43] which is not necessary for binding of Epo to target cells.[43,44]

Human Epo contains two disulfide bonds, between Cys 7 and Cys 161, and Cys 29 and Cys 33.[42,45] By the use of site-specific anti-peptide antibodies, regions of the Epo molecule probably forming part of the receptor-binding domain, have been identified.[46,47] Antibodies against peptides corresponding to residues 1–26, 40–59, 80–99 and 133–150 do not inhibit biological activity, whereas antipeptide antibodies 99–118 and 111–129 inhibit Epo activity, the inhibition being reversed by excess peptide.[46]

Knowledge of the amino acid sequence of human Epo has enabled construction of oligonucleotide probes and subsequent isolation of human,[48,49] monkey,[50] and murine,[51,52] genomic and cDNA clones for Epo. In all three species, the Epo gene exists as a single copy and is highly conserved, with the monkey and murine DNA coding sequence having a 94%[50] and 80%[52] homology, respectively with the human gene. The human Epo gene is located on chromosome 7[53–55] and more specifically by in situ hybridization, has been localized to region q11–q22.[55] Restriction fragment length polymorphisms, using either restriction enzymes Hind III or Hinf I, have been detected using Epo cDNA probes to human genetic DNA.[54,55]

Rearrangement and amplification of the Epo locus has been noted in a murine erythroleukaemic cell line which constitutively produces Epo.[56] The breakpoint was located within a 1.1 kb region upstream of an otherwise normal Epo gene and no viral sequences were detected in the immediate vicinity. Although not proven, these data are suggestive that the rearrangement leads to Epo gene transcription, and that this may have some involvement in the development of erythroleukaemia. Similar studies have yet to be reported with human erythroleukaemic cells.

CLINICAL STUDIES WITH RECOMBINANT HUMAN ERYTHROPOIETIN

The molecular cloning of the human Epo gene and its cDNA, make possible the production of large quantities of protein and its availability for use in clinical trials. An obvious use for Epo is in the correction of the anaemia associated with chronic renal failure. The anaemia associated with end stage renal disease is related to the kidneys' role as a primary source of Epo and the apparent inability of other tissues, e.g. the liver, to make a compensatory and sufficient increase in Epo production following renal dysfunction. Dialysis is unable to correct the anaemia and approximately 25% of these patients require red cell transfusions to partially correct the anaemia. Additional therapy includes anabolic androgen, vitamins and iron administration.[57]

Recombinant Epo has been administered to patients on haemodialysis intravenously several times per week (usually three) from 3–1000 Units/kg body weight.[58-63] Haemoglobin levels in most patients rose to 99–12 g/d[58,60,61,63] along with increases in reticulocyte counts and haematocrit (rising to 35% or greater)[60,63] and in many transfusion-dependent patients the need for regular red cell transfusions was abrogated.[58,60] No antibodies to the recombinant erythropoietin were detected[60,63,64] nor were toxic effects of organ dysfunction noted.[60-63] Prior to treatment, mean serum levels of Epo were 4 ± 6.4 mU/ml which rose to 33.7 ± 8.1 mU/ml during maintenance therapy (2×72 U/kg to 3×168 U/kg of recombinant Epo per week).[61]

Although no serious side effects have been noted following treatment with recombinant Epo, in some patients blood pressure has increased,[60] such that anti-hypertensive therapy was required.[62-64] In normotensive patients, blood pressure did not increase following Epo therapy.[64] The problems of hypertension appear therefore to occur primarily in previously hypertensive individuals.[65] Further trials with Epo are being performed to establish the optimum rate and extent of rise in red cells required to alleviate the anaemia in haemodialysis patients, without increasing undue risk.[66-69]

These studies suggest, however, that the use of the haemopoietic growth and differentiation regulator, Epo, will provide a useful new and naturally-occurring therapeutic alternative for the treatment of anaemia.

REFERENCES

1 Carnot P, Deflandre C. Sur l'activite hematopoietique des differents organes au cours de la regeneration du sang CR Acad Sci D 1906; 143: 432–435
2 Krantz SB, Jacobsen LO. Erythropoietin and the regulation of erythropoiesis. Chicago: University of Chicago Press, 1970
3 Graber SE, Krantz SB. Erythropoietin and the control of red cell production. Ann Rev Med 1978; 29: 31–66
4 Spivak JL, Graber SE. Erythropoietin and the regulation of erythropoiesis. Johns Hopkins Med J 1980; 146: 311–320
5 Reissmann KR. Studies of the mechanism of erythropoietic stimulation in parabiotic rats during hypoxia. Blood 1950; 5: 372–380
6 Erslev A. (1953) Humoral regulation of red cell production. Blood 1953; 8: 349–357
7 Jacobson LO, Goldwasser E, Fried W, Plzak L. Role of the kidney in erythropoiesis. Nature 1957 179: 633–634
8 Erslev AJ, Caro J, Besarab A. Why the kidney? Nephron 1985; 41: 213–216
9 Erslev AJ. Erythropoietin coming of age. N Eng J Med 1987; 316: 101–103
10 Beru N, McDonald J, Lacombe C, Goldwasser E. (1986) Expression of the erythropoietin gene. Mol Cell Biol 1986; 6: 2571–2575

11 Bondurant MC, Koury MJ. Anemia induces accumulation of erythropoietin mRNA in the kidney and liver. Mol Cell Biol 1986; 6: 2731–2733
12 Schuster SJ, Wilson JH, Erslev AJ, Caro J. Physiologic regulation and tissue localization of renal erythropoietin messenger RNA. Blood 1987; 70: 316–318
13 Koury ST, Bondurant MC, Koury MJ. Localization of erythropoietin synthesizing cells in murine kidneys by in situ hybridization. Blood 1988; 71: 524–527
14 Lacombe C, Da Silva JL, Bruneval P, et al. Peritubular cells are the site of erythropoietin synthesis in the murine hypoxic kidney. J Clin Invest 1988; 81: 620–623
15 Kurtz A, Jelkmann W, Pfuhl A, Malmstrom K, Bauer C. Erythropoietin production by fetal mouse liver cells in response to hypoxia and adenylate cyclase stimulation. Endocrinology 1986; 118: 567–572
16 Clemons GK, Fitzsimmons SL, De Manincor D. Immunoreactive erythropoietin concentrations in fetal and neonatal rats and the effects of hypoxia. Blood 1986; 68: 892–899
17 Flake AW, Harrison MR, Adzick NS, Zanjani ED. Erythropoietin production by the fetal liver in an adult environment. Blood 1987; 70: 542–545
18 Nseyo UO, Williams PD, Murphy GP. Clinical significance of erythropoietin levels in renal carcinoma. Urology 1986; 28: 301–306
19 Sherwood JB, Shouval D. Continuous production of erythropoietin by an established human renal carcinoma cell line: development of the cell line. Proc Natl Acad Sci (USA) 1986; 83: 165–169
20 Nagakura K, Ueno M, Brookins J, Beckman BS, Fisher JW. Effects of low calcium levels on erythropoietin production by human renal carcinoma cells in culture. Am J Physiol 1987; 253: 797–801
21 Kew MC, Fisher JW. Serum erythropoietin concentrations in patients with hepatocellular carcinoma. Cancer 1986; 58: 2485–2488
22 Watanobe H. Hepatocellular carcinoma associated with a rare combination of polycythemia and chronic thyroiditis. Hepatogastroenterology 1988; 35: 14–16
23 Goldberg MA, Glass GA, Cunningham JM, Bunn HF. The regulated expression of erythropoietin by two human hepatoma cell lines. Proc Natl Acad Sci (USA) 1987; 84: 7972–7976
24 Bohling T, Haltia M, Rosenlof K, Fyhrquist F. Erythropoietin in capillary hemangioblastoma. An immunohistochemical study. Acta Neuropathol 1987; 74: 324–328
25 Filmanowicz E, Gurney CW. Studies on erythropoiesis. XVI. The response to a single dose of erythropoietin in the polycythemic mouse. J Lab Clin Med 1961; 57: 65–72
26 Cotes PM, Bangham DR. Bioassay of erythropoietin in mice made polycythemic by exposure to air at reduced pressure. Nature 1961; 191: 1065–1087
27 Metcalf D, Begley CG, Williamson DJ, et al. Hemopoietic responses in mice injected with purified recombinant murine GM-CSF. Exp Hematol 1987; 15: 1–9
28 Metcalf D, Begley CG, Johnson GR, Nicola NA, Lopez AF, Williamson DJ. Effects of purified bacterially-synthesized murine Multi-CSF (IL-3) on hemopoiesis in normal adult mice. Blood 1986; 68: 46–57
29 Dunn CDR, Jarvis JH, Greenman JM. A quantative bioassay for erythropoietin using mouse fetal liver cells. Exp Hematol 1975; 3: 65–78
30 Goldwasser E, Eliason JF, Sikkema D. An assay for erythropoietin in vitro at the milliunit level. Endocrinology 1975; 97: 315–323
31 Cutler RL, Nicola NA, Johnson GR. The preparation of erythropoietin for tissue culture. Exp Hematol 1985; 13: 796–801
32 Adamson JW, Torok-Storb B, Lin N. Analysis of erythropoiesis by erythroid colony formation in culture. Blood Cells 1978; 4: 89–103
33 Egrie JC, Brown J, Lai P, Lin FK. Characterization of recombinant monkey and human erythropoietin. Prog Clin Biol Res 1985; 191: 339–350

34 Sherwood JB, Goldwasser E. A radioimmunoassay for erythropoietin. Blood 1979; 54: 885–893
35 Garcia JF, Sherwood J, Goldwasser E. Radioimmunoassay of erythropoietin. Blood Cells 1979; 5: 405–
36 Sherwood JB, Carmichael LD, Goldwasser E. The heterogeneity of circulating human serum erythropoietin. Endocrinology 1988; 122: 1472–1477
37 Dordal MS, Wang FF, Goldwasser E. The role of carbohydrate in erythropoietin action. Endocrinology 1985; 116: 2293–2299
38 Goldwasser E, Kung CK-H, Eliason J. On the mechanism of erythropoietin induced differentiation. J Biol Chem 1974; 249: 4202–4206
39 Lukowsky WA, Painter RA. Studies on the role of sialic acid in the physical and biological properties of erythropoietin. Can J Biochem 1972; 50: 909–917
40 Miyake T, Kung CK-H, Goldwasser E. Purification of human erythropoietin. J Biol Chem 1977; 252: 5558–5564
41 Jacobs K, Shoemaker C, Rudersdorf R. Isolation and characterization of genomic and cDNA clones of human erythropoietin. Nature 1985; 313: 806–810
42 Browne JK, Cohen AM, Egrie JC, et al. Erythropoietin: Gene cloning, protein structure, and biological properties. Cold Spring Harbor Symp Quant Biol 1986; 51: 693–702
43 Dordal MS, Wang FF, Goldwasser E. The role of carbohydrate in erythropoietin action. Endocrinology 1985; 116: 2293–2299
44 Goldwasser E, Kung CK-H, Eliason J. On the mechanism of erythropoietin-induced differentiation. J Biol Chem 1974; 249: 4202–4206
45 Lai PH, Everett R, Wang FF, Arakawa T, Goldwasser E. Structural characterization of human erythropoietin. J Biol Chem 1986; 261: 3116–3121
46 Sytkowski AJ, Donahue KA. Immunochemical studies of human erythropoietin using site-specific anti-peptide antibodies. Identification of a functional domain. J Biol Chem 1987; 262: 1161–1165
47 Wojchowski DM, Sue JM, Sytkowski AJ. Site-specific antibodies to human erythropoietin: Immunoaffinity purification of urinary and recombinant hormone. Biochim Biophys Acta 1987; 913: 170–178
48 Jacobs K, Shoemaker C, Ruresdorf R, et al. Isolation and characterization of genomic and cDNA clones of human erythropoietin. Nature 1985; 313: 806–810
49 Lin F-K, Suggs S, Lin C-H, et al. Cloning and expression of the human erythropoietin gene. Proc Natl Acad Sci USA 1985; 82: 7580–7584
50 Lin FJ, Lin CH, Lai PH, et al. Monkey erythropoietin gene: cloning, expression and comparison with the human erythropoietin gene. Gene 1986; 44: 201–209
51 McDonald JD, Lin FK, Goldwasser E. Cloning, sequencing, and evolutionary analysis of the mouse erythropoietin gene. Mol Cell Biol 1986; 6: 842–848
52 Shoemaker CB, Mitsock LD. Murine erythropoietin gene: cloning, expressing, and human gene homology. Mol Cell Biol 1986; 6: 849–859
53 Powell JS, Berkner KL, Lebo RV, Adamson JW. Human erythropoietin gene: high level expression in stably transfected mammalian cells and chromosome localization. Proc Natl Acad Sci USA 1986; 83: 6465–6469
54 Watkins PC, Eddy R, Hoffman N, et al. Regional assignment of the erythropoietin gene to human chromosome region 7pter—-q22. Cytogenet Cell Genet 1986; 42: 214–218
55 Law ML, Cai GY, Lin FK, et al. Chromosomal assignment of the human erythropoietin gene and its DNA polymorphism. Proc Natl Acad Sci USA 1986; 83: 6920–6924
56 McDonald J, Beru N, Goldwasser E. Rearrangement and expression of erythropoietin genes in transformed mouse cells. Mol Cell Biol 1987; 7: 365–370
57 Johnson CA, Chester MI. Pathophysiology and treatment of the anemia of renal failure. Clin Pharm 1988; 7: 117–122
58 Winearls CG, Oliver DO, Pippard MJ, Reid C, Downing R, Cotes PM. Effect

of human erythropoietin derived from recombinant DNA on the anaemia of patients maintained by chronic haemodialysis. Lancet 1986; 2: 1175–1178
59 Zins B, Drueke T, Zingraff J, et al. Erythropoietin treatment in anaemic patients on haemodialysis. Lancet 1986; 2: 1329
60 Eschbach JW, Egrie JC, Downing MR, Browne JK, Adamson JW. Correction of the anemia of end-stage renal disease with recombinant human erythropoietin. Results of a combined phase I and II clinical trial. N Engl J Med 1987; 316: 73–78
61 Stutz B, Rhyner K, Vogtli J, Binswanger U. Successful treatment of anemia in hemolysis patients using recombinant human erythropoietin. Maintenance dosage and serum concentration. Schweiz Med Wochenschr 1987; 117: 1397–1402
62 Bommer J, Alexiou C, Muller-Buhl U, Eifert J, Ritz E. Recombinant human erythropoietin therapy in haemodialysis patients—dose determination and clinical experience. Nephrol Dial Transplant 1987; 2: 238–242
63 Schaefer RM, Kurner B, Zech M, Krahn R, Heidland A. Therapy of renal anemia with recombinant human erythropoietin. Dtsch Med Wochenschr 1988; 113: 125–129
64 Casati S, Passerini P, Campise MR, et al. Benefits and risks of protracted treatment with human recombinant erythropoietin in patients having haemodialysis. Br Med J 1987; 295: 1017–1020
65 Raine AE. Hypertension, blood viscosity, and cardiovascular morbidity in renal failure: Implications of erythropoietin therapy. Lancet 1988; 1: 97–100
66 Gretz N, Lasserre JJ, Meisinger E, et al. Potential side-effects of erythropoietin. Lancet 1987; 1: 46
67 Jacquot C, Ferragu-Haguet M, Lefebvre A, Berthelot JM, Peterlongo F, Castaigne JP. (1987) Recombinant erythropoietin and blood pressure. Lancet 1987; 2: 1083
68 Bommer J, Muller-Buhl E, Ritz E, Eifert J. Recombinant human erythropoietin in anaemic patients on haemodialysis. Lancet 1987; 1: 392
69 Ahmad R, Hand M. Recombinant erythropoietin for the anemia of chronic renal failure. N Engl J Med 1987; 317: 169–170

Signal transduction pathways in mitogenesis

Enrique Rozengurt
Imperial Cancer Research Fund, Lincoln's Inn Fields, London UK

> Quiescent cells arrested in the G_0 phase of the cell cycle can be stimulated to divide by polypeptide growth factors, pharmacological agents and neuropeptides which exhibit potent synergistic effects. Bombesin-like peptides are providing valuable model mitogens to elucidate the signalling pathways leading to mitogenesis. These peptides stimulate rapid increases in ionic fluxes, inositol polyphosphate formation, activation of protein kinases and expression of proto-oncogenes. A comparison of these early molecular events with those evoked by other growth factors indicate the existence of multiple signal-transduction pathways. We propose that stimulation of cell proliferation by single or multiple factors results from the activation of separate signal-transduction pathways that cooperate to elicit the complete set of molecular events leading to mitogenesis.

The elucidation of the mechanism of action of growth factors has emerged as one of the fundamental problems in biology and may prove crucial for understanding the unrestrained proliferation of cancer cells. Many studies of growth factors have used cultured fibroblasts, such as 3T3 cells, as a model system. These cells cease to proliferate when they deplete the medium of. its growth promoting activity. Such quiescent cells can be stimulated to reinitiate DNA synthesis and cell division either by replenishing the medium with fresh serum, or by the addition of growth factors or pharmacological agents in serum-free medium.[1] Studies performed with combinations of growth factors have revealed an important aspect of their action: the existence of potent and specific synergistic interactions (see Ref. 1 for review). This finding suggested that growth factors bind to different receptors, and generate multiple intracellular signals which interact synergistically to initiate a proliferative response.

A new and intriguing development is the discovery that neuropeptides localized in neural and neuroendocrine cells of mammalian tissues can also act as growth factors for cells in culture.[2] In this context, the peptides of the bombesin family are of particular significance (see Woll and Rozengurt, this Issue). These peptides are potent mitogens for Swiss 3T3 cells[3] and may act as autocrine growth factors for small cell lung cancer.[4]

The binding of growth factors to their receptors promotes the generation of early signals in the membrane, cytosol and nucleus which lead to cell proliferation.[1] Since the initiation of DNA synthesis occurs 10 to 15h after the addition of the mitogens, it is expected that knowledge of the early events will provide clues to primary regulatory mechanisms. Here we summarize our recent studies using bombesin-like peptides for elucidating the signal transduction pathways leading to mitogenesis and compare these pathways with those activated by other growth factors. These early events in growth stimulation are depicted schematically in Figure 1.

ION FLUXES

One of the earliest events to occur after the binding of most mitogens to their receptors is an increase in the fluxes of Na^+, K^+ and H^+ across the plasma membrane (see Ref. 5 for review). Accordingly, bombesin-like peptides stimulate a rapid influx of Na^+ into Swiss 3T3 cells via an amiloride-sensitive Na^+/H^+ antiport.[6] This increases intracellular Na^+ and causes cytoplasmic alkalinization. Since the activity of the Na^+/K^+ pump is regulated by intracellular Na^+, there is a secondary stimulation of Na^+/K^+ pump activity which increases K^+ and restores the electrochemical gradient for Na^+. As discussed below, the activity of the Na^+/H^+ antiport is activated through different pathways.[6,7]

In addition to changes in monovalent ion fluxes, bombesin and structurally related peptides cause a rapid mobilization of Ca^{2+} from intracellular stores, which leads to a transient increase in the concentration of cytosolic Ca^{2+}.[6] This Ca^{2+} flux is distinct from that caused by platelet-derived growth factor (PDGF).[8,9] The mobilization of Ca^{2+} by bombesin and other mitogens may be

SIGNAL TRANSDUCTION PATHWAYS IN MITOGENESIS

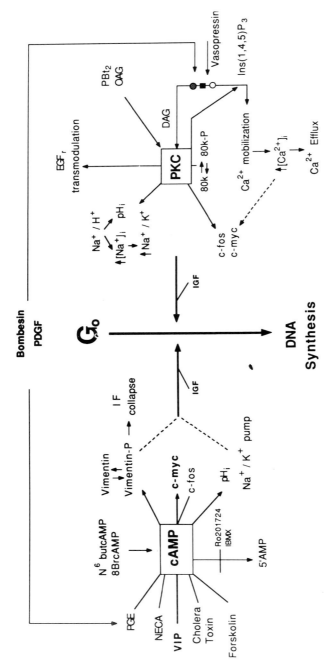

Fig. 1 Integration of early signalling events and synergistic effects elicited by growth factors, pharmacological agents and neuropeptides in quiescent Swiss 3T3 cells. Details are described throughout the text.

mediated by inositol 1,4,5-trisphosphate (Ins(1,4,5)P_3), which has been proposed to act as a second messenger in the action of many ligands that stimulate inositol lipid turnover and Ca^{2+} efflux.[10] Ins(1,4,5)P_3 is formed as a result of phospholipase C catalysed hydrolysis of phosphatidyl inositol 4,5-bisphosphate (PIP_2) in the plasma membrane, a process that also generates 1,2-diacylglycerol. Bombesin has been shown to cause enhanced inositol lipid metabolism in Swiss 3T3 cells leading to the formation of Ins(1,4,5)P_3.[8,9,11]

PROTEIN KINASE C AND INITIATION OF DNA SYNTHESIS

Protein kinase C (PKC), which is activated by diacylglycerols and is a major receptor for phorbol esters, has been implicated in the signal transduction of many short-term cellular responses (see Ref. 12 for review). Of particular interest is the evidence implicating PKC in mediating long-term responses. Phorbol esters stimulate DNA synthesis and cell division in synergy with insulin and other growth-promoting factors.[13] The mitogenic effect is mediated by high-affinity binding sites[14] which were identified as PKC. Furthermore, addition of the synthetic diacylglycerol 1-oleoyl-2-acetylglycerol (OAG) mimics the action of phorbol esters in stimulating reinitiation of DNA synthesis and cell division.[15] Another approach to testing the role of PKC in the production of biological responses is to exploit the selective removal of this enzyme caused by a prolonged pretreatment of the cells with phorbol ester. Chronic exposure to phorbol esters leads to a marked decrease in the number of specific phorbol esterbinding sites and to the disappearance of measurable PKC activity in cell-free preparations.[16,17] In parallel with this down-regulation of PKC activity, the cells become desensitized to the mitogenic effects of phorbol esters or OAG. Hence, activation of PKC is a potential pathway leading to mitogenesis.

Activation of protein kinase C in intact fibroblasts

Since activation of PKC may play a role in eliciting mitogenesis, it was of importance to test directly whether growth factors including bombesin lead to activation of this enzyme in intact, quiescent cells. A rapid increase in the phosphorylation of an acidic cellular protein with an M_r of 80 000 (termed 80K) was shown to reflect the

activation of PKC in intact fibroblasts.[18] For example, the phosphorylation of the same 80K protein is stimulated in cells by addition of:
  (i) biologically active phorbol esters;
  (ii) the synthetic diacylglycerol DAG; and
  (iii) exogenous phospholipase C, which causes phospholipid breakdown and generates diacylglycerol. Down-regulation of PKC activity prevents the increase in 80K phosphorylation by subsequent addition of phorbol esters, phospholipase C, or OAG (see Ref. 1 for review). Furthermore, the same 80K protein is phosphorylated in cell-free systems either by activation of endogenous PKC or by addition of the purified enzyme.[17] Recently a phosphoprotein closely related to 80K has been purified 3800 fold from rat brain.[19] The preparation appears homogeneous by one and two-dimensional PAGE, is an effective substrate of PKC and contains an unusually high proportion of acidic amino acids (glu, asp) and of alanine. Although the nature and role of the 80K phosphoprotein remain to be elucidated, its phosphorylation provides a specific marker for assessing which mitogenic agents activate PKC in intact cells.

Activation of protein kinase C by bombesin and other growth factors

Addition of bombesin causes a potent and rapid increase in 80K phosphorylation.[20] An enhancement in phosphorylation can be detected as early as 15 seconds after the addition of bombesin, and maximal phosphorylation is obtained in less than 1 minute. Removal of bombesin results in rapid (half-life 90s) dephosphorylation of 80K.

The 80K phosphoproteins generated in response to bombesin or phorbol 12,13-dibutyrate (PBt_2) are identical as judged by one and two-dimensional polyacrylamide gel electrophoresis and by peptide mapping.[20] Furthermore, down-regulation of PKC completely prevents the effect of bombesin on 80K phosphorylation.[20] These findings strongly suggest that bombesin rapidly stimulates PKC activity in intact and quiescent Swiss 3T3 cells. A similar conclusion was reached by Isacke et al.[21] Whether or not bombesin stimulates tyrosine phosphorylation remains controversial.[21,22]

Using the approaches outlined above it has been shown that addition of serum, PDGF and vasopressin rapidly activates PKC in quiescent Swiss 3T3 cells.[23,24] In contrast, neither insulin nor epidermal growth factor (EGF) stimulate PKC in these cells.[7,18] Hence, PKC mediates the mitogenic actions of phorbol esters, and may also play a role in the signalling of other growth factors.

G proteins and activation of PKC by bombesin

Pertussis toxin, which ADP-ribosylates and inactivates guanine nucleotide regulatory proteins (G proteins) blocks bombesin stimulation of DNA synthesis and induction of c-*myc* expression.[25] Hence, the bombesin receptor might be coupled to phospholipase C by a pertussis toxin-sensitive G protein. Experiments from our laboratory do not support this hypothesis. Pertussis toxin selectively inhibits bombesin-stimulated mitogenesis but does not interfere with polyphosphoinositide breakdown, Ca^{2+} mobilization or activation of protein kinase C.[26] The involvement of G proteins in receptor mediated responses may be studied using guanyl nucleotide analogues to control G protein activation. In several instances evidence for the existence of G proteins was obtained by introducing guanyl nucleotides into the cytosol of intact cells using permeabilization techniques that preserve the signalling mechanisms. We therefore decided to establish a permeabilization procedure in Swiss 3T3 cells in which the effect of guanyl nucleotides on bombesin-induced transmembrane signalling could be studied. We found that PBt_2 or bombesin strikingly stimulate 80K phosphorylation in Swiss 3T3 cells permeabilized with digitonin (Erusalimsky, Friedberg and Rozengurt, submitted). Furthermore, the GDP analog GDP-β-S inhibits the phosphorylation of 80K stimulated by bombesin but not by PBt_2. These results suggest that a G protein is involved in coupling the bombesin receptor to the generation of an early intracellular signal, namely the activation of PKC in Swiss 3T3 cells.

PKC, ion fluxes and transmodulation of EGF receptor

In addition to its role in stimulating cell division, PKC may also be important in coordinating the network of early events triggered by bombesin. Activation of PKC leads to increased activity of the Na^+/H^+ antiport system.[1] Stimulation of ion fluxes by bombesin is only partially inhibited, however, by PKC down-regulation suggesting that this peptide can stimulate Na^+/H^+ antiport activity by alternative mechanisms.[6] PKC activation can also inhibit Ca^{2+} mobilization, suggesting some feedback control.[8]

[^{125}I]EGF binding to specific surface receptors in Swiss 3T3 cells is markedly inhibited by bombesin and other growth factors (see Ref. 27 for review). The effect is rapid in onset and results from a decrease in the apparent affinity of the EGF receptor population for EGF. Considerable evidence implicates PKC in the regulation of EGF receptor affinity by bombesin and other transmodulating agents; the inhibition of EGF binding induced by either PBt$_2$ or bombesin is prevented by down-regulation of PKC; the EGF receptor is phosphorylated by PKC at a specific site (Thr 654) both in vitro and in vivo.[28] Thus, transmodulation of the EGF receptor may result from the covalent modification of the EGF receptor catalysed by PKC, though other mechanisms are not excluded.

CYCLIC AMP AND MITOGENESIS

Considerable evidence indicates that an increase in the cellular levels of cyclic AMP (cAMP) can act as a mitogenic signal for Swiss 3T3 cells. A variety of agents that promote cAMP accumulation in these cells, including prostaglandin E$_1$ (PGE$_1$), the adenosine agonist 5'-N-ethylcarboxamideadenosine (NECA) and cholera toxin, stimulate DNA synthesis acting synergistically with insulin, phorbol esters and other factors (see Ref. 1 for review). Similar mitogenic effects can be elicited by permeable cAMP analogues. Furthermore, PDGF, one of the most potent mitogens for fibroblasts, induces a striking accumulation of cellular cAMP in the presence of agents that reduce cAMP degradation.[29] The accumulation of cAMP elicited by PDGF is mediated by increased synthesis of E-type prostaglandins, which in turn leave the cell and stimulate cAMP synthesis through their own receptor.

Recent findings demonstrate that the neuropeptide vasoactive intestinal peptide (VIP) stimulates reinitiation of DNA synthesis when added in the presence of insulin and modulators of cAMP metabolism (i.e. forskolin or inhibitors of cAMP phosphodiesterase). The peptide, at mitogenic concentrations promotes rapid accumulation of cAMP but neither induces Ca^{2+} mobilization, nor increases the phosphorylation of the 80K protein.[30] A similar pattern of responses was also obtained with other cAMP-increasing agents. Thus, a sustained increase in cellular cAMP synergistically stimulates reinitiation of DNA synthesis in Swiss 3T3 cells.

cAMP-mediated phosphorylation in quiescent 3T3 cells

In spite of its potential importance as one of the transmembrane signalling pathways leading to mitogenesis, little is known about the phosphorylation events stimulated by cAMP in quiescent 3T3 cells. Recent results demonstrate that an elevation in the cellular levels of cAMP by forskolin increases the phosphorylation of an M_r 58 000 cellular protein in quiescent cultures of Swiss 3T3 cells.[31] The enhancement of $^{32}P_i$ incorporation into the M_r 58 000 cellular protein is detected as early as 1 min and reaches a maximum after 20 min of treatment. The phosphorylation of the M_r 58 000 protein is stimulated by other agents that cause cAMP accumulation in 3T3 cells (e.g. cholera toxin, NECA and PGE_1) and is potentiated by inhibitors of cyclic nucleotide phosphodiesterase and induced by 8BrcAMP. In contrast, the phosphorylation of 80K is not changed by any of the pharmacological agents used to increase cAMP. Thus, the stimulation of the PKC and cAMP signalling pathways can be monitored by distinct phosphorylation events.

Detergent extraction, immunoblotting and immunoprecipitation identify the M_r 58 000 phosphoprotein as vimentin, the main protein subunit of the intermediate filaments of mesenchymal cells including Swiss 3T3 cells.[31] Our studies also show that an increase in the intracellular level of cAMP induced a marked redistribution and collapse of the intermediate filaments. Recent studies raise the possibility that intermediate filaments may play a role in the transmission of information from the plasma membrane to the nucleus.[32] An attractive hypothesis is that intact intermediate filaments transmit a negative signal which restricts the initiation of the cell cycle in 3T3 cells. The redistribution induced by specific phosphorylation by cAMP dependent protein kinase might remove a constraint for the initiation of cell proliferation.

Cross-talk between protein kinase C and cAMP

While cAMP and PKC represent separate signal transduction pathways, recent results show the existence of cross-talk between these major transmembrane signalling systems. Activation of PKC by either phorbol esters or OAG markedly enhances the accumulation of cAMP in response to forskolin or cholera toxin.[33] Down-regulation of PKC blocks the enhancing effect of either PBt_2 or OAG. These findings suggest that cAMP could contribute to the signalling of growth factors that primarily act through the PKC pathway.

A salient feature of this 'cross-talk' is that it is abolished by treatment with pertussis toxin in a time and dose-dependent fashion. Since pertussis toxin does not promote cAMP accumulation in Swiss 3T3[33] it is unlikely that it acts by removing a tonic inhibitory influence on the adenylate cyclase via G_i. An attractive possibility is that a novel pertussis toxin substrate mediates the 'cross talk' between the PKC and the cAMP pathways.

The preceding findings prompted us to determine the influence of bombesin on cAMP accumulation by Swiss 3T3 cells. Bombesin causes a marked enhancement of cAMP accumulation in the presence of forskolin.[34] This effect is partially diminished by down-regulation of PKC and by the cyclo-oxygenase inhibitor indomethacin. The additive nature of these perturbations suggests that activation of PKC via 'cross-talk' and release of E type prostaglandins (like PDGF) provide two distinct pathways by which bombesin promotes enhancement of cAMP accumulation. Since down-regulation of PKC also decreases the cAMP accumulation induced by PDGF in the presence of forskolin (our unpublished results), it is likely that PDGF influences cAMP accumulation by a dual mechanism of action.

INDUCTION OF THE PROTO-ONCOGENES C-*FOS* AND C-*MYC*

In addition to the events in the membrane and cytosol described above, serum and other growth factors rapidly and transiently induce the expression of the cellular oncogenes c-*fos* and c-*myc* in quiescent fibroblasts (*see* Ref. 35 for review). Since these cellular oncogenes encode nuclear proteins it is plausible that their transient expression may play a role in the transduction of the mitogenic signal in the nucleus.

Like PDGF and other growth factors, bombesin rapidly and transiently induces the expression of the cellular oncogenes c-*fos* and c-*myc*.[25,36] Enhanced expression of c-*fos* occurs within minutes of bombesin addition and is followed by increased expression of c-*myc*. The time-course and magnitude of these effects are similar to those induced by a saturating concentration of PDGF.[36]

There is increasing evidence implicating PKC activation in the sequence of events linking receptor occupancy and proto-oncogene induction. Accordingly, bombesin-induced oncogene expression is markedly reduced by down-regulation of PKC.[35] However, direct activation of PKC by PBt_2 at saturating concentrationsrations is not sufficient to evoke a maximal increase in c-*fos* and c-*myc* mRNA levels. Addition of the Ca^{2+} ionophore A23187 at 50nM, a concentration that caused an increase in cytosolic Ca^{2+} comparable to that induced by bombesin[6] markedly enhances c-*fos* and c-*myc* induction promoted by PBt_2.[35,36] Hence, it is likely that the induction of these cellular oncogenes by bombesin is mediated by the coordinated effects of Ca^{2+} mobilization and activation of PKC but additional pathways may exist.[35]

While PKC activation increases c-*fos* and c-*myc* expression, the effect of cAMP on these proto-oncogenes has not been clearly defined.[35] Recently we found that 3T3 cells treated with forskolin exhibit a 20-fold lower level of c-*fos* mRNA than those stimulated through PKC, though they show maximal c-*myc* expression.[37] Thus, cAMP differentially controls c-*fos* and c-*myc* expression. The large induction of c-*fos* can be dissociated from cAMP-mediated mitogenesis.

EARLY SIGNALS AND SYNERGISTIC EFFECTS IN MITOGENESIS

Quiescent cells can be stimulated to recommence DNA synthesis and cell division by various polypeptide growth factors, pharmacological agents and neuropeptides which exhibit potent synergistic effects. Rozengurt[1] proposed that stimulation of cell proliferation by single or multiple factors results from the activation of separate signal transduction pathways that cooperate to elicit the complete set of molecular events leading to mitogenesis. The results discussed here and depicted schematically in Figure 1, extend this model and provide further evidence for the existence of multiple signal-transduction pathways in mitogenesis.

As summarized in Figure 1 and in Table 1, PKC and cAMP represent two separate signal-transduction pathways that can lead to mitogenesis. In the presence of insulin, activation of PKC pathway (by PBt_2 or DAG) stimulates reinitiation of DNA synthesis without early increase in cAMP. Reciprocally, an increase in the cellular level of cAMP (by multiple pharmacological agents, prostaglandins or the neuropeptide VIP) leads to DNA synthesis without early activation of PKC, Ca^{2+} mobilization or large induction of c-*fos* (Table 1). This emphasizes a crucial aspect

Table 1 Early responses elicited by various mitogens in Swiss 3T3 cells

Addition[a]	Ca^{2+} Mobilization	Na^+/K^+ pump stimulation	80K phosphorylation	58K phosphorylation	EGF receptor transmodulation	cAMP elevation	c-fos induction	c-myc induction
PBt_2/OAG	−	+	+	−	+	−	+	+
cAMP	−	+	−	+	−	+	−	+
PBt_2 + cAMP	−	+	+	+	+	+	+	+
Bombesin	+	+	+	b	+	b	+	+
PDGF	+	+	+	N.D.	+	+	+	+
EGF + Insulin	−	+	−	−	−	−	+	+

[a]The responses to each factor are indicated. cAMP was increased by a variety of agents including PGE_1, NECA, cholera toxin and forskolin.
[b]Elevation of cAMP is seen in the presence of forskolin and is indirect as explained in the text. The original data can be obtained from references in the respective sections in the text, from recent reviews (Rozengurt, 1986; Rozengurt and Mendoza, 1986; Zachary et al., 1987) and unpublished data

of the multiple signal model: many early signals play a regulatory rather than an obligatory role in the mitogenic response.[1]

Simultaneous activation of the PKC and cAMP pathways stimulates DNA synthesis in the absence of insulin or any other ligand that occupies a tyrosine kinase receptor. The synergistic effect between PKC and cAMP provides a clear example where mitogenesis is elicited by defined intracellular signal-transduction pathways (Fig. 1).

The ability of the bombesin-like peptides to induce DNA synthesis in the absence of other growth-promoting factors can be explained, at least in part, within this framework. These peptides can stimulate both signals, the PKC pathway directly and the cAMP pathway by a second, indirect mechanism. Bombesin and PDGF elicit a common set of early events in 3T3 cells (Table 1). A single system of signal transduction shared by both mitogens is, however, unlikely because the Ca^{2+} mobilizing effects of bombesin can be distinguished from those of PDGF on the basis of kinetics and sensitivity to phorbol ester inhibition.[8] Furthermore, the stimulation of Na^+ fluxes and 80K phosphorylation[23] by PDGF occur after a considerable lag period (30 s–2 min) as compared with the rapid stimulation of these events by bombesin. Additional pathways (i.e. tyrosine kinase) in the action of PDGF may exist.

Insulin added at concentrations at which it occupies the IGF_1 receptor, acts synergistically with both PKC and cAMP pathways and potently enhances mitogenesis in response to bombesin and PDGF (Fig. 1). Since insulin does not activate PKC or cAMP, it is envisaged to initiate a separate mitogenic pathway. Indeed, stimulation of DNA synthesis in 3T3 cells by insulin and EGF occurs without activation of either the PKC or cAMP pathways (Table 1), a clear demonstration of the regulatory (or redundant) nature of these pathways. In conclusion, long-term mitogenesis can be stimulated through multiple signal-transduction pathways. These alternative pathways cooperate in a synergistic fashion for transducing environmental signals from the whole organism into a mitogenic response of a specific cell.

REFERENCES

1 Rozengurt E. Early signals in the mitogenic response. Science 1986; 234: 161
2 Zachary I, Woll PJ, Rozengurt E. A role for neuropeptides in the control of cell proliferation. Dev Biol 1987; 124: 295
3 Rozengurt E, Sinnett-Smith J. Bombesin stimulation of DNA synthesis and

cell division in cultures of Swiss 3T3 cells. Proc Natl Acad Sci USA 1983; 80: 2936
4 Woll PJ, Rozengurt E. Bombesin and bombesin antagonists: studies in Swiss 3T3 cells and human small cell lung cancer. Br J Cancer 1988; 57: 579
5 Rozengurt E, Mendoza SA. Early stimulation of Na^+/H^+ antiport, Na^+/K^+ pump activity and Ca^{2+} fluxes in fibroblast mitogenesis. In: Mandel L, Benos D. eds. Current Topics in Membranes and Transport 1986; 27: 163
6 Mendoza SM, Schneider JA, Lopez-Rivas A, Sinnett-Smith JW, Rozengurt E. Early events elicited by bombesin and structurally related peptides in quiescent Swiss 3T3 cells. II. Changes in Na^+ and Ca^{2+} fluxes, Na^+/K^+ pump activity, and intracellular pH. J Cell Biol 1986; 102: 2223
7 Vara F, Rozengurt E. Stimulation of Na^+/H^+ antiport activity by epidermal growth factor and insulin occurs without activation of protein kinase C. Biochem Biophys Res Commun 1985; 130: 646
8 Lopez-Rivas A, Mendoza SA, Nanberg E, Sinnett-Smith J, Rozengurt E. The Ca^{2+}-mobilizing actions of platelet-derived growth factor differ from those of bombesin and vasopressin in Swiss 3T3 cells. Proc Natl Acad Sci USA 1987; 84: 5768
9 Nanberg E, Rozengurt E. Temporal relationship between inositol polyphosphate formation and increases in cytosolic Ca^{2+} in quiescent 3T3 cells stimulated by platelet-derived growth factor, bombesin and vasopressin. EMBO J 1988; 7: 2741
10 Berridge MJ, Irvine RF. Inositol triphosphate, a novel second messenger in cellular signal transduction. Nature 1984; 312: 315
11 Heslop JP, Blakeley DM, Brown KD, Irvine RF, Berridge MJ. Effects of bombesin and insulin on inositol(1,4,5) triphosphate and inositol(1,3,4) triphosphate formation in Swiss 3T3 cells. Cell 1986; 47: 703
12 Kikkawa U, Nishizuka Y. The role of protein kinase C in transmembrane signalling. Ann Rev Cell Biol 1986; 2: 149
13 Dicker P, Rozengurt E. Phorbol esters and vasopressin stimulate DNA synthesis by a common mechanism. Nature 1980; 287: 607
14 Collins M, Rozengurt E. Binding of phorbol esters to high affinity sites on murine fibroblastic cells elicits a mitogenic response. J Cell Physiol 1982; 112: 42
15 Rozengurt E, Rodriguez-Pena A, Coombs M, Sinnett-Smith J. Diacylglycerol stimulates DNA synthesis and cell division in mouse 3T3 cells: role of Ca^{2+}-sensitive phospholipid-dependent protein kinase C. Proc Natl Acad Sci USA 1984; 81: 5748
16 Rodriguez-Pena A, Rozengurt E. Disappearance of Ca^{2+}-sensitive, phospholipid-dependent protein kinase activity in phorbol ester-treated 3T3 cells. Biochem Biophys Res Commun 1984; 120: 1053
17 Rodriguez-Pena A, Rozengurt E. Phosphorylation of an acidic molecular weight 806000 cellular protein in a cell-free system and intact Swiss 3T3 cells: a specific marker of protein kinase C activity. EMBO J 1986; 5: 77
18 Rozengurt E, Rodriguez-Pena A, Smith KA. Phorbol esters, phospholipase C, and growth factors rapidly stimulate the phosphorylation of a Mr 80 000 protein in intact quiescent 3T3 cells. Proc Natl Acad Sci USA 1983; 80: 7244
19 Morris C, Rozengurt E. Purification of a phosphoprotein from rat brain closely related to the 80kDa substrate of protein kinase C identified in Swiss 3T3 fibroblasts. FEBS Lett 1988; 231: 311
20 Zachary I, Sinnett-Smith JW, Rozengurt E. Early events elicited by bombesin and structurally related peptides in quiescent Swiss 3T3 cells. I. Activation of protein kinase C and inhibition of epidermal growth factor binding. J Cell Biol 1986; 102: 2211
21 Isacke CM, Meisenhelder J, Brown KD, Gould KL, Gould SJ, Hunter T. Early phosphorylation events following the treatment of Swiss 3T3 cells with

bombesin and the mammalian bombesin-related peptide, gastrin-releasing peptide. EMBO J 1986; 5: 2889
22 Cirillo DM, Gaudino G, Naldini L, Comoglio PM. Receptor for bombesin with associated tyrosine kinase activity. Mol Cell Biol 1986; 6: 4641
23 Rodriguez-Pena A, Rozengurt E. Serum, like phorbol esters, rapidly activates protein kinase C in intact quiescent fibroblasts. EMBO J 1985; 4: 71
24 Rodriguez-Pena A, Rozengurt E. Vasopressin rapidly stimulated protein kinase C in quiescent Swiss 3T3 cells. J Cell Physiol 1986; 129: 124
25 Letterio JJ, Coughlin SR, Williams LT. Pertussis toxin-sensitive pathway in the stimulation of c-*myc* expression and DNA synthesis by bombesin. Science 1986; 234: 1117
26 Zachary I, Millar J, Nanberg E, Higgins T, Rozengurt E. Inhibition of bombesin-induced mitogenesis by pertussis toxin-dissociation from phospholipase C pathway. Biochem Biophys Res Commun 1987; 146: 456
27 Zachary I, Rozengurt E. Modulation of the epidermal growth factor receptor by mitogenic ligands: effects of bombesin and role of protein kinase C. Cancer Surveys 1985; 4: 729
28 Lin CR, Chen WS, Lazar CS. et al. Protein kinase C phosphorylation at Thr 654 of the unoccupied EGF receptor and EGF binding regulate functional receptor loss by independent mechanisms. Cell 1986; 44: 839
29 Rozengurt E, Stroobant P, Waterfield MD, Deuel TF, Keehan M. Platelet-derived growth factor elicits cyclic AMP accumulation in Swiss 3T3 cells: Role of prostaglandin production. Cell 1983; 34: 265
30 Zurier RB, Kozma M, Sinnett-Smith J, Rozengurt E. Vasoactive Intestinal Peptide synergistically stimulates DNA synthesis in mouse 3T3 cells: Role of cAMP, Ca^{2+} and protein kinase C. Exp Cell Res 1988; 176: 155
31 Escribano J, Rozengurt E. Cyclic AMP increasing agents rapidly stimulated vimentin phosphorylation in quiescent cultures of Swiss 3T3 cells. J Cell Physiol 1988; 137: 223
32 Geiger B. Intermediate filaments: looking for a function. Nature 1987; 329: 392
33 Rozengurt E, Murray M, Zachary I, Collins M. Protein kinase C activation enhances cAMP accumulation in Swiss 3T3 cells: inhibition by pertussis toxin. Proc Natl Acad Sci USA 1987; 84: 2282
34 Millar JBA, Rozengurt E. Bombesin enhancement of cAMP accumulation in Swiss 3T3 cells: Evidence of a dual mechanism of action. J Cell Physiol 1988; 137: 214
35 Rozengurt E, Sinnett-Smith J. Early signals underlying the induction of the proto-oncogenes c-*fos* and c-*myc* in quiescent fibroblasts: studies with peptides of the bombesin family and other growth factors. Prog Nucleic Acid Res Mol Biol 1988; 35: 261
36 Rozengurt E, Sinnett-Smith JW. Bombesin induction of c-*fos* and c-*myc* proto-oncogenes in Swiss 3T3 cells: significance for the mitogenic response. J Cell Physiol 1987; 131: 218
37 Mehmet H, Sinnett-Smith J, Moore JP, Evan GI, Rozengurt E. Differential induction of c-*fos* and c-*myc* by cyclic AMP in Swiss 3T3 cells: Significance for the mitogenic response. Oncogene Res 1988; 3: 281

Early gene induction by growth factors

J R Woodgett
Ludwig Institute for Cancer Research, London, UK

> The mechanisms by which growth factors elicit their cellular effects include the rapid transcriptional activation of a set of genes. In the past five years much has been learned of the number, identity and even function of these genetic messengers and has begun to provide a molecular basis for certain growth factor responses. The identification and characterisation of the nuclear transcription factors that stimulate expression of these genes has established the involvement of several nuclear oncogenes underscoring the importance of subversion of normal signal transduction pathways in neoplasia. Some of the immediate early genes themselves are *trans*-activators, participating in a cascade of gene induction. The current pace of progress should, in the next few years, bridge the remaining gap between the growth factor receptors and the nuclear transcription factors.

Comprehension of the pathways through which growth factors exert their effect in normal cells, and the way in which these mechanisms are disrupted in neoplastic cells is one of the central questions in biology. The synthesis of new mRNA is an absolute requirement for quiescent cells to respond to mitogenic factors indicating that transcriptional activation of genes is part of the cellular reaction.[1] Although platelet-derived growth factor (PDGF) had previously been shown to promote the synthesis of several polypeptides by 2-dimensional gel analysis,[2] the first direct demonstration that an extracellular ligand could induce gene expression involved β-interferon which was shown to increase the synthesis of RNA for two human genes.[3] These studies were followed by the finding that the expression of two protooncogenes, c-*myc* and c-*fos*, is rapidly stimulated by a variety of growth promoting agents and was a watershed in the field bringing together oncogenes, growth factors and the cell cycle.[4-9] In this review, I will describe the biology of rapidly induced genes (the 'immediate early genes') and then present an overview of the mechanisms of induction that have recently been elucidated in this fast moving field.

THE IMMEDIATE EARLY GENES

The search for genes induced by growth factors has been pursued in two ways. One is to look for changes in the levels of mRNA of a known gene after stimulation of quiescent cells with a purified growth factor or serum. The candidate genes were initially those with either a known or postulated role in cell regulation such as the proto-oncogenes. This strategy quickly led to the identification of c-*myc* and c-*fos* as targets for a variety of growth factors such as PDGF,[4-6] Epidermal growth factor (EGF),[7] serum,[8] Nerve growth factor (NGF)[9] as well as β-actin and ornithine decarboxylase and gave the first evidence for a high degree of overlap between the genetic responses to different stimulants.

To identify novel target genes for growth factor activation the strategy of differential cDNA screening has been employed. In this method cDNA is synthesized from mRNA prepared from stimulated and resting cells and each used as a probe to screen a cDNA library constructed from the stimulated cell mRNA. Plaques that hybridize with the probes derived from the stimulated cell mRNA but not (or to a lesser degree) to the resting cell probes are potential induced genes. This latter technique has been used to great effect by several groups using a selection of mitogens such as serum, PDGF, EGF, fibroblast growth factor (FGF), bombesin and phorbol esters and has resulted in the identification of over 100 inducible genes.[10-14]

Several general observations have been gleaned from these studies. One is the independence of the induction on protein synthesis, indicating that the transcriptional apparatus pre-exists in the cell and is post-translationally modified upon stimulation. The time course of activation of the genes varies considerably. For example, elevations in c-*fos* and β-actin RNA are detectable within minutes of serum stimulation, peak at 10–20 minutes and return to prestimulated levels within 2 hours. In contrast, the levels of c-*myc* do not peak until 1–2 hours after stimulation and decay over a longer period.[13,15] Bravo and colleagues have recently comprehensively catalogued the behaviour of 71 clones that are induced by serum and various growth factors.[13] They find that the clones can be grouped into classes of genes with respect to their kinetics of induction and RNA half-life. They suggest that a cohort of genes that behave like c-*fos* are required for transition from G_0 to G_1 but are not essential for passage through the rest of the cell cycle. Other genes, exemplified by c-*myc*, are required for longer periods and are perhaps involved in the transition from G_1 to S phase. Other genes are induced with longer delays and, in the case of PDGF, two of these β-fibroblast interferon and $(2'-5')$-oligoadenylate synthetase, may function to inhibit further mitogenic stimulation by the growth factor.[16]

Another characteristic of the rapidly induced genes is the superinductive effect of cycloheximide. The protein synthesis inhibitor doesn't alter the initial kinetics of induction but elevates and prolongs the maximal response. This effect is not fully understood but appears to involve inhibition of transcriptional shut-off and enhancement of RNA stability presumably by prevention of new synthesis of labile degradation enzymes. This property of cycloheximide has been exploited in the differential cloning of mRNAs to increase the sensitivity of detection.[13]

While most of the clones to inducible genes still await characterization, the limited analysis that has been performed on the gene products has generated exciting and encouraging results. These genes will be discussed in approximate order of induction.

Fos

Like most oncogenes, the function of c-*fos* has resisted analysis. Recent results, however, have demonstrated interaction of c-*fos* and v-*fos* with nuclear complexes involved in regulation of transcription and differentiation (see below).[15-19] c-*fos* is extremely sensitive to cellular conditions and can be transcriptionally activated by a wide variety of agents including stress.[4-9] Induction in fibroblasts requires the cells to be quiescent, i.e. in G_0, suggesting that *fos* is necessary for re-entry of resting cells into a state of cycling.[20]

Krox-20

This serum-induced gene was isolated by Bravo and colleagues and appears with similar kinetics to c-*fos*.[21] The predicted protein product has a molecular mass of 48kD and contains three structural motifs for zinc binding fingers. Such motifs have been observed in several DNA binding proteins such as *Xenopus laevis* transcription factor IIIA,[22] the *Drosophila melanogaster* gene *Kruppel*,[23] and the mammalian transcription factor Sp1.[24] These properties are consistent with Krox-20 being a *bona fide* transcription factor. The identification of the genes which are regulated by Krox-20 may add to the already considerable list of serum-regulated genes.

NGF1-A

This gene was isolated from PC12 cells after NGF stimulation and is induced with similar kinetics to c-*fos* except that the message persists for several days.[25] Like Krox-20, NGF1-A has three zinc finger motifs. Although there is conservation of cysteine and histidine residues in these structures, there is usually rather lower homology inbetween. Interestingly, the zinc finger regions of Krox-20 (mouse) and NGF1-A (rat) are 93% identical at the amino acid level, although this conservation is much less in the nucleotide sequence. Outside the finger repeats there is no significant homology except for the high proportion of proline, serine and threonine residues ($>40\%$). The extreme conservation of the DNA binding region of these two proteins would suggest a common DNA binding site, if not similarity of function.

KC

This gene was isolated from mouse RNA induced by PDGF.[11] Like c-*fos*, KC is rapidly and transiently expressed and is not induced in growing cells. By hybridization selection and translation, the unmodified protein product of KC is 10kD. The function of this protein is currently unknown.

JunA

This is the cellular homologue of the oncogene of avian sarcoma virus 17, v-*jun*.[26] Sequence and immunological comparisons together with DNase footprinting have established that *jun*A is very similar, if not identical, to AP-1, a transcription factor that binds to phorbol ester sensitive promoters (see below).[27-29]

JunB

This clone was isolated from mouse fibroblasts stimulated with serum or PDGF (clone 465 in Ref. 12).[30] Sequence analysis revealed significant homology in two regions to *jun*A which include a sequence conserved between *jun*A and GCN4, a yeast transcription factor, that has been shown to be a DNA binding domain.[32,33]

Myc

While the function of c-*myc* is still obscure, it is, like c-*fos*, a post-translationally-modified nuclear protein and has been postulated to be a regulator of transcription (see below).[33,34] c-*myc* is subject to stringent control at the levels of RNA transcription initiation, read-through and degradation and protein degradation.[35-37] Indeed, overexpression of c-*myc* caused by retroviral insertion or chromosomal rearrangement has been observed in a number of tumours including Burkitt lymphoma and plastocytoma. The gene has also been a target for retroviral transduction by several avian and feline RNA viruses.[38,39] In contrast to *fos* and KC, c-*myc* is inducible in sub-confluent cell cultures that are rapidly cycling, although in synchronized cultures the levels do not change throughout the cycle.[20,40] Expression of c-*myc* alone can induce quiescent cells into S-phase but the cells do not divide suggesting the requirement of other factors.[41] There is evidence that c-*myc* is involved in DNA synthesis, since it can facilitate SV40 DNA replication.[42] Additionally, antibodies to c-*myc* inhibit duplication of an autonomously replicating plasmid.[43] These features are consistent with a highly regulated, basic role for c-*myc* in the progress of the cell cycle.

JE

This gene was detected in the same way as KC, but is about 4-fold more abundant and has consequently been useful as a marker for mitogenic stimulation. Unlike c-*fos* and c-*myc*, JE expression is lineage-restricted.[20] The nucleotide sequence of JE is homologous to several cytokine genes such as M-colony stimulating factor (M-CSF) and IL-6 (also a PDGF-inducible gene),[44] although this similarity is not conserved in the predicted protein sequence.[45] The protein contains a putative cleavable hydrophobic leader sequence consistent with its similarity to the secreted cytokines.

Fra-1

This gene is one of several proteins that are antigenically related to c-*fos*.[46] The gene is induced with slower kinetics and c-*fos* and encodes a protein of 35kD.[47] This protein contains regions of amino acid homology to *fos* but is overall significantly diverged.

There are several genes that are induced later than the immediate early genes (12–18 hours), and thus outside of the scope of this review, such as proliferin (MRP), MEP, cyclin (PCNA), plasminogen activator, dihydrofolate reductase and thymidine kinase.[48] These fall into two major categories: genes involved in the synthesis of DNA and genes for secreted proteases required for dissolution of the extracellular matrix. Their delayed time course of induction may make them targets for the immediate early genes that encode DNA binding proteins (see below).

There remains the battery of immediate early genes identified by cDNA cloning, the protein products of which have yet to be characterized. Sequence analysis will help to identify DNA binding proteins with finger structures and homology to growth factors but genes not having these motifs will prove more difficult to classify. A notable absentee thus far is a protein with a homeo box domain.

MECHANISMS OF INDUCTION

The transcription factors

The isolation of inducible genes allowed the sequences upstream of the genes to be assessed for their importance in inducibility. At this point the lessons learned from studies on DNA tumour viruses played a large role in the recognition of sequence elements. Studies on the enhancer sequences of SV40 had revealed sequences that were required for transcriptional activation by, for example, phorbol esters.[49] Moreover, these sequences were protected by extracts from mammalian cells in DNase footprinting experiments implying the presence of specific DNA binding proteins. These sequences were identified in a number of other phorbol ester activated genes and were denoted TREs (TPA responsive elements).[50]

The rapidity of response and multiple sensitivities of the c-*fos* promoter have made it the subject of several studies. Interestingly, in addition to a potential TRE, the c-*fos* promoter contains an element of dyad symmetry, termed the serum response element

(SRE), which confers responsiveness to phorbol esters, serum, and EGF.[51,52] A distinct element 5' to the SRE confers inducibility to PDGF.[53] Therefore the same mitogen may utilize different sequence elements and thus different binding factors. That this is the case has been demonstrated by the purification of the factors that bind to the TRE and SRE. The TRE factor is termed AP-1, a 47kD protein.[54] The SRE factor has been isolated from Hela cells and is a 62–67kD protein termed serum response factor (SRF).[55,56] In addition the c-*fos* promoter contains a cyclic AMP responsive element (CREB) explaining induction via pathways that elevate this second messenger.[57] Cells also contain a repressor of the c-*fos* promoter: this was demonstrated by achieving induction of *fos* in quiescent cells by introduction of competing upstream *fos* promoter DNA.[58] The complexity of the c-*fos* promoter rivals only that of the DNA tumour viruses and may reflect the key position of c-*fos* in the initiation of an inductive cascade (see below).

The central role of AP-1 in transcriptional regulation has recently become clear from the realization that AP-1 is the normal cellular cognate of v-*jun*, the oncogene of avian sarcoma virus 17.[28] Thus aberrant expression or regulation of a single transcriptional regulator has the potential to relieve cells of normal cellular growth control. So what regulates AP-1? In experiments investigating the components of a nuclear complex involved in binding a sequence element in the promoter of a differentiation-sensitive gene termed aP2, the direct participation of c-*fos* was established using antiserum to *fos* protein.[17] The aP2 sequence element showed homology to TRE and c-*fos* was shown to associate with complexes that bound the TRE.[19] The climax to these experiments was the demonstration that AP-1, the TRE binding factor, is complexed to c-*fos* as judged by DNA affinity precipitation and immunoprecipitation using anti-*fos* antibodies.[59] In fact AP-1 was shown to be equivalent to a *fos*-associated protein termed p39 that had been observed, in a number of laboratories, to co-immunoprecipitate with c-*fos*. Many questions remain. For example what activates transcription of junA? Perhaps SRF will be involved. Indeed, it appears that there are hierarchies of transcriptional activation, such that a growth factor activates a pre-existing factor like SRF which then induces genes like c-*fos* which activate or modify transcriptional complexes that stimulate expression of a further bank of genes (see Fig. 1).

Further studies are required to clarify the role of c-*fos* in the transcription complex, but these findings have highlighted the *fos/jun*A complex as a prime target for transformation. As such this complex will undoubtedly be the subject of intense study. Already there is evidence that the complex can act in both negative and positive ways depending on the gene target and may interact with CREB and PDGF/*sis* sites allowing cross-regulation of the various cellular signalling pathways. The complex also contains

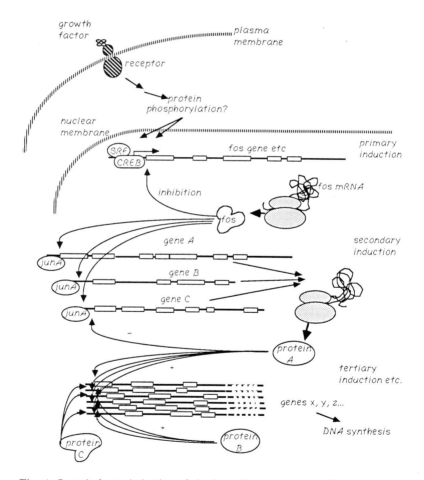

Fig. 1 Growth factor induction of the immediate early genes. Transcriptional activation of genes such as c-*fos* lead, in turn, to secondary activation of other immediate early genes (e.g. Krox-20), which can then activate further genes culminating in the cellular response.

several other proteins which are certainly prime candidates for proto-oncogenes.

FUTURE PERSPECTIVES

The identification of genes responsive to growth factor induction has allowed an investigation of the signal transduction pathway from the DNA up, as opposed to the growth factor receptors down. Some of the proteins involved in transcriptional activation have been identified. However, a link between ligand binding to its receptor and activation of the nuclear transcription complexes remains to be made. How might this gap be bridged? An obvious mechanism is via protein phosphorylation and there is increasing evidence that this means of signal transmission plays a role. Several growth factor receptors are themselves, or activate, protein-tyrosine kinases. Phorbol esters directly activate protein kinase C which is also activated via stimulation of phosphatidylinositol breakdown in the case of several growth factors such as PDGF and bombesin. Additionally, the proteins c-*myc*, SRF, AP-1/*jun*A and c-*fos* are phosphoproteins, the latter of which increases its phosphate content in response to phorbol esters.[60] One of the salient problems is thus to identify the protein kinases and phosphatases that are responsible for targeting the transcription complexes and to determine their mechanism of regulation. The relevance of the *fos*/*jun*A complex in growth control seems assured. Perhaps it will be an important target for anti-neoplastic drugs.

The elucidation of the pathways via which growth factors elicit their effects on gene induction may be difficult, but the studies completed thus far have shown that these same mechanisms are often subverted in the neoplastic state. Learning more about normal signal transduction promotes the understanding of the aberrances in neoplasia and *vice versa*.

REFERENCES

1 Baserga R. The biology of cell reproduction. Cambridge: Harvard University Press, 1985
2 Pledger WJ, Hart CA, Locatell K, Scher CD. Platelet-derived growth factor-modulated proteins: constitutive synthesis by a transformed cell line. Proc Natl Acad Sci USA 1981; 78: 4358–4362
3 Larner AC, Jonak G, Cheng Y-SE, Korant B, Knight E, Darnell JE Jr. Transcriptional induction of two genes in human cells by interferon. Proc Natl Acad Sci USA 1984; 81: 6733–6737
4 Kelly K, Cochran BH, Stiles CD, Leder P. Cell-specific regulation of the c-*myc*

gene by lymphocyte mitogens and platelet-derived growth factor. Cell 1983; 35: 603–610
5 Kruijer WJ, Cooper JA, Hunter T, Verma IM. Platelet-derived growth factor induces rapid but transient expression of the c-*fos* gene and protein. Nature 1984; 312: 711–716
6 Cochran BH, Zullo J, Verma IM, Stiles CD. Expression of the c-*fos* gene and of a *fos*-related gene is stimulated by platelet-derived growth factor. Science 1984; 226: 1080–1082
7 Bravo R, Burckhardt J, Curran T, Muller R. Stimulation and inhibition of growth by EGF in different A431 cell clones is accompanied by the rapid induction of c-*fos* and c-*myc* protooncogenes. EMBO J 1985; 4: 1193–1197
8 Greenberg ME, Ziff EB. Stimulation of 3T3 cells induces transcription of the c-*fos* protooncogene. Nature 1984; 311: 433–442
9 Kruijer W, Schubert D, Verma IM. Induction of the protooncogene *fos* by nerve growth factor. Proc Natl Acad Sci USA 1985; 82: 7330–7334
10 Linzer DIH, Nathans D. Growth-related changes in specific mRNAs of cultivated mouse cells. Proc Natl Acad Sci USA 1983; 80: 4271–4275
11 Cochran B, Reffel AC, Stiles CD. Molecular cloning of gene sequences regulated by platelet-derived growth factor. Cell 1983; 33: 939–947
12 Lau LF, Nathans D. Expression of a set of growth-regulated immediate early genes in BALB/c 3T3 cells: coordinate regulation with c-*fos* or c-*myc*. Proc Natl Acad Sci USA 1987; 4: 1182–1186
13 Almendral JM, Sommer D, Macdonald-Bravo H, Burckhardt J, Perera J, Bravo R. Complexity of the early genetic response to growth factors in mouse fibroblasts. Mol Cell Biol 1988; 8: 2140–2148
14 Edwards DR, Parfett CL, Denhardt DT. Transcriptional activation of two serum-induced RNAs in mouse fibroblasts: equivalence of one species to B2 repetitive elements. Mol Cell Biol 1985; 5: 3280–3288
15 Muller R, Bravo R, Burckhardt J, Curran T. Induction of c-*fos* gene and protein by growth factors precedes activation of c-*myc*. Nature 1984; 312: 716–720
16 Zullo JN, Cochran BH, Huang AS, Stiles CD. Platelet-derived growth factor and double-stranded ribonucleic acids stimulate expression of the same genes in 3T3 cells. Cell 1985; 43: 793–800
17 Distal RJ, Ro H-S, Rosen BS, Groves DL, Spiegelman BM. Nucleoprotein complexes that regulate gene expression in adipocyte differentiation: direct participation of c-*fos*. Cell 1987; 49: 835–844
18 Setoyama C, Frunzio R, Liau G, Mudryj M, De Crombrugghe B. Transcriptional activation encoded by the v-*fos* gene. Proc Natl Acad Sci USA 1986; 83: 3213–3217
19 Franza BR Jr, Rauscher III FJ, Josephs SF, Curran T. The *fos* complex and *fos*-related antigens recognise sequence elements that contain AP-1 binding sites. Science 1988; 239: 1150–1153
20 Rollins BJ, Morrison ED, Stiles CD. A cell cycle constraint on the regulation of gene expression by platelet-derived growth factor. Science 1987; 238: 1269–1271
21 Chavrier P, Zerial M, Lemaire P, Almendral J, Bravo R, Charnay P. A gene encoding a protein with zinc fingers is activated during G_0/G_1 in cultured cells. EMBO J 1988; 7: 29–35
22 Miller J, McLachan AD, Klug A. Repetitive Zinc-binding domains in the protein transcription factor IIIA from Xenopus oocytes. EMBO J 1985; 4: 1609–1614
23 Schuh R, Aicher W, Gaul U, et al. A conserved family of nuclear proteins containing structural elements of the finger protein encoded by *Kruppel*, a Drosophila segmentation gene. Cell 1986; 47: 1025–1032
24 Kadonaga JT, Carner KR, Masiarz FR, Tjian R. Isolation of cDNA encoding

transcription factor Sp1 and functional analysis of the DNA binding domain. Cell 1987; 51: 1079–1090
25 Milbrandt J. A nerve growth factor-induced gene encodes a possible transcriptional regulatory factor. Science 1987; 238: 797–799
26 Maki Y, Bos TJ, Davis C, Starbuck M, Vogt PK. Avian sarcoma virus 17 carries the *jun* oncogene. Proc Natl Acad Sci USA 1987; 84: 2848–2852
27 Bos TJ, Bohmann D, Tsuchie H, Tjian R, Vogt PK. v-*jun* encodes a nuclear protein with enhancer binding properties of AP-1 Cell 1988; 52: 705–712
28 Bohmann D, Bos TJ, Admon A, Nishimura T, Vogt PK, Tjian R. Human proto-oncogene c-*jun* encodes a DNA binding protein with structural and functional properties of transcription factor AP-1. Science 1988; 238: 1386–1392
29 Angel P, Allegretto EA, Okino ST, Hattori K, Boyle WJ, Hunter T, Karin M. Oncogene *jun* encodes a sequence-specific *trans*-activator similar to AP-1. Nature 1988; 332: 166–171
30 Ryder K, Lau LF, Nathans D. A gene activated by growth factors is related to the oncogene v-*jun*. 1988 Proc Natl Acad Sci USA 1988; 85: 1487–1491
31 Vogt PK, Bos TJ, Doolittle RF. Homology between the DNA binding domain of the GCN4 regulatory protein of yeast and the carboxy-terminal region of a protein encoded for by the oncogene *jun*. Proc Natl Acad Sci USA 1987; 84: 3316–3319
32 Struhl K. The DNA binding domains of the *jun* oncogene and the yeast GCN4 transcriptional activator protein are functionally homologous. Cell 1987; 50: 841–846
33 Cole MD. The *myc* oncogene: its role in transformation and differentiation. Ann Rev Genet 1986; 20: 361–384
34 Hann SR, Eisenman RN. Proteins encoded by the human c-*myc* oncogene: differential expression in neoplastic cells. Mol Cell Biol 1984; 4: 2486–2497
35 Pierchaczyk M, Yang Y-Q, Blanchard J-M, Jeanteur P, Marku KB. Posttranscriptional mechanisms are responsible for accumulation of truncated c-*myc* RNAs in murine plasma cell tumours. Cell 1985; 42: 589–597
36 Ramsey G, Evan GI, Bishop JM. The protein encoded by the human proto-oncogene c-*myc*. Proc Natl Acad Sci USA 1984; 81: 7742–7746
37 Bentley D, Groudine M. A block to elongation is largely responsible for decreased transcription of c-*myc* in differentiated HL-60 cells. Nature 1985; 321: 702–706
38 Alitalo K, Ramsey G, Ohlsson S, Colby WW, McGrath JP, Levinson AD. Identification of nuclear proteins encoded by viral and cellular *myc* oncogenes. Nature 1983; 306: 274–277
39 Levy LS, Gardner MB, Casey JW. Isolation of a feline leukaemia provirus containing the oncogene *myc* from a feline lymphosarcoma. Nature 1984; 308: 853–856
40 Thompson CB, Challoner PB, Neiman PE, Groudine M. Levels of c-*myc* oncogene mRNA are invariant throughout the cell cycle. Nature 1985; 314: 363–366
41 Cavalieri F, Goldfard M. Growth factor-deprived BALB/c 3T3 murine fibroblasts can enter the S phase after induction of c-*myc* gene expression. Mol Cell Biol 1987; 7: 3554–3560
42 Classon M, Henriksson M, Sumegi J, Klein G, Hammaskjold M-L. Elevated c-*myc* expression facilitates the replication of SV40 DNA in human lymphoma cells. Nature 1987; 330: 272–274
43 Iguchi-Ariga SM, Itani T, Kiji Y, Ariga H. Possible function of the c-*myc* product: promotion of cellular DNA replication. EMBO J 1987; 6: 2365–2371
44 Kohase M, Henriksen-DeStephano D, May LT, Vilcek J, Sehgal PB. Induction of *beta* 2-interferon by tumour necrosis factor: a homeostatic mechanism in the control of cell proliferation. Cell 1986; 45: 659–666

45 Rollins BJ, Morrison ED, Stiles CD. Cloning and expression of JE, a gene inducible by platelet-derived growth factor and whose product has cytokine-like properties. Proc Natl Acad Sci USA 1988; 85: 3738–3742
46 Franza BR, Sambrucetti LC, Cohen DR, Curran T. Analysis of *fos* protein complexes and *fos*-related antigens by high resolution two-dimensional gel electrophoresis. Oncogene 1987; 1: 213–221
47 Cohen DR, Curran T. *fra*-1: a serum-inducible, cellular immediate-early gene that encodes a *fos*-related antigen. Mol Cell Biol 1988; 8: 2063–2069
48 Denhardt DT, Edwards DR, Parfett CLJ. Gene expression during the mammalian cell cycle. Biochim Biophys Acta 1986; 865: 83–125
49 McKnight S, Tjian R. Transcriptional selectivity of viral genes in mammalian cells. Cell 1986; 46: 795–805
50 Angel P, Imagawa M, Chiu R, et al. Phorbol ester-inducible genes contain a common *cis* element recognised by a TPA-modulated *trans*-acting factor. Cell 1987; 49: 729–739
51 Treisman R. Identification of a protein-binding site that mediates transcriptional response of the c-*fos* gene to serum factors. Cell 1986; 46: 567–574
52 Greenberg ME, Siegried Z, Ziff EB. Mutation of the c-*fos* gene dyad symmetry element inhibits serum inducibility of transcription in vivo and the nuclear regulatory factor binding in vitro. Mol Cell Biol 1987; 7: 1217–1225
53 Hayes TE, Kitchen AM, Cochran BH. Inducible binding of a factor to the c-*fos* regulatory domain. Proc Natl Acad Sci USA 1987; 84: 1272–1276
54 Lee W, Mitchell P, Tjian R. Purified transcription factor AP-1 interacts with TPA-inducible elements. Cell 1987; 49: 741–752
55 Treisman R. Identification and purification of a polypeptide that binds to the c-*fos* serum response element. EMBO J 1987; 6: 2711–2717
56 Prywes R, Roeder RG. Purification of the c-*fos* enhancer-binding protein. Mol Cell Biol 1987; 7: 3482–3489
57 Bravo R, Neuberg M, Burckhardt J, Almedral J, Wallich R, Muller R. Involvement of common and cell type-specific pathways in c-*fos* gene control: stable induction by cAMP in macrophages. Cell 1987; 48: 251–260
58 Sassone-Corsi P, Verma IM. Modulation of c-*fos* gene transcription by negative and positive cellular factors. Nature 1987; 326: 507–510
59 Rauscher III FR, Cohen DR, Curran T et al. *Fos*-associated protein p39 is the product of the *jun* protooncogene. Science 1988; 240: 1010–1016
60 Barber JR, Verma IM. Modification of *fos* proteins: phosphorylation of c-*fos*, but not v-*fos*, is stimulated by 12-tetradecanoyl-phorbol-13-acetate and serum. Mol Cell Biol 1987; 7: 2201–22

Growth factor receptors

M D Waterfield
Ludwig Institute for Cancer Research, Middlesex Hospital/University College Branch, London, UK

> The initial interaction of growth factors with their target cells is mediated by specific high affinity cell surface receptors. The structural and functional diversity found in growth factors is more limited at the receptor level where receptors for structurally and functionally distinct factors seem to share structural motifs and employ a restricted number of signal transduction and second messenger systems. In many cases the receptors for particular factors remain to be characterized, but rDNA techniques offer the hope that all receptors can eventually be defined in structural detail. As yet understanding of the signal transduction mechanisms remains limited but when unravelled this may offer routes for artificial modulation of growth factor action.

An ever increasing number of structurally distinct polypeptide growth factors or growth regulators are being characterized as will be evident from reading the chapters in this book. The ability to define the structure of a polypeptide that exerts a complex biological response was for many years dependent on the isolation of the factor from a large amount of biological material using an assay that made it possible to monitor the fractionation process. This was, and is, often a complex and virtually impossible task for rare factors. Having sufficient pure factor of known structure it was then possible to define and perhaps isolate the unique cell surface receptor with which the factor bound and triggered its biological response. The limitations on the isolation of factors and their receptors imposed by their rarity has largely been overcome by the introduction of recombinent DNA techniques. Through the deduction of a partial amino acid sequence or in some cases, solely by monitoring a biological response induced by an expressed cDNA clone, it is now possible to deduce the complete predicted amino acid sequence of a factor and subsequently to produce this factor in large amounts. The availability of the biologically active factor allows the definition of the receptor and opens up the possibility of purifying the receptor polypeptide for further study, including cDNA cloning to predict the receptor amino acid sequence. In some cases, the receptor itself can be characterized at the DNA level through the monitoring of its unique ligand stimulated biological activity which is encoded by a particular cDNA clone and hence deduce a putative structure prior to characterization of the receptor polypeptide. The majority of the receptor structures discussed in this chapter have been deduced through the combination of protein chemistry and rDNA techniques and it is to be expected that in the future, structural and functional details of the majority of the growth factors and their receptors will be deduced through similar approaches. This chapter outlines what we have learnt from the structures deduced thus far and how this helps in understanding the function of receptors in the signal transduction cascade initiated by growth regulators.

DIVERSITY OF GROWTH FACTOR AND RECEPTOR STRUCTURES

The elucidation of the structures of a large number of different growth factors has shown that they exhibit great diversity in their amino acid sequences. A comparison of the deduced sequences shows that only a limited number can be assigned to gene families encoding homologous factors. Where sufficient information is available, it appears that homologous factors may, in at least one case (EGF family, see Burgess, this Issue), interact with the same receptor or may, in other cases, interact with distinct receptors. For the EGF family, the two related human genes for epidermal growth factor (EGF), transforming growth factor alpha (TGFα) and the homologous gene found in vaccinia viruses (VVGF), all encode factors which interact with the same receptor. This may also be the case for the transforming growth factor β family (TGFβ) (at present thought to have at least 3 related genes) and for the fibroblast growth factor family (FGF) (at present thought to have 5 related genes), although there is insufficient data on their receptors to answer this question at present. In the case of insulin and the insulin like growth factors (IGFs) and for the platelet derived growth factors (PDGF) AA, AB and BB, there appears to be two distinct receptors which may however share binding sites for these related factors although with distinct affinities. It is perhaps to be expected that in evolution the duplication and diversification of both the growth factor and its receptor genes could, at different times, generate single or multiple related factors for the same receptor or perhaps unrelated receptors. The expression of related factors which interact with the same receptors at different times in developement could provide one type of control of growth factor initiated responses. The majority of the growth factors appear to be unique genes. This may only reflect the lack of information about related genes, only further experimental evidence will clarify this point. In many cases, the terminology used reflects lineage specificities in functions or the cell type of origin. Thus in the case of the colony stimulating factors (CSFs), it is their ability to promote differentiation and proliferation particularly of granulocyte and macrophage lineages which is shared rather than features of their primary structures. As far as is known for the CSFs, the receptors for these factors may be as diverse in structure as the factors themselves. Similarities in the nomenclature of the interleukins (numbers one to six) reflects their function in the immune and haemopoietic systems rather than implying homologies in their structures and indeed as is true from the CSFs, there may be an equivalent diversity in their receptor structures.

The diversity of growth factor structures suggests that a similar diversity in recepter structures might exist. In fact a lower degree of diversity is found in the structural features of receptors because they share common signal transduction systems. Thus the receptors for PDGF (AB) and CSF-1 are homologous while their ligands are quite distinct in structure. In this case, structural motifs from at least two distinct gene families appear to have been used in the evolution of both PDGF and CSF-1 receptors. For their external domains the immunoglobulin domain has been copied five times through a process of gene duplication and mutated to provide the ligand binding domains while the cytoplasmic regions have incorporated tyrosine kinase domains. Structurally diverse growth factors such as EGF and insulin also have receptors which share common structural motifs with each other in their ligand domains and with the receptors for PDGF and CSF-1 in their cytoplasmic domains. The common use of a kinase domain by several receptors which have distinct external domains would imply similarities in their signal transduction mechanisms. For other factors such as NGF, IL1 and IL2, the analysis of their receptors suggests that novel and perhaps unique mechanisms exist for these and other factors. This may, however, simply reflect the lack of data on receptors for other factors—we shall have to wait and see. In subsequent sections the diversity and similarities in receptor structure and function will be examined in detail. An outline of the receptor signal pathways is shown in Figure 1.

RECEPTORS LINKED TO G PROTEINS

A large numbers of receptors which transduce an extraordinary variety of different physiological responses are known to be linked to a family of GTP binding or G proteins which serve to amplify and regulate the intracellular responses activated by specific receptors.[1] The majority of these physiological activities are not normally directly involved in proliferative cellular responses, however, synergistic responses can occur in the presence of their respective ligands and various growth factors.[2] Indeed it is clear that some growth factors acting alone may exert their effects via G proteins. Examples of well characterized physiological responses are those of epinephrine which, through binding to the β-adrenergic receptor will activate G_s and hence adenylate cyclase to raise intracellular cAMP concentrations and modulate the phosphorylation of enzymes that mediate glycogen breakdown. Agents which promote sustained increases in cAMP levels (prostaglandins acting through their receptors, cholera toxin by activating G_s or forskolin by activating adenylate cyclase) can cause synergistic proliferative responses with growth factors.[2] A number of small peptides which modulate growth regulation may be linked more directly to the G-protein pathways. The neurohypophyseal hormone vasopressin, bombesin and the structurally related gastrin releasing peptide (GRP) and the neuromedins can all influence the growth of certain cells in culture. Indeed, in the case of GRP it is thought that autocrine responses to abnormal synthesis of this factor could be involved in the growth of human small cell lung cancer cells (see chapter by Woll & Rozengurt). For these small peptides and for other growth factors, including perhaps PDGF, the receptors are thought to be linked to a putative G protein that can activate phospholipase activity to generate a series of inositol phosphates which mobilize intracellular calcium and also to generate the second messenger diacylglycerol that can activate protein kinase C. The common events which follow involve changes in phosphorylation of enzymes that form part of

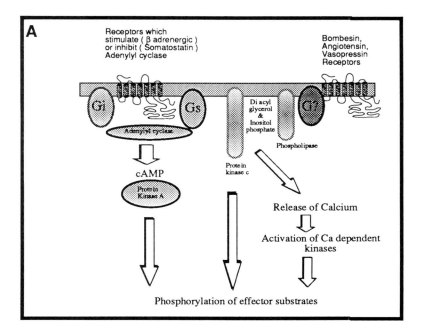
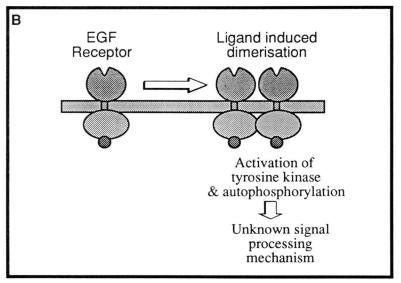

Fig. 1 Mechanisms of growth signal transduction
(a) Receptors linked through G proteins to protein kinases.
(b) The EGF receptor, a typical ligand activated tyrosine protein kinase.

intracellular cascades mediated by the diverse activated protein kinases.

The structure of the receptors for GRP, vasopressin and the neuromedins remains unclear at present. There are suggestions that the bombesin (GRP) receptor may be similar in size[3] to the β-adrenergic, substance K, muscarinic acetylcholine angiotensin and serotonin receptors. These proteins form a family of receptors having similar structural organization with seven putative transmembrane alpha helical segments. We shall have to wait and see whether this ever growing family of G protein linked receptors will include important growth factor receptors.

RECEPTORS WITH CYTOPLASMIC TYROSINE KINASES

The discovery by Cohen that EGF stimulated a protein tyrosine kinase activity which was an integral part of the receptor and which could phosphorylate the receptor itself provided a novel insight into the possible signal transduction mechanisms used by growth factor receptors (reviewed in Ref. 4). It was, of course, the discovery that the transforming proteins $pp60^{v\text{-}src}$ and $pp150^{v\text{-}abl}$ were tyrosine kinases that provoked the search for this activity and the subsequent demonstration that the truncated EGF receptor could be a transforming protein[5] provided an enormous stimulus for further characterization of this family of receptor kinases.

The basic structural motif that links this family of receptors is the tyrosine kinase domain which is homologous to that of the prototype kinase of $pp60^{c\text{-}src}$.[6] There are now 9 distinct genes encoding tyrosine kinases which lack transmembrane polypeptide sequences and have no external domains which could bind a ligand (*src, yes, FYN, fgr, HCK, LYN, LYK, abl* and *fes*). These kinases are modified (myristylated) so that they can be associated with membranes. A new leucocyte tyrosine kinase *ltk* having a transmembrane domain but lacking a significant external domain has recently been described.[7] This kinase may be involved in T cell receptor signal transduction. It is possible that all these enzymes may modulate receptor signals through their interaction with receptors or with G proteins and other regulators. Currently tyrosine kinase domains have been found in the EGF, PDGF, insulin, IGF I and CSF-1 receptors and in the receptor like proteins *c-kit, NEU, RET, c-ros, TRK, MET* and the drosophila

EGF and insulin receptors and 7-less protein which lacks a known ligands (see Fig. 2).

The basic features of the receptor and *src* kinase catalylic domains include a sequence of 250–300 amino acids which has regions of great conservation interspersed with stretches of variable sequences including deletions and insertions relative to the prototype *src* sequence.[6] A concensus sequence Gly-X-Gly-X-X-Gly with an invariant lysine residue located 14–23 residues C-terminal is thought to be involved in nucleotide binding. Indeed modification or mutation of this lysine inactivates the kinase. Amino and C-terminal to the kinase domain are additional stretches of sequence which link the kinase to the transmembrane region or are regulatory domains. In the case of the EGF receptor (and c-NEU) a 200 amino acid domain lies C-terminal to the kinase and contains the major (P_1) and minor (P_2 and P_3) in vivo tyrosine phosphorylation sites. For the PDGF, CSF-1 and c-kit receptors there is an additional insert within the kinase domain that may confer some

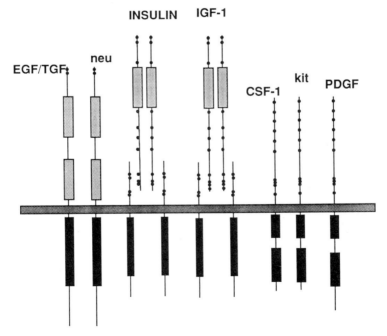

Fig. 2 Models of the ligand activity tyrosine protein kinases.
The hatched boxes and black dots indicate cysteine rich homologous regions.
The black boxes represent the tyrosine kinase region.

sub-group specific function to these receptors (see Fig. 3). The role of the tyrosine kinase in receptor signal transduction remains obscure. It is clear that ligand binding will activate the kinase and that the receptors themselves become phosphorylated. Studies with purified EGF receptors suggest that the phosphorylation is an autophosphorylation event, however it may be that in vivo an intermolecular phosphorylation takes place and is important in modulation of receptor functions[8]. In the case of the insulin receptor phosphorylation of tyrosine 1146, 1150 and 1151 will activate the kinase which then becomes ligand independent. A tyrosine located at a homologous site in $pp60^{v-src}$ when phosphorylated increases kinase activity and mutation of the equivalent tyrosine in the PDGF receptor abolishes kinase activity. For the EGF receptor phosphorylation at the homologous tyrosine seems non-functional while phosphorylation at the major C-terminal tyrosine (P_1) acceptor site appears to have only a small effect on the kinase activity. In the case of all the *src* family kinases there is a regulatory tyrosine at the C-terminus which has a negative effect

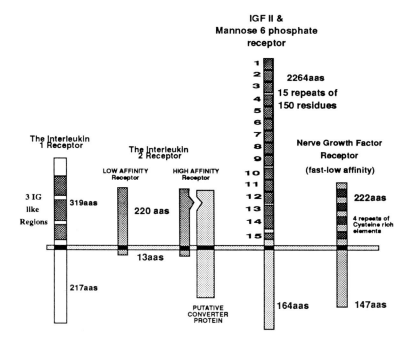

Fig. 3 Receptors which use as yet unknown signal transduction mechanisms. (IG—immunoglobulin).

on the kinase and is deleted in the formation of the transforming proteins. This site is not autophosphorylated but modified by a distinct kinase. The regulation and role of the tyrosine kinase in signal transduction remains unclear and the search for non-receptor substrates which might mediate signal transduction has not been rewarding. The only process where the kinase has recently been shown to be involved is receptor internalisation which is not essential for signal transduction.

The interaction of the ligand and receptor in most cases results in internalisation and down regulation of the receptors—a process which through the use of mutant EGF receptors has been shown to be kinase dependent[8] and could be mediated by autophosphorylation.

At this time we are still left with the tyrosine kinase enzyme function which is common to many receptors and to the *src* family proteins which cannot be linked into a cascade connecting receptors with the modulation of gene expression that is involved in the initiation of DNA synthesis and cell proliferation.

THE LIGAND BINDING DOMAIN OF THE TYROSINE KINASE RECEPTORS

The interaction of different growth factors with their receptors is mediated by the external domain of these glycoproteins. Through a combination of protein chemistry and cDNA cloning the structures of fourteen receptor like proteins have now been established. As yet the ligands for six of these are unknown, the receptors having in most cases been discovered as transforming proteins or as genes related to those of known receptors or in the case of the drosophila 7-less protein through analysis of mutant developmental genes.

The receptors can be divided into four different groups based on the conservation of particular structural motifs.[9] The EGF receptor group at present consists of the human and drosophila EGF receptors and the human *c-NEU* (or *ERB-B2* and *HER-2*) and rat *c-neu* (or *erb-b2* and *her-2*) proteins. The external domains contain conserved amino acid sequences some of which have a large number of regularly spaced cystine—probably cystine residues (*see* Figs 2 & 3). Applying structure prediction techniques has made it possible to define putative subdomains within the structures[10] (*see* chapter by McDonald, Murray-Rust and Blundell). The insulin and IGF1 receptors share many common stretches of sequence in their external domains. These receptors are processed from a single chain precursor to form disulphide linked homodimers of α and β chains. A single cysteine rich domain is located in the α chain.

The PDGF (AB) receptor[11] group includes the CSF-1 receptor[12] (human and feline) and the feline *c-kit* protein which was discovered as the transforming protein *v-kit*[13] and for which no ligand is yet known. These receptors have distinct external domains from that of the EGF and insulin groups. In this case, gene duplication has led to the evolution of a structure which seems to have 5 repeats distantly related to the immunoglobulin v-region primordial domain. The structural features of this domain have been used many times by different cell surface receptors (e.g. IL-1 and IL-6 receptors, T-cell receptor, Thy-1, IgA receptor etc.). As mentioned previously the CSF-1 and PDGF ligands do not appear to be related, showing how evolutionary a common protein domain gene can be used to form distinct ligand binding pockets. The external domains of those receptors which as yet lack ligands (*MET*[14], *TRK*[15], *RET*[16], *c-ros*[17], 7-less[18]) do not fit within the 3 groups described above. As more receptor like proteins are discovered, the shared features of further groups may be revealed.

RECEPTORS WITH UNIQUE STRUCTURES

The structure of the receptors for some growth factors do not have any features which provide clues to their relationship to known protein structures or to receptors where some idea about their signal transduction mechanisms exists. These include the IL-1, IL-2, NGF and IGF II receptors (see Fig. 3).

The IL-1 receptor has an external domain with three immunoglobulin like domains, a transmembrane domain and a cytoplasmic domain of unique sequence 319 amino acids long.[19] The IL-2 receptor[20] structure defines a protein with an external ligand binding domain of 220 amino acids, a transmembrane domain and a small cytoplasmic domain of 13 amino acids. Recently it has been proposed that this receptor is linked to a 'converter' protein to provide a transmembrane signal transduction mechanism. The NGF receptor[21] has an external domain of 222 amino acids linked via a transmembrane domain to a cytoplasmic region of 147 amino acids. Nothing is known of the function of this domain. The IGF II receptor[22] is particularly interesting because it appears identical to the mannose-6-phosphate receptor. Further details of the function of this receptor in binding two distinct ligands remain to be established so that its unusual apparent dual role can be understood. Preliminary analysis of the receptor for TGFβ indicates there are three different binding proteins of 53 000 (I), 73 000 (II) and 300 000 (III) MW which are ubiquitously expressed on cells. The 53 000 protein could be involved in transduction of the growth inhibitory signal. At present the detailed structure of these receptors is unknown.

The structures of many other receptors have yet to be established. In some cases, the molecular size has been determined, the protein partly purified and cDNA cloning is in progress. For other receptors present in low numbers on rare cells a great deal more ingenuity will be required to characterize their structures. Undoubtedly, the problems will be overcome and we can expect many new surprises to come from these experiments.

SIGNAL TRANSDUCTION

The binding of a growth factor to its receptor must generate a signal that is amplified and transduced to activate cytoplasmic regulatory proteins which in turn alter gene expression and induce a mitogenic effect. For those receptors linked to G-proteins it is clear that amplification and generation of second messengers can be mediated by cAMP, by cGMP, by phospholipase activation, calcium mobilization or by generation of the second messenger diacylglycerol with activation of protein kinase C or finally by the modification of ion channel proteins.

For the tyrosine kinase receptors there is no clear understanding of the transduction pathway at present. It is now recognized that the interaction of many growth factors initiates rapid effects on gene transcription—as many as 60–100 genes being activated and others deactivated within 15–60 minutes of ligand binding. In some cases, these gene products are recognized as transcription factors or proteins that modulate such factors (*see* Woodgett, this issue). The details of the activation pathways which link these events to the receptors remain to be established.

How does the signal cross the membrane? For these receptors where we know structural details it appears that the single transmembrane domains they possess cannot themselves transduce a signal such as that conveyed by an ion channel because they have only amino acids with uncharged side chains in this domain. The sole mechanism available seems in this case to be physical movement of one domain with respect to the other to induce a conformational change. In this case it is necessary to invoke push-pull, rotational or other mechanisms to induce conformational changes that could activate for example the tyrosine kinase. At present it seems likely that receptor dimerisation provides a better alternative explanation. Thus a ligand induced change in the receptor's external domain would induce dimerisation and force the apposition of two receptor internal domains and allow inter-receptor phosphorylation to occur at least in the case of the tyrosine kinase receptors. What appears next is currently unknown.

REFERENCES

1. Casey PJ, Gilman AG. G Protein involvement in receptor-effector coupling. J Biol Chem 1988; 263: 2577–2580
2. Rozengurt E. The mitogenic response of cultured 3T3 cells: integration of early signals and synergistic effects in a unified framework. In: Cohen P, Houslay M, eds. Amsterdam: Elsevier, 1985
3. Kris RM, Hazan R, Villines J, Moody TW, Schlessinger J. Identification of the bombesin receptor on murine and human cells by cross linking experiments. 1987; J Biol. Chem. 262: 11215–11220
4. Carpenter G. Receptors for epidermal growth factor and other polypeptide mitogens. Rev Biochem 1987; 56: 881–915
5. Downward J, Yarden Y, Mayes E, Scrace G, Totty N, Stockwell P, Ullrich A, Schlessinger J, Waterfield M. Close similarity of epidermal growth factor receptor and v-erb-B oncogene protein sequences. Nature 1984; 307: 521–527
6. Hanks SK, Quinn AM, Hunter T. The protein kinase family: conserved features and deduced phylogeny of the catalytic domains. Science 1988; 241: 42–52
7. Ben-Neriah Y, Bauskin AR. Leucocytes express a novel gene encoding a putative transmembranes protein-kinase devoid of an extracellular domain. Nature 1988; 333: 672–676
8. Schlessinger J. The epidermal growth factor receptor as a multifunctional allosteric protein. Biochemistry 1988; 27: 3119–3123
9. Yarden Y, Ullrich A. Molecular analysis of signal transduction by growth factors. Biochemistry 1988; 27: 3113–3118
10. Bajaj M, Waterfield MD, Schlessinger J, Taylor WR, Blundell T. On the tertiary structure of the subcellular domain of the epidermal growth factor and insulin receptors. Biochem Biophys Acta 1987; 916: 220–226
11. Yarden Y, Escobedo JA, Kuang W-J et al. Structure of the receptor for platelet-derived growth factor helps define a family of closely related receptors. Nature 1986; 323: 226–232
12. Sherr CJ, Rettenmier CW, Sacca R, Roussel MF, Look AT, Stanley R. The c-fms proto-oncogene is related to the receptor for the mononuclear phagocyte growth factor CSF-1. Cell 1985; 41: 665–676
13. Feihua Q, Ray P, Brown K, Barker PE, Jhanurov S, Ruddle F, Besmer P. Primary structure of c-kit: relationship with the CSF-1/PDGF receptor kinase family—oncogenic activation of v-kit involves deletion of extracellular domain and C terminus. EMBO J 1988; 7: 1003–1011

14 Park M, Dean M, Kaul K, Braum MJ, Gouda MA, Vande Woude G. Sequence of MET proto-oncogene cDNA has features characteristic of the tyrosine kinase family of growth-factor receptors. Proc Natl Acad Sci USA 1987; 84: 6379–6383
15 Martin-Zanca D, Hughes S, Barbacid M. A human oncogene formed by he fusion of truncated tropomyosin and protein tyrosine kinase sequences. Nature 1986; 319: 743–748
16 Takahashi M, Cooper GM. ret Transforming gene encodes a fusion protein homologous to tyrosine kinases. Mol Cell Biol 1987; 7: 1378
17 Neckameyer WS, Wang L.-H. Nucleotide sequence of Avian Sarcoma Virus UR2 and comparison of its transforming gene with other members of the tyrosine protein kinase oncogene family. J Virol 1985; 53: 879–884
18 Bowtell DDL, Simon MA, Rubin GM. Nucleotide Sequence and Structure of the sevenless gene of *Drosophila melanogaster*. Genes Dev 1988; 2: 620–634
19 Simms JE, March CJ, Cosman D et al. cDNA Expression cloning of the IL-1 Receptor, a Member of the Immunoglobulin Superfamily. Science 1988; 241: 585–589
20 Smith KA. Interleukin-2: Inception, Impact and Implications. Science 1988; 240: 1169–1176
21 Radeke MJ, Misko TP, Hsu C, Herzenberg LA, Shooter EM. Gene transfer and molecular cloning of the rat nerve growth factor receptor. Nature 1987; 325: 593–597
22 Morgan DO, Edman JC, Standing DN, Fried VA, Smith MC, Roth RA, Rutter WJ. Insulin like growth factor II receptor as a multifunctional binding protein. Nature 1987; 239: 301–307

Structure-function relationships of growth factors and their receptors

Neil McDonald
Judith Murray-Rust
Tom Blundell
Laboratory of Molecular Biology, Department of Crystallography, Birkbeck College, London, UK

The primary amino acid sequences of several receptor tyrosine kinases have recently made it possible to deduce similarities in the molecular organization of these large multidomain proteins. This has allowed a classification of these receptors into three groups (*see* Waterfield this Issue and for review in Ref. 1). Class I includes the EGF receptor and the *neu* proto-oncogene, Class II includes the insulin and insulin-like growth factor 1 (IGF-1) receptors, and Class III the platelet derived growth factor (PDGF) and the colony stimulating factor 1 (CSF-1) receptors. The conformation of the ligands for the Classes I and II receptors have been defined using X-ray diffraction, 2-D nuclear magnetic resonance (NMR) and knowledge based modelling procedures. It seems that the ligands are more diverse in sequence than the receptor tyrosine kinases so they cannot be classified as rigorously. However, certain features are common to all growth factors (so far defined) which form compact, globular structures and this allows a discussion of possible interactions between the ligand and receptor; but in the absence of a molecular structure for any of the receptors, we can only review biochemical evidence and deductions from predictive and modelling studies. Various models for the signal transduction process are discussed in the light of current work on receptor interactions.

HORMONE AND GROWTH FACTOR STRUCTURES

The structural stability which characterizes many polypeptide growth factors reflects the internal stabilization contributed by the core of the molecule, the high proportion of disulphide cross-linking and also their surface interactions with solvent. The relative inflexibility introduced by these effects compared to smaller hormones, such as glucagon, suggests the structures observed by physical techniques—either from a crystal lattice or in solution—are similar to the structure presented to the receptor.

Ideally the investigation of structure-function relationships would be centred on a three-dimensional structure of a ligand-receptor complex, but until quite recently this has not been realizable because of the limited quantities of receptor available for study. Instead the efforts of several laboratories have concentrated on defining the biologically active conformation of the growth factors, using chemical and molecular genetic experiments to modify the native molecule. In this way the importance of distinct structural areas of the ligand in the formation of the receptor-bound conformation can be deduced. It is important that modifications made should not alter the overall tertiary structure of the molecule, otherwise functionally important areas of the protein may be affected even though they may be distant from the altered site. It is therefore necessary to characterize the changes made to the native conformation using biophysical methods, such as circular dichroism and fluorescence.

INSULIN

The first hormone structure defined using X-ray crystallography was porcine insulin[2,3] and more recently the structures of human, hagfish and bovine insulin have also been solved.[4-6] An insulin precursor molecule is first synthesized and later converted to insulin by removal of the C peptide chain to give a correctly folded monomer made up of an A and a B chain. The A chain consists of two helical regions (residues A1–A7 and A13–A19), connected by an extended loop whilst the B chain contains an alpha-helix (B9–B19), a sharp turn and then an extended flexible strand from B24–B30 (see Fig. 1). On dimerization these strands from the two B chains form a less flexible antiparallel beta-sheet.

Examination of sequence variations (there are approximately 40% invariant residues) between different species and a compari-

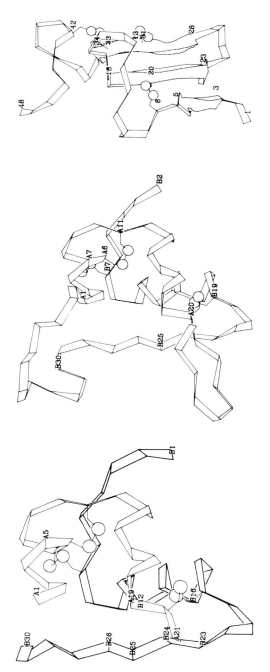

INSULIN IGF-1 EGF

Fig. 1 A schematic representation of the main chain polypeptide backbone for insulin, IGF-1 and des 49–53 EGF (coordinates of EGF courtesy of I Campbell). Key residue alpha carbon atoms are labelled and the cystine residues are drawn as circles. The picture was produced using a program written by A M Lesk and K D Hardman.[48]

son of biological activities led to the suggestion that an area including both the amino and carboxy terminal of the A chain (Gly A1, Val A3, Glu A4, Val A19 and Asn A21) and adjacent B chain residues (Val B12, Phe B24 and Phe B25) was involved in receptor binding.[7] The B chain residues include several hydrophobic residues involved in the monomer–monomer interaction on insulin dimerization, and this led to a proposal that a similar mechanism may be responsible for insulin receptor binding.[8] However, the affinity for receptor binding is 1000-fold greater than that for insulin dimerization, suggesting that additional or slightly different interactions are involved. Structural modifications have generally supported this view. Removal of the last five amino acids of the B chain causes a loss of potency but maintenance of full agonism. However activity falls to near zero for desoctapeptide insulin, but is restored when Phe B24 is replaced. Amidation of the despentapeptide and desheptapeptide insulin also restores full activity and indicates that the charge requirement at this end of the molecule is critical. Since most modifications to either end of the A chain cause serious loss of activity the complete A-chain is probably required for the retention of a native conformation.

Overall, both polar and hydrophobic residues at both ends of the A chain and at the carboxy terminus of the B chain, which are brought into close proximity by the insulin fold, contribute to the dimer interactions and therefore (by analogy), to the receptor binding.

Both insulin-like growth factors (IGF-I and II) are single chain molecules which have connecting C peptides similar to that of proinsulin and an additional D peptide extension to their A chain carboxy termini. Both of these C and D peptides seem to lie close to the proposed insulin receptor binding region and may explain their reduced insulin receptor affinity. A model for both IGFs, based on the conserved hydrophobic core of insulin and the 50% sequence similarity with insulin, was built in 1978.[9] This suggested that at least some of the proposed receptor binding region in insulin was conserved in the IGFs—of particular note are residues Phe B24, Phe B25 and Tyr B26 in insulin which are conserved as Phe, Tyr and Phe for both IGFs. Attempts to differentiate the biological effects of the IGFs and insulin have been difficult because of the cross-reactivity these ligands show for each other's receptors.

The IGFs bind with high affinity to the insulin receptor and the type I and II IGF receptors as well as to two classes of soluble binding proteins present in serum.

Modifications to IGF-1 at the amino terminus have shown that the structural determinants for binding to the insulin and type I IGF receptors are different from those of the type II IGF receptor and the serum binding proteins (which do not bind insulin). These derivatives show a reduced affinity only for the latter two molecules. Changes in the putative receptor binding region for IGF-1 such as the mutation of the Phe 24 to leucine or serine (found in a naturally occurring insulin), results in a decreased affinity of this derivative for both the insulin and type I IGF receptors and supports the view that IGF-1 has a similar receptor binding region to insulin. The coupling of the A chain of insulin to the B chain IGF-1 has been reported[11] and has indicated the C terminal octapeptide of the A chain of IGF-I to be primarily involved in the mitogenic response of this molecule.

Insulin-like molecules are also found in molluscs (MIP)[12] and in silkworms (PTTH or bombyxin).[13] Their amino acid sequences are consistent with an insulin-like core, although the receptor binding regions would seem to be quite different.

EPIDERMAL GROWTH FACTOR

Epidermal growth factor is a single-chain polypeptide of 53 residues containing three disulphide bonds which define three looped regions from residues 1–20, 14–31, and 32–53 (see Fig. 1). The recent determination of the solution structure of human EGF[14,16] and mouse EGF[15,17] using two dimensional nuclear magnetic resonance techniques has shown EGF to have a globular structure with its tertiary structure organized as two domains. In the first domain, the major feature is a turn[18-25] followed by a beta-hairpin with an antiparallel beta-sheet structure.[25-29,34-38] There is a small hydrophobic core contributed by residues Pro 7, Tyr 10, Tyr 13, His 22 and Tyr 29. The second domain contains a double hairpin structure with a hydrophobic core comprising Val 34, Ile 35, Tyr 37, Trp 49 and Trp 50. Human EGF has recently been crystallized and full X-ray analysis is now underway.[17]

An analysis of sequence variations of EGFs from different species and a comparison with related growth factors, such as TGFα (transforming growth factor alpha), and VVGF (vaccinia virus growth factor) shows 20% sequence homology with only a few residues being completely conserved. These include all six cystines and residues Tyr 13, Gly 36, Tyr 37, Gly 39, Arg 41 and Leu 47 (using human EGF sequence assignments). This indicates that the second domain is the most conserved, with several conserved residues lying spatially close to each other. All these related proteins have similar biological activities and seem to bind with high affinity to the EGF receptor.

Earlier work producing modified EGF analogues implicated the beta-sheet residues 20–31 in EGF receptor binding,[18] though doubts have been cast on these results because synthetic peptides were used in the studies. More recent work (see Burgess, this Issue) has shown that truncations to both mouse EGF and TGFα at the carboxy terminus involving residue Arg-48, gave equipotent EGF and TGFα analogues. Loss of residue Leu-47 from mouse EGF (using selective proteolysis and site specific mutation) and also mutation of Asp-47 and Leu-48 in TGFα,[19-21] resulted in a large reduction of EGF receptor affinity and potency, implicating this region in receptor recognition or in the maintainence of a biologically active conformation. Corresponding work on human EGF has shown different results on the role and flexibility of the C-terminus. An equivalent truncation to residues 1–48 for human EGF has reduced binding affinity but preserved similar mitogenic activity, suggesting that this region is involved in receptor binding.[16,22,23] However this result may be due to the instability of the 1–48 EGF truncation resulting in a heterogeneous preparation of this analogue. Removal of residue Leu-47 using proteolysis produced large changes in receptor affinity, similar to mouse EGF. Alterations to the amino terminus has a very limited effect on affinity or activity, though changes to the residue Phe-15 in TGFα, also lowered receptor affinity, so this area may be important. Further work investigating both the sequence and the tertiary structure close to these important regions will help to confirm these findings.

EGF-like domains are found in many other proteins including TGFα, VVGF, SVGF (Shope virus growth factor), the low density lipoprotein receptor, tissue plasminogen activator, coagulation factors VII, IX and X, protein S, protein C and the EGF precursor domains (for review see Ref. 24). Despite variation in sequence between loops, a common EGF fold seems likely for all these structures. Indeed this structure may be a common motif for mediating protein–protein interactions, with several of these molecules being involved in cell surface interactions in an analogous way to EGF, but with differing specificities.

In summary, both the EGF and insulin ligand families appear to interact with their respective receptors through extensive surface regions which are easily perturbed and only brought together by the characteristic tertiary fold of the protein. The small size of the growth factors with respect to their receptors, suggests that most residues would be buried after the formation of a ligand–receptor complex, so the separation of areas of the ligand necessary for molecular recognition from those required for signal transduction is a complex task. To date no full antagonists have been found for insulin or EGF. However it is clear that the biological activity resides in a spatial grouping within the molecule rather than a contiguous sequence of amino acids.

RECEPTOR STRUCTURE

Growth factor receptors can be divided into an external ligand binding domain and an intracellular tyrosine kinase domain. These are connected physically and functionally through the cell membrane by a short membrane spanning region. The functional integrity of these domains has been emphasized by experiments involving the construction of hybrid receptors. These chimeras are formed by coupling an extracellular domain of one receptor to the cytoplasmic domain of another. Several such chimeric molecules have been shown to be active receptors with a ligand specificity dependent on the extracellular domain coupled.[25,26] The recent expression of stable, soluble ligand binding domains and active kinase domains for both the EGF[27,28] and insulin receptors,[29,30] has confirmed this view. It is hoped that these studies will provide material suitable for X-ray analysis which will avoid the inherent problems of crystallizing intrinsic membrane proteins. In the absence of a full X-ray structure of any of these receptor systems, there is still a need for a molecular model for the design and interpretation of experimental work and we shall discuss a possible model for both domains in this section.

EXTRACELLULAR DOMAIN

The extracellular domain comprises about half the total receptor sequence and contains one high affinity binding site per receptor monomer based on stoichiometric quantitation of ligand required to saturate the receptor. Several N-linked glycosylation sites are present and have been shown to be important for the acquisition of a ligand binding site.[31,32] Another important feature is the presence of cystine-rich regions which are assumed to form disulphide bonds although the exact disulphide content has not been quantified. The unusually high protease resistance of the receptor may well be a result of this cross-linking, or could arise from the compact folding of separate subdomains in these regions which add stability to the structure.

We have proposed a model for these extracellular domains based on sequence alignment and secondary structure predictions for the EGF, *neu* proto-oncogene, insulin and IGF-1 receptors.[33] Extensive similarity is seen between the human EGF-receptor, drosophila EGF receptor homologue, *v-erb* B oncogene product and the *neu* gene product, and separately between the insulin and IGF-1 receptors. Our alignment of these two subgroups together shows low but significant homology within the cystine-rich subdomains and the more variable subdomains which preceed them.

Our model (Figs. 2 and 3) shows an alignment of two large variable regions for all the receptors discussed, which suggested that they contained a conserved hydrophobic pattern in addition to a highly conserved glycine residue. The large variable regions (L1 and L2) consist of four or five motifs, each with a predicted short α-helix-turn-β-strand pattern. The loops joining these conserved motifs are highly variable. In the EGF-receptor, drosophila EGF-receptor homologue and *neu* gene product, each L subdomain is followed by a cystine-rich region S. Similarities between the L1, L2 and S1, S2 regions have suggested that an ancestral gene encoding the L-S was duplicated to give the observed L_1–S1 L2–S2 repeat. The second L domain is not followed by a second S cystine region in the insulin and IGF-1 receptors. In other gene duplicated repeats, such as those in bacterial ferredoxins, the two halves do not form separate globular clusters, but fold in a cooperative way with the repeated chain fold having two fold symmetry, like that of a dimer. Thus the ancestral L-S gene may well have encoded a protein tending to form a molecular dimer long before gene duplication doubled the chain length. In this way a gene duplication event may have taken advantage of a structural adaption that had already occurred. One efficient way to produce a binding cleft is to bind the specific ligand between two globular subunits that associate about a two fold axis, hence forming an extended recognition site.

Evidence supporting our model has been reported. Firstly circular dichroism studies on a secreted soluble EGF-receptor extracellular domain[28] support the presence of α and β secondary structure. Also studies of affinity labelled receptor subjected to

EGF receptor

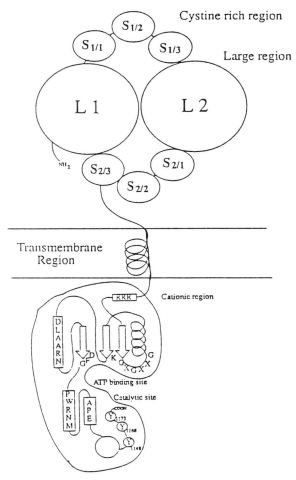

Fig. 2 A simplified representation of the EGF receptor, showing the large (L) subdomains and small (S) subdomains in the external domains in a symmetrical arrangement about a two-fold axis. The intracellular tyrosine kinase domain shows the βαβ nucleotide binding motif and residues thought to be involved in ATP binding. Also shown are the major autophosphorylation sites (Y) and sequences specific to all tyrosine kinase domains (which are boxed).

Insulin and IGF-1 receptors
Single monomer of the dimeric complex

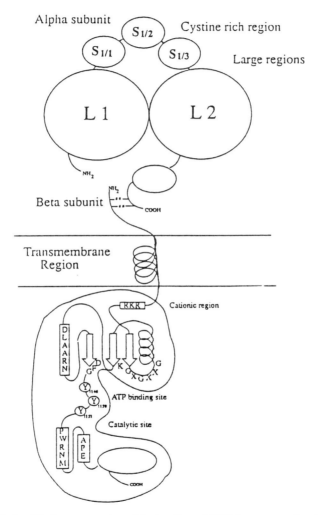

Fig. 3 A simplified representation of the insulin and IGF-1 receptors, showing the large (L) subdomains and small (S) subdomains in the external domains in a symmetrical arrangement about a two-fold axis. The intracellular tyrosine kinase domain shows the $\beta\alpha\beta$ nucleotide binding motif and residues thought to be involved in ATP binding. Also shown are the major autophosphorylation sites (Y) and sequences specific to all tyrosine kinase domains (which are boxed).

fragmentation showed EGF to be attached to a receptor fragment containing the entire L2 subdomain.[34]

To date only limited modifications within extracellular subdomains have been tested. Partial deletions from the amino terminus of the EGF receptor result in a reduced affinity to EGF. The *v-erb* B gene product is a truncated chicken EGF receptor that contains almost no extracellular domain, does not bind EGF and has a constitutively active kinase domain.[35]

THE TRANSMEMBRANE DOMAIN

A single transmembrane region of 23–26 residues couples the extracellular ligand binding domain to the catalytic tyrosine kinase domain. There is no conservation of specific sequences within the transmembrane regions, though the sequences are all highly hydrophobic. There are also several basic residues at the cytoplasmic end of the putative transmembrane stretch, which are thought to act as a 'stop' transfer function for the insertion of the polypeptide chain into the membrane. The transmembrane stretch, is thought to form an α-helix, since 20 amino acids are sufficient to cross the 30 Å cell membrane, though a 3–10 helix which is more extended with three residues per turn, would require only 14 amino acids. Helical structures have been confirmed for several transmembrane polypeptides (including alamethicin, melittin and more recently gramicidin A[36]), and would seem to be energetically stable.

THE INTRACELLULAR DOMAIN

The intracellular domain has a protein tyrosine kinase function with a conserved ATP-binding site. At least 65 putative kinase sequences have been identified and share extensive sequence homology even between different classes.[37] The kinase domains contain from 250 to 300 amino acids (30Kd), and analysis of conserved sequences as well as truncations of these domains has helped in defining their molecular boundaries. Several features are common to all receptor tyrosine kinases: (i) an ATP-binding site; (ii) sequences which confer tyrosine kinase specificity, i.e. allowing phosphoryl transfer specifically to tyrosine residues; (iii) sequences determining substrate specificity that control which intracellular proteins can be phosphorylated, (iv) autophosphorylation sites (tyrosine side chains), which may serve in regulating the kinase activity towards exogenous substrates.[38,39]

The ATP-binding site is separated from the cell membrane by about 50 residues which contain a highly positively charged region that is thought to interact with the phospholipid bilayer. Two sections to the ATP-binding region have been suggested.[40] Firstly an N terminal region, comprising a putative β-strand-α-helix-β-strand region, the two strands lying parallel and adjacent. This contains the GlyXGlyXXGly sequence motif, where the glycines are essential in the formation of a tight turn between β-strand 1 and the α-helix. This stabilizes the interactions between the α-helix dipole and the negatively charged γ-phosphate group. The second β-strand ends with a conserved lysine residue which is predicted to form a salt bridge with an oxygen atom on the γ-phosphate of ATP. Mutation of this lysine in both the EGF[41] and the insulin receptors[42] leads to the abolition of ligand induced kinase activity and mitogenic response.

The C terminal region of the ATP-binding site contains a third β-strand with a Asp-Phe-Gly sequence present in all kinases. The aspartic acid side chain may form a hydrogen bond with the amino group at position 6 of the adenine ring, and the phenylalanine side chain could form a hydrophobic interaction with the adenine ring.

Sequence comparison of all known and presumptive serine/threonine and tyrosine kinases have shown unique stretches of sequence conserved in serine/threonine kinases, and different sequences conserved for all tyrosine kinases. The sequences lie on the amino terminal side of a conserved Ala-Pro-Gly sequence which follows 20 residues after the ATP binding site and may well be involved in determining the specificity of the amino acid side chain to be phosphorylated (see Fig. 2).

A model based on this discussion is shown in Figure 2 where a possible arrangement of the EGF and insulin receptor structures is presented. Several features have been defined in detail using knowledge-based modelling procedures. Overall these multidomain proteins show a close molecular organization with even closer homologies in their intracellular kinase domains than for the ligand-recognition site. This may reflect strong evolutionary constraints against changes within these domains.

MODELS FOR RECEPTOR LIGAND BINDING AND SIGNAL TRANSDUCTION

Two possible models for receptor ligand binding can be distinguished

The most probable model would involve the larger non-cystine rich domains, L1 and L2 as previously mentioned. Alternatively an interaction of the growth factor with the cystine rich domains may occur, possibly involving disulphide exchange. This is less likely in view of the structural importance of these cystines in the ligands three-dimensional structure.

It is likely that the ligand-receptor interaction will principally involve hydrophobic contacts and contributions from hydrogen bonding possibly with the exclusion of solvent, leading to significant conformational change in both growth factor and receptor. This would follow an induced-fit mechanism[43] to attain the receptor-bound ligand conformation. This is in contrast to the receptor selecting a minor conformer population present in solution as happens with glucagon. The conformational change is likely to lead to allosteric effects, which are probably essential for any mode of signal transduction.

Signal transduction may take place through intramolecular or intermolecular allosteric mechanisms. In the first case ligand binding would induce a conformational change in the receptor that could alter the positioning of the transmembrane alpha-helix with respect to the unbound receptor state, and this would lead to activation of tyrosine kinase function within receptor monomers.[44] Ligand binding might induce either rotational or translational movement of the helix. Rotation would require that the receptor be constrained from free rotation on both sides of the membrane. However cell membranes are fluid systems, with freely diffusing and rotating molecules including growth factor receptors, so that a mechanism involving this type of movement is unlikely. Translational movement, a 'push-pull' mechanism, may be used, though the lack of sequence conservation of the transmembrane region makes this mode of signal propagation less attractive.

An intermolecular allosteric mechanism of signal transduction would involve receptor aggregation, most likely dimerization.[45] This is a common feature of other ligand-receptor complexes subject to endocytosis, for example the LDL receptor.[46] After ligand binding, receptors can be seen to cluster on the cell surface prior to internalization. However dimer formation may be a consequence of ligand binding, rather than a prerequisite for kinase activation and hence signal transduction. Many other systems have their allosteric activity mediated by symmetrical oligomers that serve to enhance the signal and increase the sensitivity of the system. Thus the activation of the kinase could affect the association state of the receptor, leading to increased dimer formation. This would bring the kinase domains of both monomers close together enabling a bimolecular phosphorylation and activation mechanism. The finding that the insulin receptor associates as a dimer would also satisfy this requirement.[47]

REFERENCES

1 Yarden Y, Ulrich A. Receptor tyrosine kinases. Ann Rev Biochem 1988; 57: 443–478
2 Blundell TL, Cutfield JF, Cutfield SM et al. Atomic positions in rhombohedral 2-zinc insulin crystals. Nature 1971; 231: 506–511
3 Baker EN, Blundell TL, Cutfield JF et al. The structure of 2Zn pig insulin crystals at 1.5 A resolution. Philos Trans R Soc London [Biol] 1988; 319: 369–456
4 Chawdhury SA, Dodson EJ, Dodson GG et al. The structure of human insulin. Diabetologia 1983; 25: 460
5 Cutfield JF, Cutfield SM, Dodson EJ et al. The structure and biological activity of hagfish insulin. J Mol Biol 1979; 132: 85–90.
6 Smith GD, Duax WL, Dodson EJ et al. The structure of des-Phe B1 insulin. Acta Crystallogr 1982; B38: 3038–3032
7 Pullen RA, Lindsay DG, Wood SP et al. Receptor-binding region of insulin. Nature 1976; 231: 506–511
8 De Meyts PE, Van Obberghen J, Roth A, Wollmer A, Brandenberg D.Mapping of the residues responsible for the negative cooperativity of the receptor-binding region of insulin. Nature 1978; 273: 504–509
9 Blundell TL, Bedarkar S, Rinderknecht E, Humbel RE. Insulin-like growth factor: a model for tertiary structure accounting for immunoreactivity and receptor binding. Proc Natl Acad Sci USA 1978; 75: 180–184
10 Cascieri MA, Chicchi GG, Applebaum J, Hayes NS, Green BG, Bayne ML. Mutants of human insulin-like growth factor I with reduced affinity for the type I insulin-like growth factor receptor. Biochemistry 1988; 27: 3229–3233
11 King GL, Kahn CR, Samuels B, Danho W, Bullesbach EE, Gattner HG. Synthesis and characterisation of molecular hybrids of insulin and insulin-like growth factor 1. The role of the A-chain extension peptide. J Biol Chem 1982; 257: 10869–10873
12 Smit AB, Vreugdenhil E, Ebberink RHM, Geraerts WPM, Klootwijk J, Joosse J. Growth-controlling molluscan neurons produce the precursor of an insulin-related peptide. Nature 1988; 331: 535–538
13 Nagasawa H, Suzuki A, Ishizaki H. Amino acid sequence of a prothoraciotropic hormone of the silkworm Bombyx mori. Proc Natl Acad Sci USA 1986; 83: 5840–5843
14 Cooke RM, Wilkinson AJ, Baron et al. The solution structure of human epidermal growth factor. Nature 1987; 327: 339–341
15 Montelione GT, Wuthrich K, Nice EC. et al. The solution structure of murine epidermal growth factor. Proc Natl Acad Sci USA 1987; 84: 5226–30

16 Makino K, Morimoto M, Nishi M et al. Proton nuclear magnetic resonance study on the solution conformation of human epidermal growth factor. Proc Natl Acad Sci USA 1987; 84: 7841–7845
17 Higuchi Y, Morimoto Y, Horinaka A, Yasuoka N. Tertiary structure of mouse epidermal growth factor determined by two-dimensional NMR. J Biochem 1988; 103: 905–6
18 Komoriya A, Hortsch M., Meyers C, Smith M, Kanety H, Schlessinger J. Proc Natl Acad Sci USA 1984; 81: 1351–5
19 Burgess A, Lloyd CJ, Smith S et al. Murine epidermal growth factor: structure and function. Biochemistry 1988; 27: 4977–4985
20 Ray P, Moy FJ, Montelione GT et al. Expression and site-directed mutagenesis of epidermal growth factor gene. Biochemisty 1988; 27: 7289–7295
21 Lazar E, Watanabe S, Dalton S, Sporn MB. Transforming growth factor alpha: mutation of aspartic acid 47 and leucine 48 results in different biological activities. Mol Cell Biol 1988; 8: 1247–1252
22 Hollenberg MD, Gregory H. Epidermal growth factor-urogastrone: biological activity and receptor binding of derivatives. Mol Pharmacol 1980; 17: 314–320
23 Gregory H, Thomas CE, Young JA, Willshire, Garner A. The contribution of the C-terminal undecapeptide sequence of urogastrone-epidermal growth factor to its biological action. Regul Pept 1988; 22: 217–226
24 Apella E, Weber IT, Blasi F. Structure and function of epidermal growth factor-like regions in proteins. FEBS Lett 1988; 231: 1–4
25 Reidel H, Dull TJ, Schlessinger J, Ullrich A. A chimaeric receptor allows insulin to stimulate tyrosine kinase activity of epidermal growth factor receptor. Nature 1986; 324: 68–70
26 Riedel H, Schlessinger J and Ullrich A. A chimeric, ligand-binding v-erbB/EGF receptor retains transforming potential. Science 1987; 236: 197–200
27 Greenfield C, Patel G, Clark S, Jones N, Waterfield MD. Expression of the human EGF receptor with ligand-stimulatable kinase activity in insect cells using a baculovirus vector. EMBO J 1988; 7: 139–46
28 Greenfield C, Haley F, McDonald NQ, Blundell TL, Waterfield MD. 1988 (Manuscript in preparation)
29 Ellis L, Sissom J, Levitan A. Truncation of the ectodomain of the human insulin receptor results in secretion of a soluble insulin binding protein from transfected CHO cells. J Mol Rec 1988; 1: 25–31
30 Ellis L, Levitan A, Cobb MH, Ramos P. Efficient expression in insect cells of a soluble, active human insulin receptor protein-tyrosine kinase domain by use of a baculovirus vector. J Virol 1988; 62: 1634–1639
31 Slieker LJ, Lane MD. Post-translational processing of the epidermal growth factor receptor. J Biol Chem 1985; 260: 687–690
32 Olson TS, Bamberger MJ, Lane MD. Post-translational changes in tertiary and quaternary structure of the insulin receptor. J Biol Chem 1988; 263: 7342–7351
33 Bajaj M, Waterfield MD, Schlessinger J, Taylor W, Blundell TL. On the tertiary structures of the extracellular domains of the EGF and insulin receptors. Biochem Biophys Acta 1987; 916: 220–226
34 Lax I, Burgess WH, Bellot F, Ullrich A, Schlessinger J, Givol D. Localisation of a major receptor-binding domain for epidermal growth factor by affinity labeling. Mol Cell Biol 1988; 8: 1831–1834
35 Bargmann CI, Weinberg A. Oncogenic activation of the Neu-encoded receptor protein by point mutation and deletion. EMBO J 1988; 7: 2043–2052
36 Langs DA. Three dimensional structure of the uncomplexed form of the transmembrane ion channel peptide Gramicidin A. Science 1988; 241: 188–191
37 Hanks SK, Quinn AM, Hunter T. The protein kinase family: conserved features and deduced phylogeny of the catalytic domains. Science 1988; 241: 42–52

38 Tornquist HE, Avruch J. Relationship of site specific β-subunit tyrosine autophosphorylation to Insulin activation of the Insulin receptor protein kinase activity. J Biol Chem 1988; 263: 4593–4601
39 Downword J, Waterfield MD, Parker P. Autophosphorylation and protein kinase C phosphorylation of the Epidermal Growth Factor Receptor. J Biol Chem 1985; 260: 14538–14546
40 Sternberg MJE, Taylor WR. Modelling the ATP-binding site of oncogene products, the epidermal growth factor receptor and related proteins. FEBS Lett 1984; 175: 387–91
41 Moolenaar WH, Bierman AJ, Tilly BC et al. A point mutation at the ATP-binding site of the EGF-receptor abolishes signal transduction. EMBO J 1988; 7: 707–710
42 Ebina Y, Araki E, Taira M et al. Replacement of lysine residue 1030 in the putative ATP-binding region of the insulin receptor abolishes insulin- and antibody-stimulated glucose uptake and receptor kinase activity. Proc Natl Acad Sci USA 1987; 84: 704–708
43 Koshland DE. Application of a theory of enzyme specificity to protein synthesis. Proc Natl Acad Soc USA 1958; 44: 98–104
44 Staros JV, Cohen S, Russo MW. In: Cohen P, Maunslay MD eds. Molecular Mechanisms of Transmembrane Signalling. New York: Elsevier 1985: pp. 253–278
45 Schlessinger J. The epidermal growth factor as a multifunctional allosteric protein. Biochemistry 1988; 27: 3119–3123
46 Goldstein JL, Anderson RGW, Brown MS. Coated pits, coated vesicles and receptor-mediated endocytosis. Nature 1979; 279: 679–685
47 Massague J, Pilch PF, Czech MP. Electrophoretic resolution of three major insulin receptor structures with unique subunit stoichiometries. Proc Natl Acad Sci USA 1980; 77: 7137–7141
48 Lesk AM, Hardman KD. Methods in Enzymology 1985; 115: 381–390

Altered growth regulation in cancer

M D Waterfield
Ludwig Institute for Cancer Research, Middlesex Hospital/University College Branch, London, UK

> The cell regulation pathways initiated by growth factors may be subverted at several distinct levels in cancer cells. The abnormal production of a growth factor may, through action on its receptor, stimulate aberrant growth. The need for the factor can also be bypassed in several ways. This can occur through the expression of abnormal receptors which no longer require their ligand to generate a signal or through the activation of post receptor processes at key points in the intracellular pathways which normally transduce and modulate the receptor signal. Studies of oncogenes have shown that they may function as abnormal Growth Factors or abnormal receptors, induce expression of potential signal regulators or encode proteins which modulate gene transcription. Such studies offer new clues to mechanisms involved in the causation of cancer.

The reasons for focussing attention on the role of growth factors in cancer cells are now perhaps obvious. This has however not always been the case, and several developments over the last ten years have been responsible for a shift in emphasis within the cancer research field that has resulted in a detailed dissection of the pathways triggered by growth factors which may be subverted in cancer cells.

Amongst the key observations which focused attention on growth factors were results which showed that certain transformed or tumour derived cell lines required less serum as a supplement to support their growth in tissue culture compared to normal cells. From the work of Temin, Todaro and others emerged the concept that the reduced requirement for serum resulted from *de novo* synthesis of growth factors by the cells themselves. The term

Autocrine was coined to describe this phenomenon and *Paracrine* to describe the local synthesis of a factor by a distinct but adjacent cell[1] (*see* Fig. 1).

The further analysis of tumour cell growth factors, through fractionation of conditioned media, has resulted in the isolation of the transforming growth factors α^2 and $\beta^{3,4}$ and indeed of several other growth regulators. Particularly important was the recognition that the so called transforming growth factors were normal gene products. A further stimulus to the study of the potential role of autocrine growth factor production in cancer cells came from the observations that the *sis* oncogene encodes the platelet derived growth factor (PDGF)[5,6] and that the *int* 2 [7] and *hst* [8] oncogenes could encode fibroblast growth factor (FGF)[9,10] like polypeptides. Much of the work on these factors was carried out using fibroblasts which are easy to grow in tissue culture and which have been used extensively by tumour virologists to study transformation. The ability also to obtain and culture haemopoietic cells easily, which are continuously produced in the mature animal and consequently distinct from most adult cells that do not normally proliferate, has made it possible to isolate lineage specific colony-stimulating factors and a variety of lymphokines whose role in normal and cancer cells is under detailed investigation. These are dealt with in other chapters. Unfortunately, the major tumours found in man are of epithelial origin and these cells have proved difficult to grow in tissue culture. Consequently study of the factors characterized thus far is limited to particular cell types and a number of important regulators may await characterization.

The study of oncogenes has provided further clues to mechanisms of growth factor signal subversion. First it was recognized that the signal pathways triggered by growth factors could be turned on and the effects of the growth factor mimicked by expression of an altered receptor encoded by an oncogene that induced ligand independent signalling. Secondly it was shown that oncogenes and tumour promoters could activate post receptor functions which would normally only be triggered when receptors bind their ligands showing that the whole cascade of growth factor induced intracellular events could be susceptible to subversion at key points in cancer cells. These observations have given a coherent framework for investigation of growth factor and oncogene action which will be outlined here.

ABNORMAL SYNTHESIS OF GROWTH FACTORS

The ability of certain transformed and tumour derived cells to produce factors which enable them to reduce their dependence on serum compared to normal cells growing in tissue culture could be explained if the conversion to a cancer cell involved the synthesis of growth factors normally found in serum or of specific 'transforming' factors. The analysis of conditioned media from tumour cells has resulted in the purification of several diverse growth regulators and, except in certain specific cases where the factors are encoded by oncogenes (see below) these factors have been found to be normal gene products that can also be produced by normal cells. The characterization of the transforming growth factors (α and β) from the conditioned media of RNA tumour virus transformed fibroblasts serves as a good example of the isolation of novel factors that proved to be normal factors rather than tumour specific transforming factors.[2-4] One major characteristic of transformed

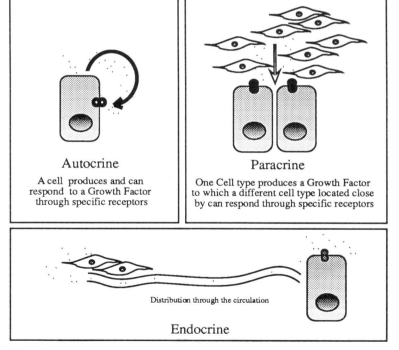

Fig. 1 Different mechanisms for delivery of growth factors and hormones to target cells.

cells is their ability to form colonies in semi-solid media, a property which could be conferred on normal cells (Rat 1 fibroblasts) by the addition of conditioned media from the transformed cells. The fractionation of such media revealed two novel factors which were both required to confer the ability to grow in semi-solid media to the normal cells—they were named *transforming* growth factors (TGFs) α and β. As is described in detail in chapters by Burgess and Hsuan (this Issue) TGFα is a member of the EGF family and acts through the EGF receptor while TGFβ (which may have two or more related genes) is a bipotential regulator that can stimulate proliferation of some cells and inhibit growth of others. In both cases, the factors can be produced by normal cells and are synthesized as structurally identical proteins by the tumour cells. These results suggest that it could be abnormal factor synthesis, perhaps in the wrong place at the wrong time, which allows certain tumour cells to acquire the altered growth properties which are dependent on these factors.

The effect of activation of growth factor production on transformation was vividly illustrated by the observation that the oncogene sis encoded the B chain of platelet derived growth factor. PDGF is the major mitogen for connective tissue cells which is released into serum from platelets and is unique in that it can act as a mitogen on its own for certain fibroblasts (Swiss 3T3 cells). The realization that Simian Sarcoma Virus (SSV), which was isolated from a monkey osteosarcoma, contained an oncogene (*sis*) which encoded PDGF came from sequence studies of the viral genome and of the purified growth factor PDGF[5,6]. This was the first discovered function for an oncogene and the realization that cellular transformation could be mediated by the synthesis of this growth factor provided what appeared to be solid support for the role of *autocrine* growth factor synthesis in the conversion of a normal to a cancer cell. Subsequent work suggests that the viral encoded factor interacts with PDGF receptors in the endoplasmic reticulum and on the cell surface thus turning on the cascade of events which the normal factor triggers through its receptor (*see* Heldin & Westermark, this issue). These results raised the possibility that other oncogenes may encode growth factors. This has proved to be the case for only 3 other oncogenes. Recent work suggests that mouse mammary tumour virus can activate, through promoter insertion, the *int-2* gene[7] which appears to encode a member of the fibroblast growth factor gene family. The related oncogenes *hst/KS3* and *FGF5* have been detected using the 3T3 transfection assay in human cancer DNAs (a total of five genes FGFa[9], FGFb[10], int-2[7], hst[8]/KS3 and FGF5[11] have now been assigned to this family). It has however proved extremely hard to find the expression and secretion of the putative growth factors. It is fascinating that the *int-2* and *hst* genes appear to be almost next to each other on the chromosome. A distinct oncogene, *int-1*[12], which could also encode a putative growth regulator can also be activated by promoter insertion by MMTV. The coding regions of these genes are not altered in their conversion to oncogenes, reinforcing the concept that abnormal synthesis rather than the production of altered factors is important.

The role of the *sis* and FGF related oncogenes in transformation of cells in culture and as oncogenes in experimental animals is still under active investigation. It is clear that SSV and MMTV can produce tumours in animals but it remains unclear whether other events besides the activation of *sis* and *int-2* are necessary to induce these tumours.

To examine the potential for other factors to induce a transformed phenotype through constitutive expression and possibly autocrine action, the factors EGF,[13] TGFα,[14] and basic FGF to which a signal peptide had been added[15] (and GM-CSF[16] and CSF-1[17] see Owen Jenkinson this issue) have been expressed in normal cells using various vectors. Such altered expression was shown to produce several of the characteristics of the transformed phenotype in 3T3 or Rat 1 cells. The expression of these factors also increased the tumourgenicity of the cells. The importance of an autocrine mechanism has proved difficult to establish experimentally because the ligand-receptor interaction can occur intracellularly, presumably during biosynthesis. Similar difficulties exist in examining tumour derived cell lines. The role of bombesin (or GRP) in small cell lung cancer[18] could involve an autocrine mechanism which is discussed in detail in the chapter by Woll and Rozengurt.

The experimental studies summarized here and examined in detail in other chapters in this Issue show that abnormal growth factor production through autocrine or paracrine mechanisms could be important as one step in the multi-step conversion of a normal human cell to a cancer cell. As yet little definitive evidence exists to show a clear autocrine effect for growth factors in human cancers.

At this point it is perhaps relevant to emphasis the potential inhibitory effect of growth factors in cell growth. Clearly TGFβ

can selectively inhibit development and proliferation of certain cell types perhaps most notably, epithelial, endothelial, hemopoietic, lymphoid and neuroectodermal cells.[19,20] In the case of epithelial cells, from which the majority of human tumours are derived, the further evaluation of the role of this regulator will be most interesting. As yet, it is not known whether defective synthesis of TGFβ could play a role in tumour production but recent work implicating the loss of TGFβ receptors in retinoblastoma cell lines which correlates with the response of the normal retinal and tumour cells to TGFβ could be of great importance.[21] Further work will explore this facet of the function of TGFβ and other growth regulators such as the myeloid leukaemia inhibitory factors which can act as negative modulators of cell growth and development.

SUBVERSION OF RECEPTOR STRUCTURE AND FUNCTION

The action of a growth factor on target cells requires receptor expression. Abnormal display of a functional receptor in a cell that can interpret the signal it generates could result in abnormal cell development and proliferation.

The determination of the structure of the EGF receptor revealed a distinct mechanism for generating a receptor signal in cells in the absence of ligand.[5] Through a comparison of the receptor amino acid sequence with known oncogene sequences it became clear that avian erythroblastosis virus (AEV) had acquired a portion of the EGF receptor gene. Thus the AEV oncogene *erb-b* could express a truncated receptor on the surface of infected cells. The acquisition by AEV of only the middle segment of the receptor gene means that the expressed transforming protein has a truncated external domain which can no longer bind ligand and a shortened and mutated C-terminus.[5] The mechanism of signal transduction by the EGF receptor remains unclear (reviewed in ref. 22; and *see* chapter on 'Growth factor receptors') and hence it is difficult to confirm the suggestion that the truncated receptor generates a ligand independent transformation signal. The infection of chickens with AEV rapidly induces erythroblastosis and subsequently the formation of sarcomas. Cells from both types of tumours express truncated receptors. EGF receptors are not normally expressed on the erythroid lineage and if an EGF signal is generated through expression of the altered receptor then it must be assumed that erythroid cells have the cellular machinary to transduce a mitogenic effect. The analysis of the changes necessary to convert a normal EGF receptor to a transforming protein have yet to unravel the relevance of the external and internal truncations and C-terminal mutations for the mechanisms which generate the different types of tumours. It seems that the expression of receptors with truncation of only the ligand binding domain can result in erythroblastosis since avian leukosis virus (ALV) can induce erythroblastosis in chickens through insertional mutagenesis of the EGF receptor gene. Further C-terminal truncation and mutation which has taken place during acquisition of the *erb-b* gene by AEV seems necessary for this virus to induce sarcomas. Mutagenesis studies have not been able to pinpoint the effects of C-terminal truncation to specific alterations such as the loss of the major in vivo autophosphorylation site P1 (reviewed in Refs. 22 and 23).

The demonstration by Sherr that the feline oncogene *v-fms* encoded a truncated and mutated CSF-1 receptor provided a second clear demonstration that an altered receptor could act as a transforming protein.[24] Detailed analysis of *c-fms* and *v-fms* shows that elimination of a C-terminal regulatory tyrosine residue and also a mutation(s) in the external domain that may mimic activation by ligand are necessary to generate the transforming protein.[25] Besides these two receptors, where the ligand is known, a number of other oncogenes which encode putative receptors have been described. Closely related to the *fms* protein is *kit* for which a ligand is not known. Drastic DNA rearrangements resulting from manipulations of cells (or DNA) in the laboratory have resulted in the isolation of the *MET* and *TRK* oncogenes (*see* chapter on 'Growth factor receptors'). In these oncogenes, sequences derived from other genes have replaced regions of the receptor proteins, presumably causing activation of the receptor signal transduction mechanisms. A much smaller change, involving mutation of a single nucleotide, which can be induced through transplacental chemical carcinogenesis by N-nitrosomethylurea in rats, is sufficient to induce a mutation which converts a valine to glutamic acid residue in the transmembrane region of the EGF receptor related proto-oncogene *neu*[26] (also known as *HER-2* or *erb-b2*) to generate a transforming protein. Other altered potential receptors are encoded by the *mas* oncogene which encodes a protein that resembles members of the β-adrenergic receptor family and appears to encode angiotensin receptor, the *ros* oncogene which encodes a protein that resembles the insulin receptor and finally the *RET* oncogene which appears to be unique at present.

These results demonstrate that a number of receptors or potential receptors, for which we don't know the ligands, can be mutated to generate what seem to be ligand independent transforming proteins. It remains unclear how many receptors of the hundreds (or more) which exist can be converted to transforming proteins. Since these altered receptors have been found to be encoded by retroviral oncogenes, have been induced by chemical carcinogenesis or generated by laboratory manipulation of cells, it is important to establish whether such changes can occur in human cancers.

Analysis of the limited number of receptors for which we have the probes has shown that drastic re-arrangements of receptor genes are infrequent. The most complete analysis carried out thus far concerns the EGF and *c-NEU* (or *erb-b2* or *HER-2*) genes where hundreds of primary tumours and cell lines, albeit of limited types, have been examined. Amplification of the EGF receptor gene is common in squamous tumour cell lines and also occurs in a number of squamous primary tumours. Only in certain brain tumours has the gene been shown to be re-arranged. The *HER-2* gene is also amplified in a limited number of mammary tumours. Analysis at the protein level also reveals over-expression induced without gene amplification for both the EGF receptor and *NEU* proteins presumably by altered receptor mRNA transcription or translation or through altered receptor processing. Surveys of large numbers of tumours are required to establish the prognostic significance of these results (reviewed in Ref. 27).

The effects of overexpression of normal receptors has been investigated experimentally. It seems clear that overexpression of both EGF receptor in the presence of ligand and of the *c-NEU* protein (perhaps also in the presence of an unknown ligand) can induce some of the properties of transformed cells. The overexpression of *c-NEU* seems to be more transforming than similar expression of the EGF receptor. A great deal more work on the role of altered receptors and abnormal expression levels of receptors in cancer cells and the investigation of primary tumours is clearly needed to evaluate the relevance of receptor subversion in the human disease.

ALTERED INTRACELLULAR SIGNAL MODULATION PATHWAYS

Cells in serum or in the body are exposed to a number of growth regulators which acting through different receptors and distinct second messenger functions can induce synergistic growth responses. Rozengurt (this Issue) has shown using the Swiss 3T3 system how the stimulation of the cAMP, inositol phosphate and tyrosine kinase receptor second messenger (?as yet unknown) pathways can be stimulated, inhibited or transmodulated with either growth factors, drugs of known specificity or other agents to influence the response of a cell to several different growth regulators.

In the context of synergistic responses and of particular relevance to cancer studies are the phorbol esters, long known to exert effects on growth and differentiation, and to act as tumour promoters. The identification of protein kinase C as the phorbol ester receptor (and the realization that there are a family of PKCs) together with the knowledge that growth factors such as bombesin or PDGF can presumably through phospholipase activation generate the PKC activator diacylglycerol emphasizes the way in which tumour promoters could bypass receptor stimulated activation of PKC (reviewed in Ref. 28).

SUBVERSION OF GROWTH FACTOR INTRACELLULAR SIGNAL CASCADES

A large number of distinct growth factors, acting through a smaller but extensive series of receptors, use a limited number of second messenger systems to turn on shared cascades of intracellular regulators which alter gene expression and stimulate DNA synthesis (*see* Fig. 2). Within these cascades a number of oncogenic proteins have been located. NGF, EGF, PDGF and many other factors will induce a rapid (15 min) induction of *c-fos* (and perhaps as many as 60–100 other genes) and a slower (1 h) induction of *c-myc*. These pathways can be subverted by expression of the *v-fos* and *v-myc* oncogenes presumably by generating persistent rather than transient signals. Recently it has been shown that *v-jun* encodes a transcription factor with which *fos* can interact and that a subset of genes can thus be modulated at the transcriptional level. The mechanism by which different receptors can activate *fos*, *myc* and other proto oncogenes is as yet unclear (see

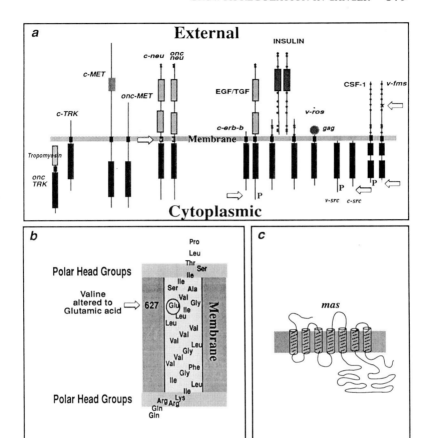

Fig. 2 Subverted receptors as transforming proteins

(a) The normal tyrosine kinase receptors and their truncated or mutated transforming counterparts are shown with arrows indicating specific important alterations involving particular amino acids or loss of phosphorylation sites.

(b) The site of mutation in the transmembrane region of rat onc-*neu* which involves conversion of a valve to a glutamic acid residue.

(c) The *mas* oncogene which is the angiotensin receptor. This receptor has seven transmembrane helices.

chapter by Balkwill, this Issue)—perhaps because we have yet to fully understand the signal transduction mechanisms.

REFERENCES

1 Sporn MB, Todaro GJ. Autocrine secretion and malignant transformation of cells. N Engl J Med 1980; 303: 878–880

2 Sporn MB, Roberts AB. Autocrine growth factors and Cancer. Nature 1985; 313: 745–747
3 Massague J. The TGF-β family of growth and differentiation factors. Cell 1987; 49: 437–438
4 Sporn MB, Roberts AB, Wakefield CM, de Crombrugghe B. Some recent advances in chemistry and biology of transforming growth factor b. J Cell Biol 1987; 105: 1039–1045
5 Waterfield MD, Scrace GT, Whittle N et al. Platelet-derived growth factor is structurally related to the putative transforming protein p28^{sis} of Simian Sarcoma Virus. Nature 1983; 301: 35–39
6 Doolittle RF, Hunkapillar MW, Hood LE et al. Simian Sarcoma Virus is derived from the gene encoding a platelet derived growth factor. Science 1983; 221: 273–277
7 Smith R, Peters G, Dickson C. Multiple RNAs expressed from the int-2 gene in mouse embryonal carcinoma cell lines encode a protein with homology to fibroblast growth factors. EMBO J 1988; 4: 1013–1022
8 Taira M, Yoshida T, Mujagawa K, Sakamoto H, Terada M, Sugimura T. cDNA sequence of human transforming gene hst and identification of the coding sequence required for transforming activity. Proc Natl Acad Sci USA 1987; 84: 2980–2984
9 Abraham JA, Mergia A, Whang JL et al. Nucleotide sequence of a bovine clone encoding the angiogenic protein basic fibroblast growth factor. Science 1986; 233: 545–548
10 Abraham JA, Whang JC, Tumulo A et al. Human basic fibroblast growth factor: nucleotide sequence and genomic organisation. EMBO J 1986; 5: 2523–2528
11 Zhan X, Hu X, Goldfarb M. Mol Cell Biol; In Press
12 Rijsewiji F, Schuermann M, Wagenaar E, Parren P, Weigel D, Nusse R. The Drosophila Homology of the Mouse Mammary Oncogene int-1 is identical to the segment polerity gene wingless. Cell 1987; 50: 649–657
13 Stern DF, Hare DL, Cecchim MA, Weinberg RA. Construction of a Novel Oncogene based on Synthetic Sequences encoding Epidermal Growth Factor. Science 1987; 235: 321–324
14 Rosenthal A, Lindquist PB, Bringman TS, Goeddel DV, Derynck R. Expression in Rat Fibroblast of a Human Transforming Growth Factor αcDNA Results in Transformation. Cell 1986; 46: 301
15 Rogelj S, Weinberg RA, Fanning E, Klagsbrun M. Basic Fibroblast growth factor fused to a signal peptide transforms cells. Nature 1988; 331: 173–175
16 Lang RA, Metcalf D, Gough NM, Dunn AR and Gouda TD. Expression of a Hemopoietic Growth Factor cDNA in a Factor-dependent cell line results in Autonomous Growth Tumorigenicity. Cell 1985; 43: 531–542
17 Rettenmier CW, Roussel MF, Ashmum RA, Ralph P, Price K, Sherr CJ. Synthesis of membrane-bound Colony-stimulating Factor 1 (CSF-1) and Down modulation of CSF-1 receptors in NIH 3T3 cells Transformed by Cotransfection of the Human CSF-1 and c-fms (CSF-1 Receptor) genes. Mol. Cell Biol 1987; 7: 2378–2387
18 Cuttitta F, Carney DN, Mulshire J et al. Bombesin-like peptides can function as autocrine growth factors in human small-cell lung cancer. Nature 1985; 316: 823–826
19 Massague J. The TGF-β family of growth and differentiation factors. Cell 1987; 49: 437–438
20 Sporn MB, Roberts AB, Wakefield LM, de Crombrugghe B. Some recent advances in the chemistry and biology of TGFβ. J Cell Biol 1987; 105: 1039–1045
21 Kimchi A, Wang X-F, Weinberg RA, Cheifetz S, Massague J. Absence of

TGFβ receptors and growth inhibitory responses in retinoblastoma cells. Science 1988; 240: 196–199
22 Yarden Y, Ullrich A. Molecular Analysis of Signal Transduction by Growth Factors. Biochemistry 1988; 27: 3113–3118
23 Schlessinger J. The Epidermal Growth Factor as a Multifunctional Allosteric Protein. Biochemistry 1988; 27: 3119–3123
24 Sherr CJ, Rettenmier CW, Sacca R, Roussel MF, Look AT, Stanley R. The c-fms proto-oncogene product is related to the receptor for the mononuclear phagocyte growth factor CSF-1. Cell 1985; 41: 665–676
25 Roussel MF, Dull TJ, Rettenmier CW, Ralph P, Ullrich A, Sherr CJ. Transforming potential of the c-fms proto-oncogene (CSF-1 receptor). Nature 1987; 325: 549–552
26 Bargmann CI, Weinberg RA. Oncogenic activation of the neu-encoded receptor protein by point mutation and deletion. EMBO J 1988; 7: 2043–2052
27 Waterfield MD. Subversion of growth receptor action in cancer. In: Franks LM, Teich N, ed. The Cellular and Molecular Biology of Cancer. Oxford: Oxford Science Pubs, 1988
28 Kikkawa U, Nishizuka Y. The role of protein kinase C in transmembrane signalling. Ann Rev Cell Biology 1986; 2: 149–179

Haemopoietic growth factors: their role in acute myeloblastic leukaemia

N G Testa
T M Dexter
Paterson Institute for Cancer Research, Christie Hospital and Holt Radium Institute, Manchester, UK

> The chromosome alterations specifically associated with leukaemia are found largely in the regions where the genes for the haemopoietic growth factors (as well as other regulatory molecules or their receptors) are located, indicating a crucial role of the growth factors in leukaemogenesis. However, growth factor genes *per se* do not generally induce leukaemia when inserted into normal haemopoietic cells, although they will do so if they are inserted into immortalized haemopoietic stem cell lines. The response of AML cells to these growth factors is extremely heterogeneous, and the tilting of the balance between self-reproduction (leading to perpetuation of the leukaemic process) and differentiation ('death' of the malignant cells) depends on several parameters, on the type and combination of factors to which the cells are exposed, with IL-3 and GM-CSF tending to favour self-renewal, and G-CSF and M-CSF tending to favour differentiation. These findings open the possibility to consider the use of growth factors to control the leukaemic process, although such treatments should be approached with considerable caution, and on an individual patient basis.

The haemopoietic growth factors, a family of glycoproteins first described in the sixties, play a crucial role in the survival, development, proliferation and maturation of normal haemopoietic cells. These molecules, originally called colony-stimulating factors (CSFs) because of their capacity to stimulate the formation of colonies of haemopoietic cells in vitro in soft gel systems have in the recent past been purified and molecularly cloned. The availability of recombinant growth factors has allowed the investigation of their roles in the control of normal haemopoiesis (see Dexter, this Issue).[1-3] The end result of this complex regulation of cell production, with the considerable overlap of target cells for the different CSFs (each acting through its own specific high affinity receptor)[3] is the fine tuning of the production of the different types of mature haemopoietic cells in normal steady state and the prompt and adequate response to haemopoietic stress. The important observation that bone marrow cells from untreated patients with acute myelobastic leukaemia (AML) are dependent on CSFs for proliferation in vitro[4,5] led to experiments designed not only to test the role of growth factors in the development of the leukaemic process, but also to test the possibility of using the knowledge so acquired in the therapeutic control of leukaemia.

HAEMOPOIETIC GROWTH FACTORS AND ACUTE MYELOBLASTIC LEUKAEMIA

Chromosome abnormalities

Cytogeneticists have been aware for a long time of chromosomal alterations which appear to be specifically associated with human leukaemia. Deletions and translocations in the long arm of chromosome 5 are often found in AML and in the myelodysplastic syndromes which may precede it. It therefore aroused considerable interest when a cluster of regulatory genes were located to chromosome 5 (Table 1).[6-8] Not only the genes for IL-3, GM-CSF and M-CSF are located in the q23–q33 region, but the c-*fms* normal cellular protooncogene, thought to code for the M-CSF receptor, is in close proximity.[9] Also, the genes coding for the receptor for platelet-derived growth factor, and the epithelial growth factor are located close by. It is not difficult to envisage that alterations in that area of chromosome 5, where such a cluster of growth-regulatory genes are located, are likely to be crucial to the development of leukaemia. A relatively high frequency of deletions in the 5q region (5q- syndrome) occurs in patients with primary myelodysplasia with refractory anaemia and abnormal megakaryocytes. Deletions in the bands 5q23–q31 are considered to be

Table 1 The location of growth factor genes

Factor	Chromosome location	Chromosomal alterations common in leukaemia
IL-3, GM-CSF, M-CSF	Chromosome 5 (q23–q33)	Deletions and translocations (in AML and myelodysplasia), monosomy 5 (in secondary AML)
G-CSF	Chromosome 17 (q21–q22)	Translocations 15; 17, iso17q (in acute promyelocytic leukaemia)
EPO	Chromosome 7 (q11–q22)	Monosomy 7 (in myelodysplasia and secondary AML)

See text for references
IL-3: Interleukin 3; G: granulocyte; M: macrophage; CSF: colony stimulating factor; Epo: erythropoietin.

critical, suggesting that the role of genes located in this area are more likely to play a critical role in the pathogenesis of the disorders.[6,7] The variability in the breakpoints observed in chromosome 5 suggest that the loss of a critical DNA sequence may be essential for malignant transformation, either by the reduced level of a gene product, or by allowing the expression of a recessive allele in the homologous chromosome. Mutations involving c-*fms* (coding for the M-CSF receptor) may also contribute to provide growth stimulatory signals in the absence of a ligand, as will be detailed below. It is also worthy of notice that in secondary AML, developed after intense chemotherapy for a primary malignancy, monosomy 5 is frequently observed leading to the suggestion that this lesion may be a marker of mutagen-induced leukaemia.

The gene coding for G-CSF has been located to the q21–q22 region of chromosome 17, proximal to the breakpoint in the translocation (15;17) which may be observed in acute promyelocytic leukaemia.[10,11] The protooncogene c-*erbB*-2 is also located in chromosome 17. This protooncogene is related to the oncogene v-*erbB*, which has close homology with the epidermal growth factor receptor[12], and which induces erythroleukaemia in chickens.[13] The protooncogene c-*erbA* (homologous to the thyroid hormone receptor)[14] and the gene for nerve growth factor receptor are also localized in the proximity.

The gene for erythropoietin (Epo), the growth factor essential for erythroid cell production, has been located in q11–q12 in chromosome 7[15]. Again, monosomy 7 is seen in myelodysplasia in childhood and in secondary AML.

Of course, the abnormalities described are usually observed at diagnosis, when the bone marrow and the circulating cells are already grossly abnormal. Although the likely important role of growth factors in the development of the leukaemic process may be inferred from those findings, they teach us little about the early steps involved in the development of leukaemia. However, evidence from experimental systems indicate that growth factors may play important roles in the early stages of leukaemogenesis.

Experimental induction of leukaemia

The introduction of the GM-CSF gene (using retroviral vectors) into factor-dependent, non-leukaemic, murine stem cell lines resulted in leukaemia when the cells were inoculated into mice. The infected cells synthesized and secreted GM-CSF, and grew independently of exogenous CSF.[16] However, the target cells were already immortalized and blocked in their ability to undergo normal differentiation, and it is likely that the GM-CSF insertion was only the last step in the unknown process leading to leukaemia. This concept is supported by recent data which indicate that insertion of the coding sequence of IL-3 into normal fetal liver cells results in the production of immortal cell lines, which secrete IL-3, but which are not tumourigenic. However, the same procedure carried out on factor-dependent haemopoietic cell lines resulted in tumourigenesis. These results indicate that production of IL-3, probably by progenitor cells, leads to apparently normal proliferation and maturation, but the same process in cells already immortalized leads to neoplasia. Therefore, it would appear that growth factor-independency, by itself, is not sufficient to convert normal into malignant cells, and that further steps are required.

An alternative approach has been to infect murine cells with the v-*fms* oncogene (related to c-fms, which encodes the M-CSF receptor). This oncogene acts promiscuously as a tyrosine kinase refractory to ligand-induced degradation and can transform haemopoietic cells not belonging to the mononuclear phagocyte lineage. Mice engrafted with the infected cells developed myeloproliferative disorders and clonal erytholeukaemias or B-cell lymphomas.[18] Thus, v-*fms* expression can play a role in the transformation of several haemopoietic lineages, including those that may not normally express the c-*fms* coded M-CSF receptor.

Evidence for a very early alteration in the response of progenitor cells (CFC) to growth factors has come from experiments in which kittens were infected with a strain of feline leukaemia virus which causes an acute myeloproliferative disease resembling AML in humans.[19] As early as 10 days after infection there was a marked expansion of GM-CFC, with incidences up to 10 times higher than normal. This expansion was accompanied by an altered (more sensitive) response to CSF, and was not accompanied by abnormalities in the BFU-E, which remained normal both in incidence and in sensitivity to growth factors. So far, no evidence of increased levels of CSFs in the bone marrow or of autocrine production of CSFs by the colony-forming cells has been obtained. Whether the abnormalities found are due to an early change in the sensitivity to growth factors (through increased numbers or sensitivity of receptors, or their abnormal activation?) or due to a capacity for autocrine production of growth factors leading to apparently autonomous growth has not been determined. Clearly, however, such changes are likely to be of crucial importance in the early stages of leukaemogenesis.

Effects of growth factors on leukaemic cells

The proliferative response of AML cells to growth factors is extremely heterogeneous. As reviewed by Lowenberg et al.,[20] the in vitro susceptibility to CSFs (measured by the formation of colonies of blast cells in vitro) and the number of receptors per cell, are of the same order as those found in normal CFC. The leukaemic cells respond to growth factors with similar phenomena to those shown by normal cells, including induction of colony formation, increased cell survival and stimulation of DNA synthesis (Table 2). However, due to the heterogeneity in the leukaemic cell population, what is important for the understanding and the eventual control of the disease is to learn how, in the blast cells, the balance between self-renewal and differentiation is affected leading

Table 2 Effects of growth factors on AML cells

Effect (in vitro)	Growth factor
Induction of colony formation	IL-3, GM-CSF, GM + G-CSF
Stimulation of DNA synthesis	IL-3, GM-CSF
Enhanced cell survival	IL-3, GM-CSF (M-CSF, Epo rarely)
Enhanced survival of CFC	GM-CSF
Induction of differentiation	G-CSF & M-CSF (others rarely)

Data taken from references 20, 21.
IL-3; interleukin 3; CSF: colony-stimulating factor; G: granulocyte; M: macrophage; Epo: erythropoietin; CFC: colony-forming cells.

to the perpetuation of the leukaemia. The first four effects listed in Table 2 will favour an imbalance biased towards cell renewal. It is known that blast colony formation in vitro and cell renewal of leukaemic cells in suspension culture is enhanced by IL-3, GM-CSF and G-CSF (the latter usually in combination with other factors), although again extreme variability is observed in individual cases.[21] G-CSF has the capacity to induce differentiation (which may be equated to leukaemic cell 'death') in experimental leukaemia in mice.[22] Similar results may be observed in human leukaemia.[20,23] Indications of granulocyte or moncyte maturation may also be obtained on rare occasions after in vitro treatment with IL-3 or GM-CSF. Maturation will perhaps be found more frequently after M-CSF, known to be a strong inducer of mature macrophage cell function.[3]

The variability shown by the leukaemic cells in their response to growth factors raises the question of why some leukaemic cells, which may be normal in terms of ligand-receptor binding, do not respond with normal maturation, and may lead to the search for abnormalities in the signal transduction mechanism.

Another question to be addressed is the synthesis and release of CSFs by the leukaemic cells themselves. Both G-CSF and GM-CSF genes (with an altered structure) have been detected in a few cases of AML, although none seemed to have been expressed.[24] Also, autocrine secretion of GM-CSF, which was neutralized by an anti-GM-CSF antibody has been reported in AML.[25]

EFFECT OF STROMAL REGULATORY CELLS ON LEUKAEMIA

The inductive microenvironment provided by stromal cells found in the bone marrow and grown in long-term bone marrow cultures favours the proliferation of normal haemopoietic cells over that of leukaemia cells in experimental systems and in patients. (Reviewed by Testa *see* Ref. 26.) Cultures of bone marrow from mice with T cell leukaemia or from patients with chronic myelocytic leukaemia (CML) or AML, facilitate the selective growth of normal haemopoietic cells and may not promote the survival or growth of the leukaemic cells. In the murine system, the marrow cells taken from leukaemic mice and subsequently grown in vitro have the ability to reconstitute normal haemopoiesis in the haemopoietic system of lethally irradiated recipients.

In cultures of marrow cells from patients with CML, disappearance of the Ph chromosome and re-establishment of normal haemopoiesis has been observed.[27] Again, although the response, specially in AML, is variable, the results have been encouraging enough to allow clinical trials using cultured bone marrow cells (biologically 'purged' from leukaemic cells in the cultures) for autologous bone marrow transplantation as treatment for AML.[26]

The reason for the selective 'death' of leukaemic cells in long-term culture is not known. Haemopoietic growth factors, such as G-CSF and M-CSF are produced within the stromal regulatory layer, and that may lead to differentiation ('death') of the leukaemic cells. Significantly, IL-3, which may favour cell renewal over differentiation, has not been detected in those cultures.[28] The interaction between production of growth factors (some yet unknown?), their binding to molecules in the extracellular matrix (themselves cell-bound?), and their interaction with stroma cell-bound normal stem cells work together to regulate normal haemopoiesis.[28] Subtle alterations in the ability of leukaemic cells to interact with marrow stromal cells are likely to play a role in their death in culture and the use of appropriate combinations of haemopoietic growth factors (perhaps together with other growth modulators) may well improve this therapeutic approach to the treatment of AML.

REFERENCES

1 Metcalf D. The granulocyte-macrophage colony stimulating factors. Science 1985; 229: 16–22
2 Dexter TM. The message in the medium. Nature 1984; 309: 746–747
3 Nicola N. Why do hemopoietic growth factor receptors interact with each other? Immunol Today 1987; 8: 134–140
4 Iscove NW, Senn JS, Till JE, McCulloch EA. Colony formation by normal and leukemic human marrow cells in culture: effect of conditioned medium from human leukocytes. Blood 1971; 37: 1–15
5 Metcalf D, Moore MAS, Sheridan JW, Spitzer G. Responsiveness of human granulocytic leukemic cells to colony stimulating factor. Blood 1974; 43: 847–859
6 LeBeau M, Epstein ND, O'Brien SJ et al. The interleukin-3 gene is located on human chromosome 5 and is deleted in myeloid leukemias with a deletion of 5q. Proc Natl Acad Sci USA 1987; 84: 5913–5917
7 LeBeau MM, Westbrook CA, Diaz MO et al. Evidence for involvement of GM-CSF and FMS in the deletion (5q) in myeloid disorder. Science 1986; 231: 984–987
8 Pettenati MJ, LeBeau MM, Lemons RS et al. Assignment of CSF-1 to 5q33.1: Evidence for clustering of genes regulating haemotopoiesis and for their involvement in the deletion of the long arm of chromosome 5 in myeloid disorders. Proc Natl Acad Sci USA 1987; 84: 2970–2974
9 Sherr CF, Rettenmier CW, Sacca R, Roussel MF, Look AT, Stanley ER. The c-fms proto-oncogene product is related to the receptor for the mononuclear phagocyte growth factor, CSF-1. Cell 1985; 41: 665–676

10 Tweardy DJ, Cannizzaro LA, Palumbo AP et al. Molecular cloning and characterization of a cDNA for human granulocyte colony-stimulating factor (G-CSF) from a glioblastoma multiforme cell line and localization of the G-CSF gene to chromosome band 17q21. Oncogene Res 1987; 1: 209–220
11 Simmer RN, Webber LM, Shannon MF et al. Localisation of the G-CSF gene on chromosome 17 proximal to the breakpoint in the t(15;17) in acute promyelocytic leukemia. Blood 1987; 70: 330–332
12 Dounward J, Yarden Y, Mayes E, Scrace G et al. Close similarity of epidermal growth factor receptor and v-erbB oncogene protein sequences. Nature 1984; 307: 521–527
13 Graf T, Beug H. Role of v-erbA and v-erbB oncogenes of avian erythroblastosis virus in erythroid cells transformation. Cell 1983, 34: 7–9
14 Weinberger C, Thomsson C, Ong ES, Lebo R, Gruol DJ, Evans RM. The c-erb-A gene encodes a thyroid hormone receptor. Nature 1986; 324: 641–646
15 Law ML, Cai GY, Lin FK et al. Chromosomal assignment of the human erythropoietin gene and its DNA polymorphism. Proc Natl Acad Sci USA 1986; 83: 6920–6924
16 Lang RA, Metcalf D, Gough NM, Dunn AR, Gonda TJ. Expression of a hemopoietic growth factor cDNA in a factor dependent cell line results in autonomous growth and tumorigenicity. Cell 1985; 43: 531–542
17 Wong PMC, Chung SW, Nienhuis AW. Retroviral transfer and expression of the interleukin-3 gene in hemopoietic cells. Genes Dev 1987; 1: 358–365
18 Heard JM, Roussel MF, Rettenmeir CW, Sherr CS. Mutilineage hematopoietic disorders uinduced by transplantation of bone marrow cells expressing the V-FMS oncogene. Cell 1987; 51: 663–673
19 Testa NG, Onions DE, Lord BI. Pre-leukaemic abnormalities caused in cats by infection with a new isolate of Feline Leukaemia Virus (FeLV AB/GM). Hematologica 1988; 73: 317–320
20 Lowenberg B, Delwel R, Touw I, 1989. Hematopoietic growth factors and progenitor cells in human acute leukaemia. In: Dexter TM, Garland J, Testa NG, eds. Molecular and cellular biology of hemopoietic growth factors. New York: Dekker, 1989; In press
21 Miyauchi J, Kelleher C, Yang YC et al. The effects of three recombinant growth factors, IL-3, GM-CSF and G-CSF on the blast cells of acute myeloblastic leukaemia maintained in short term suspension culture. Blood 1987; 70: 657–663
22 Metcalf D. Regulator-induced suppression of myelomonocytic leukemic cells: clonal analysis of early cellular events. Int J Cancer 1982; 30: 203–210
23 Souza LM, Boone TC, Gabrilove J et al. Recombinant human granulocyte colony-stimulating factor; effects on normal and leukaemic cells. Science 1986; 232: 61–65
24 Cheng GYM, Kelleher CA, Miyanchi, J et al. Structure and expression of genes of GM-CSF and G-CSF in blast cells from patients with acute myeloblastic leukemia. Blood 1988; 71: 204–208
25 Young DC, Griffin JD. Autocrine secretion of GM-CSF in acute myeloblastic leukaemia. Blood 1986; 68: 1178–1181
26 Testa NG, Coutinho L, Chang J, et al. The use of cultured bone marrow cells for autologous transplantation in patients with acute myeloblastic leukaemia. Haematol Blood Transfus 1987; 31: 75–78
27 Eaves C, Coulumbel L, Dube I, Kalousek J, Cashman J, Eaves AC. Maintenance of normal and abnormal haemopoietic cell populations in long-term cultures of CML and AML marrow cells. In: Cronkite EP, Dainiak N, McCaffrey RP, Palek J, Quesenberg PJ, eds. Hematopoietic stem cell physiology. New York: Liss, 1985; pp. 403–413
28 Dexter TM, Ponting ILO, Roberts RA et al. Growth and differentiation of haemopoietic stem cells. J Gen Physiol 1988; In press

Clinical use of growth factors

M H Bronchud[1]
T M Dexter[2]

Cancer Research Campaign Department of Medical Oncology [1], Christie Hospital and Holt Radium Institute, and Department of Experimental Haematology [2], Paterson Institute for Cancer Research, Manchester, UK

> Cellular proliferation and differentiation in the living organism are regulated, at least in part, by a complex network of interacting peptides, or growth factors. The purification and molecular cloning of these growth factors has now led to the exciting task of ascertaining their physiological role in vivo and to verify their value as therapeutic substances worthy of clinical use. Rigorous methods of drug evaluation are required to prove the efficacy and safety of these new biological agents, particularly now that so many of them are being produced by the new genetic engineering techniques. Haemopoietic growth factors and growth factors involved in the regulation of the immune response have been more extensively studied clinically and are discussed in this section.

Molecularly cloned and purified growth factors have been used in a limited number of clinical situations. The safety of these recombinant products has not to be taken for granted, and concern about it has prompted a number of quality control criteria and toxicology studies,[1] which include testing for undesirable impurities, such as residual proteins from the host organism, usually *Escherichia coli*, pyrogens, contaminating viruses and foreign DNA. Toxicology studies in experimental animals are also hampered by the potential species-specificity of many of the actions of these growth factors and by the inadequacies of conventional criteria of toxicity, e.g. LD_{50}, when applied to these biological agents. The main objectives of these clinical trials are summarized in Table 1.

REGENERATION OF NORMAL TISSUES

Anaemia of chronic disease and end-stage renal failure: erythropoietin

Erythropoietin is mainly produced by the kidney and patients in chronic renal failure are often anaemic. Two clinical trials[2,3] have now fully confirmed that recombinant erythropoietin can correct the anaemia of end-stage renal failure avoiding the problems of sensitisation to transplantation antigens, infection with cytomegalovirus or other viruses, and iron overload associated with repeated blood transfusions. In addition a sense of well-being is usually restored to the patient and there is also an improvement in the clotting defect of uraemia.[4] More importantly, the treatment is well tolerated, although influenza-like symptoms of short duration can occur in some patients and hypertension may develop, perhaps as a result of the increase in blood volume or blood viscosity. In most studies the hormone has been given intravenously three times

Table 1 Potential clinical use of growth factors

I-*Regeneration of normal tissues*
  1-Anaemia of chronic diseases: erythropoietin
  2-Chemotherapy-induced neutropaenia: myeloid growth factors
  3-Epithelial regeneration: epidermal growth factor
  4-Others: bone fractures (bone cell differentiation and growth factors) and peripheral neuropathies (nerve growth factors)

II-*Immunotherapy of cancer*
  1-Interferons
  2-Interleukin-2
  3-Tumour necrosis factor
  4-Myeloid growth factors

III-*Stimulation of scarring (to enhance wound healing)*
  1-Platelet-derived growth factor
  2-Fibroblast growth factors

IV-*Correction of growth factor deficiencies: replacement therapy*
  1-Anaemia of chronic renal failure: erythropoietin
  2-Dwarfism: human growth hormone (and somatomedins)
  3-Cyclic neutropaenia: myeloid growth factors

V-*Control of abnormal proliferation: anti-growth factors*
  1-Inhibitors of growth factor synthesis (cyclosporin A)
  2-Negative growth factors (e.g. transforming growth factor beta)
  3-Monoclonal antibodies (to growth factors or growth factor receptors)
  4-Synthetic antagonists
  5-Crinotoxins (conjugates of growth factors to potent cellular toxins)

a week at 75–450 IU/kg body weight weekly, but other modes of administration are currently being explored. Strictly speaking, the use of recombinant erythropoietin in chronic renal failure should be regarded as *replacement therapy* as a relative deficiency of this growth factor exists in these patients. However, encouraging results are also expected in on-going clinical trials in patients with anaemia of chronic disease, like in rheumatoid arthritis and cancer, where there is no clear deficit of erythropoietin production. In addition recombinant erythropoietin in high doses stimulates platelet formation in vitro[5] and in animals,[6] and combined with other haemopoietic growth factors may be of help in regenerating bone marrow following chemotherapy or bone marrow transplantation.

Chemotherapy-induced neutropaenia: myeloid growth factors

Four myeloid colony-stimulating factors (CSF's) have now been produced by recombinant DNA technology (*see* Dexter, this issue): multi-CSF or interleukin-3 (IL-3), granulocyte-macrophage colony-stimulating factor (GM-CSF), granulocyte colony-stimulating factor (G-CSF) and macrophage colony-stimulating factor (M-CSF). They are all glycoproteins, but the extended carbohydrate portion of each molecule seems not to be needed for their biological activity. Each CSF has a corresponding specific membrane receptor and granulocyte-macrophage progenitor cells are known to simultaneously coexpress receptors for more than one CSF, although cross-modulation of these receptors can occur following the binding of one type of receptor by its specific CSF.[7] Recombinant GM-CSF has been produced in both glycosylated (eukaryotic) and unglycosylated (bacterial) forms. Recombinant G-CSF is available in unglycosylated form only.

When recombinant GM-CSF was given by continuous intravenous infusion to monkeys, a significant increase in the leukocyte count was observed, reaching a level seven times above the preinfusion average after approximately eight days of infusion. In this case, a mixture of eosinophils, neutrophils, lymphocytes and monocytes was seen.[8] In further work it was reported that recombinant GM-CSF can shorten the period of neutropaenia after autologous bone marrow transplantation in primates.[9]

G-CSF produced a dose-dependent increase in peripheral leucocytes in monkeys, but, in this case (and unlike GM-CSF) only an increase in neutrophils was seen.[10] Of great significance was the observation that G-CSF, given following cytotoxic therapy to monkeys and mice, accelerated recovery from the chemotherapy-induced leukopaenia. However, when monkeys were treated with G-CSF for six days prior to chemotherapy it was found that, in spite of an initial eight-fold increase in peripheral neutrophils, G-CSF treatment failed to prevent post-chemotherapy neutropaenia. These encouraging animal studies soon led to the first clinical trials.

The first published clinical trial with GM-CSF demonstrated dose-dependent increases in circulating leucocytes in patients with acquired immunodeficiency syndrome (AIDS) and bone marrow failure.[11] The drug was given by a single intravenous infusion, followed 48h later by continuous intravenous therapy and after 14 days all patients had normal or above normal circulating leucocyte counts. In many patients, however, the number of peripheral eosinophils significantly exceeded the number of mature neutrophils. This relative lack of leucocyte specificity of GM-CSF has also been observed in other clinical trials,[12,13] but no consistent effects on platelet counts or red blood cells have been reported, suggesting that the multi-lineage effect seen in vitro is, for some reason, not manifest in vivo. However, some increase in platelet counts and reticulocytes has been reported in some patients with myelodysplastic syndromes[12] treated with GM-CSF.

In general, these growth factors are more effective and better tolerated when given by continuous, rather than bolus, intravenous infusion. This is probably a reflection of their relatively short half-life, and it also emphasizes the strict dependence of growth factor responsive cells on the continuous presence of circulating hormone. Perhaps the main problem with GM-CSF is its relative toxicity. Fever is a frequent complication,[14] and so is bone pain, which has been called *medullary pain* because it is experienced in the lower back, hip areas, ribs, shoulders and sternum.[12] It can be severe and it has also been described, in a mild to moderate form, by patients receiving recombinant G-CSF when given by single, but not continuous, intravenous infusion.[15] The more worrying side-effect of GM-CSF is a *capillary-leak syndrome* seen at doses of 30 µg/kg/day and above, and manifested by erythroderma, fluid retention with pleural effusions, generalized oedema and renal dysfunction.[13] Although the pathogenesis of this toxicity is not known, it has been suggested that it reflects activation of macrophages and lymphocytes. In addition, it has been reported that GM-CSF treatment can lead to a decreased mobility of circulating neutrophils[16], which could decrease their protective effect against infections.

In contrast, recombinant G-CSF when given by continuous infusion to patients with small cell lung cancer produced a more specific increase in peripheral neutrophils, which were shown to be normal in tests of their mobility and phagocytic activity.[17] In this trial, the clinical value of G-CSF was shown by a considerable reduction in the period of absolute neutropaenia (median of 80%) with a return to normal or above normal, neutrophil counts within two weeks after day 1 of chemotherapy (Fig. 1). Probably as a result of this, the number of severe infections was significantly reduced. Although the neutrophil nadir induced by the chemotherapy was not prevented by G-CSF, recovery was considerably speeded up. In addition, no side effects related to G-CSF therapy were found and two main biological effects were observed:

(a) an early fall in peripheral neutrophils, within the first hour, followed by a rapid release of mature neutrophils into the circulatory pool;

(b) stimulation of proliferation and differentiation of neutrophil precursors in the bone marrow with a mean of 20% increase in bone marrow cellularity, probably representing the expansion of the neutrophil precursor cell pool.[18]

A similar leucocyte specificity was found in other trials with bolus injections of G-CSF, but at high doses some increase in peripheral monocytes was also found.[15,19] In all clinical trials with G-CSF so far reported no dose-limiting toxicity has been found and it has proved useful in reducing the neutropaenia associated with the following cytotoxics: doxorubicin, ifosfamide, etoposide, melphalan, methotrexate, vinblastine, cisplatin, cyclophosphamide and BCNU. Relatively little has yet been reported regarding the protective effect of GM-CSF in chemotherapy-treated patients, however in a preliminary report of GM-CSF given to sarcoma patients receiving chemotherapy the number of neutrophils at nadir was not significantly different than controls, although the total leucocyte blood count was slightly higher.[20] G-CSF is also being used as *replacement* therapy in clinical trials on the rare, but interesting, condition of cyclic neutropaenia. Cytotoxics are also employed in the treatment of chronic inflammatory disorders, e.g. aggressive forms of rheumatoid arthritis or cryptogenic fibrosing alveolitis, and the concomitant use of myeloid growth factors might also be of use in these situations.

One concern when using growth factors in the management of

cancer patients is that the growth factors might promote the growth of the cancer cells themselves. This explains why no clinical trials of myeloid growth factors have yet been done in myeloid leukaemias, since many primary cultures of myeloid leukaemias in man and mouse remain strictly dependent on exogenous CSF for survival and proliferation.[21] Results with

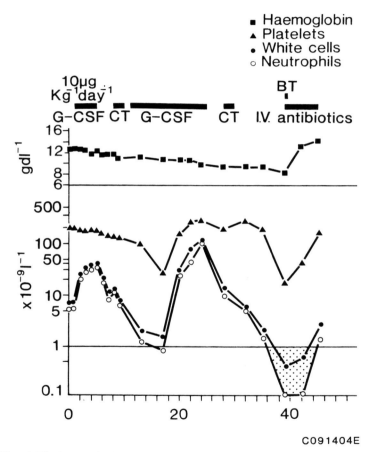

Fig. 1 The haematological profile in one patient treated with recombinant human G-CSF given by continuous infusion and intensive chemotherapy is shown. The increase in total white blood cells produced by G-CSF was due to a specific increase in peripheral neutrophils and, when chemotherapy (CT) was followed by G-CSF the period of absolute neutropaenia (shaded area) was virtually abolished. In contrast, when the patient received the same chemotherapy without G-CSF she became severely neutropaenic requiring admission for intravenous antibiotics and a blood transfusion (BT).

established tumour cell lines are of less clear relevance (since they may bear little resemblance to primary tumours), but, for example, GM-CSF has been shown to promote the growth of cell lines derived from osteosarcoma and breast carcinoma origin.[22]

It has been suggested that the clinical use of combinations of growth factors could prove more useful than individual growth factors on their own, and indeed in mice there seems to be a synergy between interleukin-1 and G-CSF.[23] Other combinations, e.g. M-CSF and G-CSF, might also prove useful, and the addition of a megakaryocyte growth factor or high dose erythropoietin to a myeloid growth factor could improve platelet recovery.

Finally, recombinant human IL-3 has recently become available, and when administered to primates it causes an increase in eosinophil, platelets and reticulocyte counts. A synergistic effect was noted when an infusion of IL-3 in primates was followed by an infusion of GM-CSF.[24] Clearly, this and other combinations, e.g. IL-3 and G-CSF, need to be tested in controlled clinical studies.

IMMUNOTHERAPY OF CANCER

For many years a search has been made to find T-cell specific responses against human tumours but, in general, this has led to disappointing results. Moreover, solid tumours are usually also resistant to natural killer cells (NK). A clinically effective *magic bullet*, to home in on cancer tissue while sparing normal cells, remains to be found in spite of the monoclonal antibody revolution. Several other agents, with immunoregulatory and pro-liferative or anti-proliferative activities have also been studied. Interferons were, at one stage, unrealistically expected to be widely successful. Although they have some antitumor activity in renal cell carcinoma, non Hodgkin's lymphoma, chronic myeloid leukaemia and myeloma, their routine clinical use will probably remain restricted to rare conditions such as hairy-cell leukaemia, and perhaps condylomata acuminata.[25] Non MHC-restricted cytotoxicity for tumour cells has recently been found in a number of previously unrecognized lymphocyte cell types which appear to be stimulated by interleukin-2 (IL-2). The main ones are: lymphokine-activated killer cells (LAK) and tumour-infiltrating lymphocytes (TIL).[26] The use of IL-2, with or without concomitant administration of LAK cells or TIL cells, has now been reported in a number of clinical trials. The best results have shown responses in 20–30% of patients, particularly with renal cell carcinomas and melanomas, for which no satisfactory therapy exists.[27,28] However, there were few complete remissions and the toxicity was at times severe, with fever, rigors, hypotension, fluid retention and renal impairment often requiring admission to the intensive care unit. These side-effects probably reflect the complexity of the lymphokine cascade, of which IL-2 is a major component.[29] For example, IL-2 induces the production of other lymphokines, like γ-interferon and tumour necrosis factor (TNF). The latter, also known as cachectin, is a primary mediator of the lethal effect of endotoxin and can produce haemorrhagic necrosis of experimental tumours. Unfortunately, most human cancers are highly resistant to its toxic effects.[30]

CONTROL OF ABNORMAL PROLIFERATION: ANTI-GROWTH FACTORS

The proliferative changes that occur after tissue injury generally play a protective role. Thus, granulation tissue forms a barrier to bacteria and their toxins, or replaces dead tissue by fibrous tissue. In some cases the fibrous tissue itself may be deleterious for the organism, leading to fibrosis or shrinkage of the organ, as in cirrhosis of the liver. There are several growth factors, produced by platelets or inflammatory cells, which are known to influence the proliferation and differentiation of fibroblasts at the sites of tissue injury: platelet-derived growth factor and interleukin-1 (IL-1) are two examples. Inhibitors of IL-1 activities are currently being characterized[31] and could have a potential therapeutic role. Similarly, inhibitors of IL-2 production, like cyclosporin A, are powerful immunosuppressive agents.[32] The existence of negative growth factors has long been suspected (e.g. *chalones*), and it has now become apparent that some growth factors can have a negative growth effect in vitro.[33] Another class of growth inhibitors would be molecular conjugates of potent toxins with growth factors. They could be called *crino-toxins* because growth factors can act in an endocrine, paracrine or autocrine fashion. One example is the recently reported diphtheria toxin-IL-2 fusion protein.[34] Monoclonal antibodies to growth factor receptors or synthetic antagonists are also attracting the attention of major research institutions, as one obvious potential application of these anti-growth factors would be the treatment of cancer.

REFERENCES

1 World Health Organisation. Quality control of biologicals produced by recombinant DNA techniques. Bull WHO 1983; 61: 879–911
2 Winearls CG, Oliver DO, Pippard MJ, Reid C, Downing MR, Cotes PM. Effect of human erythropoietin derived from recombinant DNA on the anaemia of patients maintained by chronic haemodialysis. Lancet 1986; 2: 1175–1178
3 Eschbach JW, Egrie JC, Downing MR, Browne JK, Adamson JW. Correction of the anemia of end-stage renal disease with recombinant human erythropoietin: results of a phase I and II clinical trial. N Engl J Med 1987; 316: 73–78
4 Casati S, Passerini P, Campise MR, Graziani G, Cesana B, Perisic M, Ponticelli C. Benefits and risks of protracted treatment with human recombinant erythropoietin in patients having haemodialysis. Br Med J 1987; 295: 1017–1020
5 Sakaguchi M, Kawakita M, Matsushita J, Shibuya K, Koishihara Y, Takatsuki K. Human erythropoietin stimulates murine megakaryopoiesis in serum free culture. Exp Hematol 1987; 15: 1028–1034
6 Berridge MV, Carter JM, Fraser JK. Effects of recombinant human erythropoietin on platelet production in the rat. Blood 1987; 70 (Suppl 1): 348a
7 Walker F, Nicola NA, Metcalf D, Burgess AW. Hierarchical down-modulation of hemopoietic growth factor receptors. Cell 1985; 43: 269–276
8 Donahue RE, Wang EA, Stone DK et al. Stimulation of haematopoiesis in primates by continuous infusion of recombinant human GM-CSF. Nature 1986; 321: 872–875
9 Nienhuis AW, Donahue RE, Karlsson S, et al. Recombinant human granulocyte-macrophage colony-stimulating factor shortens the period of neutropenia after autologous bone marrow transplantation in a primate model. J Cli Invest 1987; 80: 573–577
10 Welte K, Bonilla MA, Gillio AP et al. Recombinant human granulocyte colony-stimulating factor: effects on hematopoiesis in normal and cyclophosphamide-treated primates. J Exp Med 1987; 165: 941–948
11 Groopman JE, Mitsuyasu RT, DeLeo MJ, Oette DH, Golde DW. Effect of recombinant human granulocyte-macrophage colony-stimulating factor on myelopoiesis in the acquired immunodeficiency syndrome. N Engl J Med 1987; 317: 593–598
12 Vadhan-Raj S, Keating M, LeMaistre A et al. Effects of recombinant human granulocyte-macrophage colony-stimulating factor in patients with the myelodysplastic syndromes. N Engl J Med 1987; 317: 1545–1552
13 Brandt SJ, Peters WP, Atwater SK et al. Effect of recombinant human macrophage colony-stimulating factor on hematopoietic reconstitution after high dose chemotherapy and autologous bone marrow transplantation. N Engl J Med 1988; 318: 869–876
14 Peters WP, Shogan J, Shpall EJ, Jones RB, Kim CS. Recombinant human granulocyte-macrophage colony-stimulating factor produces fever. Lancet 1988; i: 950
15 Morstyn G, Campbell L, Souza LM et al. Effect of granulocyte colony stimulating factor on neutropenia induced by cytotoxic chemotherapy. Lancet 1988; i: 667–672
16 Peters WP, Brandt SJ, Atwater SK et al. Effect of recombinant human granulocyte-macrophage colony-stimulating factor on hematopoietic reconstitution and granulocyte function following high does chemotherapy and autologous bone marrow transplantation. Proc Am Soc Clin Oncol 1988; 7: 160 (Abstract No 616)
17 Bronchud MH, Scarffe JH, Thatcher N et al. Phase I/II study of recombinant human granulocyte colony-stimulating factor in patients receiving intensive chemotherapy for small cell lung cancer. Br J Cancer 1987; 56: 809–813
18 Bronchud MH, Potter MR, Morgenstern G et al. In vitro and in vivo analysis of

the effects of recombinant human granulocyte colony-stimulating factor in patients. Br J Cancer, 1988; 58: 64–69

19 Gabrilove JL, Jakubowski A, Scher H et al. Effect of granulocyte colony-stimulating factor on neutropenia and associated morbidity due to chemotherapy for transitional cell carcinoma of the urothelium. N Engl J Med 1988; 318: 1414–1422

20 Antman K, Griffin J, Elias A et al. Effect of rGM-CSF on chemotherapy induced myelosuppression in sarcoma patients. Proc Am Soc Clin Oncol 1988; 7: 160 (Abstract No 619).

21 Metcalf D. The molecular biology and functions of the granulocyte-macrophage colony-stimulating factors. Blood 1986; 67: 257–267

22 Dedhar S, Galloway P, Eaves C. Human granulocyte-macrophage colony-stimulating factor is a growth factor for a variety of cell type of non-hemopoietic origin. Proc Am Soc Clin Oncol 1988; 29: 51 (Abstract No 201)

23 Moore MAS, Warren DJ. Synergy of interleukin-1 and granulocyte colony-stimulating factor: in vivo stimulation of stem call recovery and hemopoietic regeneration following 5-fluorouracil treatment of mice. Proc Natl Acad Sci USA 1987; 84: 7134–7138

24 Donahue RE, Seehra J, Norton C et al. Stimulation of hematopoiesis in primates with human interleukin-3 and granulocyte-macrophage colony-stimulating factor. Blood Abstract 1987; 70: 133a

25 Merigan TC. Human interferon as a therapeutic agent. N Engl J Med 1988; 318: 1458–1460

26 Rosenberg SA. Immunotherapy of cancer using interleukin-2: current status and future prospects. Immunol Today 1988; 58–62

27 Rosenberg SA, Lotze ML, Muul L et al. A progress report on the treatment of 157 patients with advanced cancer using lymphocyte-activated killer cells and interleukin-2 or high dose interleukin-2 alone. N Engl J Med 1987; 316: 889–897

28 West WH, Tauer KW, Yannelli JR et al. Constant-infusion recombinant interleukin-2 in adoptive immunotherapy of advanced cancer. N Engl J Med 1987; 316: 898–905

29 Dinarello CA, Mier JW. Lymphokines. N Engl J Med 1987; 317: 940–945

30 Beutler B, Cerami A. Cachectin: more than a tumor necrosis factor. N Engl J Med 1987; 316: 379–384

31 Oppenheim JJ, Kovacs EJ, Matsushima K, Durum SK. There is more than one interleukin-1. Immunol Today 1986; 7: 45–56

32 Bunjes D, Hardt, C, Rollinghoff M, Wagner A. Cyclosporin A mediates immunosuppression of primary cytotoxic T-cell responses by impairing the release of interleukin-1 and interleukin-2. Eur J Immunol 1981; 11: 657–661

33 Knabbe C, Lippman ME, Wakefield LM et al. Evidence that transforming growth factor beta is a hormonally regulated negative growth factor in human breast cancer cells. Cell 1987; 48: 417–428

34 Bacha P, Williams DP, Waters C, Williams JM, Murphy JR, Strom TB. Interleukin-2 receptor-targeted cytotoxicity. J Exp Med 1988; 167: 612–622

Index

A

Acquired immunodeficiency syndrome (AIDS), 593
Activins, 331, 427
Acute myeloblastic leukaemia (AML), 582–589
  chromosome abnormalities, 583–584
Altered growth regulation in cancer, 570–581
Angiogenesis, 447
Anti-growth factors, 597
Apoptosis, 357
Autocrine motility factor (AMF), 482, 489

B

B cells
  activation, 374–377
  differentiation factors (BCDFs), 371–388
    BCDF-2 or IL-5, 345–346, 364–365
    multiple activities, 381–383
    proliferation factors, 377–378
    responses, regulation of, 374–381
    factors which inhibit, 381
    stimulatory factor-1 (or IL-4), 364
  growth factors (BCGFs), 371–388
BAIRD A & WALICKR P A: Fibroblast growth factors (FGFs), 438–452
BALKWILL F R: Tumour necrosis factor (TNF), 389–400
BCGF see B cell differentiation factors
Bombesin, 492–504, 516, 519–520
  PKC, 519–521
Bovine collagen inducing factor (polyergin), 426
Bradykinin, 492–504
BRL see buffalo rat liver cells
BRONCHUD M H & DEXTER T M: Clinical use of GFS, 590–599
Buffalo rat liver cells (BRL), 323
BURGESS A W: Epidermal growth factor and transforming growth factor alpha, 401–424

C

Cachectin see tumour necrosis factor
'Cachexin' (or TNFα), 366–367
Calcium mobilization, 492–504
  mitogenesis, 524–526
CALLARD R: Cytokine regulation of B-cell growth and differentiation, 371–388
Cancer
  abnormal synthesis of GFs, 572–574
  clinical use of GFs, 590–599
  signal modulation pathways, 578
  small cell ling (SCLC), 501–504
CD see cluster differentiation antigens
Cell adhesion molecules (CAMs), 488
CFU cells, 338–340, 346
Cholera toxin, 521
Chronic renal failure, 591–592
CLEMMONS D R: Structural and functional analysis of insulin-like growth factors, 465–480
Clinical use of GFs, 590–599
  anti-growth factors, 597
  CSFs, 592–596
  immunotherapy, 596
  regeneration of normal tissues, 591–596
Cluster differentiation antigens (CDs), 352–357, 361–363, 365, 372, 373
Colony-forming cells (CFC), 585–586
Colony stimulating factors (CSFs), 340–347, 361–362, 364–366, 372–374, 391, 429, 582–589
  receptors, 543, 546–547
Cyclic AMP
  mitogenesis, 521–526
Cyclosporin A, 362
Cytokine regulation of B-cell growth and differentiation, 371–388
Cytotoxic conjugates, 419
Cytotoxic/suppressor cells (or CD8 cells), 363

D

Da cells (transformed lymphomona cell-line), 324
DAG see diacylglycerol
Daunomycin, 419
DEXTER T M: Haemopoietic growth factors, 337–349
DEXTER T M see also BRONCHUD M H or TESTA N G
DIA see differentiation inhibitory factor
Diabetes, 447, 474
Diacylglycerol (DAG), 519, 524, 544, 578

Differentiation inhibitory factor (DIA), 323–325

E

Early gene induction, 529–540
  immediate, 530–534
  mechanisms, 534–537
Epstein-Barr virus (EBV), 378
EGF *see* Epidermal growth factor
Embryogenesis, growth factors in, 319–336
Embryonic stem cells (ES), 322–324
Endorphin (beta), 503
Eosinophil differentiation factor, 345–346
Eosinophil-CSF (or IL-5), 364–365
Epidermal growth factor and transforming growth factor α, 401–424
Epidermal growth factor (EGFs), 401–424, 481, 493, 516
  biological effects, 406–411
  biosynthesis and tissue distribution, 402–404, 405
  cancer, 416–418
  clinical & industrial uses, 418–419
  discovery & characterization, 401–402
  gastric ulcers, 419
  genes, homologies & structure, 412–416
  in vitro, 407–409
  in vivo, 409–411
  receptor, 546
Erythropoietin (Epo), 506–514, 581–588
  assays for, 508–509
  clinical use, 591–592
  extrarenal production, 507–508
  physiology, 506–507
  production by transformed cells, 508
  structure & gene cloning, 509–511

F

FELDMANN M, LONDEI M & HAWORTH C: T cells and lymphokines, 361–370
Fibroblast growth factors (FGF), 325–328, 330–332, 438–452
  biological functions, 441–446
  discovery, 438
  embryonic development, 446
    activities & regulation, 448–450
  modulation of endocrine response, 442–445
  neurology, 445–446
  pathophysiology, 446–448
  pleitropic activities, 440
  receptors, 542
  tissue repair, 441–442
  family, 439–441
Fluorescence activated cell sorter (FACS), 346
Follicle stimulating hormone, FSH, 427, 428
Forskolin, 521, 523, 525, 544

G

G proteins, 492, 504
  PKC, 519
Gastrin, 503
Gene induction by Gfs, early, 529–540
GHERARDI E *see* STOKER M
Growth factor receptors, 541–553
  diversity of structures, 542–543
Growth factors in embryogenesis, 319–336
Growth hormone, 321–322, 469, 473
Growth regulation
  in cancer, 570–581

H

Haemopoiesis, role of GFs in, 340–341
Haemopoietic GFs *see also* colony-stimulating factors
Haemopoietic growth factors (IL-3), 337–349, 365–366
  evolutionary/structural relationships, 344–345
  synergistic activities, 345–347
  their role in acute myeloblastic leukaemia, 582–589
Haemopoietic system, 337–340
Haemopoietin-1 (or IL-1), 346
HAWORTH C *see* FELDMANN M
HEATH J K & SMITH A G: Growth factors in embryogenesis, 319–336
HELDIN C-H & WESTERMARK B: Platelet-derived growth factor: A family of isoforms that bind to two distinct receptors, 453–464
Helper T cells (or CD4 T cells), 363, 371, 379
Heparin, 325, 439
Hepatocyte stimulating factor (or IL-6), 365
HILDA *same as* LIF
HLA *see* human leucocyte antigen
HSUAN J J: Transforming growth factors β, 425–437

Human interleukin for Da cells
  (HILDA) see LIF
Human leucocyte antigen (HLA), 362

I
IGFs see insulin-like growth factors
IL see interleukin
Immunoglobulin isotype selection,
  379–380
Immunotherapy, 596–597
INFs see interferons
Inhibins, 331, 427
Insulin, 543
Insulin-like growth factors (IGFs),
  320–322, 427
  binding proteins, 473–475
  in vivo actions, 477–478
  receptors, 471–472
    structural characterization, 466–468
    synthesis & secretion, 468–471
    target cell actions, 475–477
Interferon B2 (or IL-6), 365
Interferons (IFNs), 361–363, 366,
  372–373, 375, 377, 379, 389, 394
  gene expression, 529
Interleukins (ILs), 340–347, 350,
  361–368, 372–388, 389, 409, 440
  receptors, 543
Introduction, 317–318

J
JENKINSON E J see OWEN J J T
JOHNSON G R: Erythropoietin,
  506–514

K
Kaposi's sarcoma, 325, 440

L
Leukaemia, acute myeloblastic,
  582–589
  effects of GFs, 586–587
  experimental induction, 585–586
  stromal cells, 587–588
Leukaemia, chronic myelocytic,
  587–588
Leukaemia inhibitory factor (LIF),
  324–325
LONDEI M see FELDMANN M
Low density lipoprotein (LDL)
  receptor, 413
LT see lymphotoxin
Luteinizing hormone, 410
Lymphocyte maturation (T), 350–360

Lymphocyte ontogeny
  (B), signals in, 358–359
  (T), signals in, 350–357
Lymphokine production, 363
Lymphotoxin (LT), or TNFβ),
  361–364, 366–367, 393–394, 397

M
Mast cells, 364
McDONALD N, MURRAY-RUST J
  & BLUNDELL T: Structure-
  function relationships of growth
  factors and their receptors, 554–569
Mechanisms of early gene induction,
  535
Mesoderm induction, 327
MIS see Mullerian inhibitory substance
Mitogenesis, signal transduction
  pathways in, 515–528
  early signals & synergistic effects,
    524–526
Mouse mammary tumour virus
  (MMTV), 326
Models
  receptor ligand binding, 565–567
Moloney murine sarcoma virus
  (MMSV), 404
MMTV see Mouse mammary tumour
  virus
Mullerian inhibiting substance
  (MIS), 331, 427
Myeloid cell GFs, 345
Myeloid leukaemia inhibitory
  factors, 575
Myelomonocytic leukaemia cell line,
  341

N
Natural killer cells (NK), 361,
  363–364, 367–368
Nerve growth factor (NGF), 401, 481
  receptors, 543
Neuromedins, 493
Neuropeptides as growth regulators,
  492–505
  receptor antagonists, 498–500
  small cell lung cancer (SCLC),
    501–503
Neuropeptides as growth regulators
Nippostrongylus brasiliensis, 380
NK cells see natural killer cells
Non-tumorigenic mouse mammary
  epithelial cell line (NMuMG), 417
Normal rat kidney (NRK) fibroblasts,
  408, 430–431

O

OWEN J J T & JENKINSON E J: Regulatory factors in lymphoid development, 350–360

P

PDGF *see* platelet-derived growth factor
PKC *see* protein kinase C
Plasmacytoma growth factor BSF-2 (or IL-6), 365
Plasmodium berghei, 395
Plasmodium falciparum, 395
Platelet-derived growth factor: A family of isoforms that bind to two distinct receptors, 453–464
Platelet-derived growth factors (PDGF), 408, 427, 430–431, 433, 453–464, 481, 489, 494, 516
  autocrine & paracrine effects in normal cells, 459
  autocrine & paracrine effects in tumours, 458–459
  cAMP, 521, 523
  in vivo, 460
  isoforms, 454
  receptor activation, 456–457
  receptors, 455–456, 542–549
  SSV-transformation, 457
Polyergin (bovine collagen inducing factor), 426
Pre-T & Pre-B cells, 338, 341, 358–359
Prostaglandins, 407, 410
  cAMP, 520
Protein kinase C (PKC), 578
  cAMP, 522–523
  EGF receptor, 520
  mitogenesis, 517–526
Proto-oncogenes, 529–540, 554

R

Receptors, 541–553
  CSF, 554
  IGF, 554, 563
  PDGF, 554
  signal transduction, 551–552
  structural diversity, 542–543
  structure-function relationships, 554–569
  with cytoplasmic tryosine kinases, 546–549
  with unique structures, 550–551
  TNF, 391
Regulatory factors in lymphoid development, 350–360

Rheumatoid arthritis, 367
ROZENGURT E: Signal transduction pathways in mitogenesis, 515–528
ROZENGURT E *see also* WOLL P J

S

Sarcoma growth factor (SGF), 402, 404
Scatter factor and other regulators of cell mobility, 481–491
Scatter factor, 481–491
  action on epithelial cells, 484–485
  embryonic development, 487–488
  fibroblasts, 486
  growth, 486
  motility, 488–490
  purification & characteristics, 482–483
  specificity of action, 487
Septic shock, 367
Signal transduction pathways
  altered in cancer, 578–579
  mechanisms, 545
  models, 565–567
  mitogenesis, 515–528
    ion fluxes, 516–518, 520–521
Protein kinase C & DNA synthesis, 517–521
  proto-oncogenes, 523–524
Simian sarcoma virus (SSV), 453, 457
Small cell lung cancer (SCLC), 501–504
SMITH A G *see* HEATH J K
Somatomedins *see* insulin-like growth factors
STOKER M & GHERARDI E: Scatter factor and other regulators of cell mobility, 481–491
Structural and functional analysis of insulin-like growth factors, 465–480
Structural/evolutionary relationships, 344–345
Structure-function relationships
  EGF, 558–560, 562
  extracellular domain, 560–564
  hormones & GF, 555
  insulin, 555–558, 563
  intracellular domain, 564–565
  models, 565–567
  receptors, 560, 554–569
  subversion in cancer, 575–578
  transmembrane domain, 564
Structure-function relationships of growth factors and their receptors, 554–569
Substance K, 503
Substance P, 500–504

Synergistic activities, 362, 364
  mitogenesis, 524–526

T

T cell
  growth factor (or IL-2), 363
  function, 363
  growth, regulation of, 362
  replacing factors (TRF), or IL-5 & IL-6, 372, 379, 381
T cells and lymphokines, 361–370
T helper cells (Th), 371, 379
TESTA N G & DEXTER T M: Haemopoietic growth factors: Their role in acute myeloblastic leukaemia, 582–589
TGFs see transforming growth factors
Th see T helper cells
Thyroid hormone, 410
Thyrotropin (TSH)
TNF see tumour necrosis factor, 372, 379
Transforming growth factors (TGFs), 322, 328–332, 401–424, 425–437
  alpha (TGFα), 328, 401–424
    biological effects, 406–411
      in vitro, 407–409
      in vivo, 409–411
    biosynthesis and tissue distribution, 403–405
    cancer, 416–418
    clinical & industrial uses, 418–419
    discovery & characterization, 402
    genes, homologies & structure, 412–416
  beta (TGFβ), 328–332, 361, 368, 425–437
    biosynthesis & structure, 426–427
    cellular differentiation & growth inhibition, 432–433
    cellular transformation, 429–431
    mitogenic properties, 431–432
    prospects, 434
    receptors, 427–429
Tryosine kinase receptor
  ligand binding domain, 549–550
Trypanosoma brucei, 396
Tumour necrosis factor (TNF), 361–368, 372, 377–378, 389–400
  action, 393–395
  anticancer activity, 397–398
  as a GF, 392
  bone & cartilage, 394–395
  cachexic state, 396
  cytotoxic activities, 392–393
  history, 390
  immune disorders, 396–397
  infectious disease, 395
  molecule & LT, 390
  receptors, 391

U

Urogastrone see EGF

V

Vaccinia viruses (VVGFs), 542
Vasoactive intestinal peptide (VIP), 492–504
Vasopressin, 492–504
Vegetal pole cells, 327
  DNA synthesis, 521

W

WALICKE P A see BAIRD A
Wasting, pathology of, 367
WATERFIELD M D: Altered growth regulation in cancer, 570–581
WATERFIELD M D: Introduction, 317–319
WESTERMARK B see HELDIN C-H
WOLL P J & ROZENGURT E: Neuropeptides as growth regulators, 492–505
WOODGETT J R: Early gene induction, 529–540